D1252962

Beyond Anthrax

Larry I. Lutwick · Suzanne M. Lutwick
Editors

Beyond Anthrax

The Weaponization of Infectious Diseases

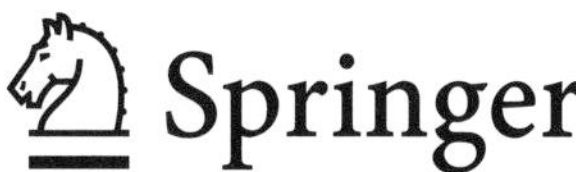

Editors
Larry I. Lutwick
VA New York Harbor Health Care System
Division of Infectious Diseases
SUNY Downstate Medical School
Brooklyn, NY, USA
larry.lutwick@va.gov

Suzanne M. Lutwick
Director of Grant Development
Hackensack University Medical Center Foundation
Hackensack, NJ, USA
slutwick@humed.com

ISBN: 978-1-58829-438-8 e-ISBN: 978-1-59745-326-4
DOI: 10.1007/978-1-59745-326-4

Library of Congress Control Number: 2008934792

Printed on acid-free paper

springer.com

Piglet sidled up to Pooh from behind.
"Pooh," he whispered. "Yes, Piglet?"
"Nothing," said Piglet, taking Pooh's paw.
"I just wanted to be sure of you."

This book is dedicated to those whom we always want to be sure of:
Our parents and siblings and
Talora and Zev,
Rachel and Robert,
Zach and Mollie,
Arielle and Talal,
Nina and...

May all of you be able to spend playfully exploring the world of Pooh without any interference by the contents of this text. And to a best friend who is looking down upon us, still not a sports fan, Steve Straus.

Larry Lutwick
Suzanne Lutwick

Preface

> "If there is one thing the history of evolution has taught us it's that life will not be contained. Life breaks free, expands to new territory, and crashes through barriers, painfully, maybe even dangerously."
>
> – Dr. Ian Malcolm, "*Jurassic Park*" (1993)

> "The most merciful thing in the world, I think, is the inability of the human mind to correlate all its contents. We live on a placid island of ignorance in the midst of black seas of infinity, and it was not meant that we should voyage far. The sciences, each straining in its own direction, have hitherto harmed us little; but some day the piecing together of dissociated knowledge will open such terrifying vistas of reality, and of our own frightful position therein, that we shall either go mad from the revelation or flee from the deadly light into the peace and safety of a new dark age."
>
> – H.P. Lovecraft, "*The Call of Cthulhu*" (published 1928)

Howard Phillips Lovecraft was an American author of horror, fantasy, and science fiction. His major inspiration and invention was overt cosmic horror, and he is often regarding as one of the most influential horror writers of the twentieth century, exerting widespread and indirect influence, and frequently compared to Edgar Allan Poe. The above quotation begins the story and could be applied to more modern times, nearly 80 years since the story's publication in "Weird Tales." Of course, it is easy to argue that the sciences have no longer "harmed us little" with such developments of nuclear bombs and other weapons of mass destruction (WMDs). Among the WMDs (as the media enjoys calling them) are those of the biological variety. It is these agents that serve as the basis of this textbook.

"*Beyond Anthrax, The Weaponization of Infectious Diseases*" has been in development for a number of years and is meant as a primer for clinicians and epidemiologists on a variety of agents, organisms, or toxins, which are generally considered at the forefront of potential use in a biological attack from a rouge nation or radical group. In the aftermath of the September 11 World Trade Center attacks, a number of cases of inhalational anthrax were diagnosed in the eastern United States, specifically the New York City metropolitan area and Washington, DC, although the first case was diagnosed in Florida. The finding of a disease such as anthrax outside of its general geographic area with an uncommon presentation (inhalation rather than cutaneous exposure) is the factor that raises the red flag of a possible bioterrorist attack. In this case, the spores of *Bacillus anthracis* were found to have been weaponized to increase infectivity and placed (by a person still unknown) in the mail. The letters, by processing in post office facilities or by opening at the final destination, delivered a deadly message producing inhalation anthrax in 11 individuals with a 45% case fatality rate [1]. Much information has been published regarding anthrax as a biological agent, and for reasons of space and minimizing repetition regarding this disease, the text will start beyond anthrax and discuss the remaining Category A agents as well as delve into a number of the diseases placed in Category B. It will suffice to say, however, that the anthrax incident has demonstrated what terrorism really does in getting a huge bang for its buck; that is, for a small number of cases, the outbreak caused major disruption to much of the fiber of this country changing some of it forever.

Before going forward, we must take stock of reality and not just jump, willy-nilly, on to the Lovecraftian slippery slope of the inevitability of something evil occurring fashioned by the hand of some bad person. No doubt, the possibility of the use of biological warfare has always existed millennia before the acceptance of the Germ Theory, a short century or so ago. Many of these events are discussed in Stuart Handysides' introductory chapter on the history of the topic. It is, to this point, useful to refer to the John Snow [2] Memorial Outbreak Scoreboard during the last decade or so. In doing so, our evil task doers are clearly trounced in overall numbers of cases and outbreaks by Mother Nature (MN), the world's most devious bioterrorist.

Although aided by humankind, MN has fashioned newly recognized diseases such as SARS (severe acute respiratory syndrome) [3] like a Golem out of the virtual molecular mud and has facilitated diseases such as monkey pox [4] and West Nile virus [5] unknown on a continent to appear there.

Furthermore, she has assisted in the production of multidrug resistant organisms [6,7] in a healthcare arena where fully sensitive ones had been present. Additionally, and certainly last but not least, MN continues to percolate new strains of influenza A including the current H5N1 avian strain [8] that threaten to win the primary race for next pandemic candidate. Although the diseases forthcoming in this text may be formidable opponents in the future, it remains a solid wager that infectious disease clinicians, epidemiologists, and public health personnel will have their hands soiled with many more threats than that are contained here.

Following the Stuart Handysides (former Medical Editor of Communicable Disease and Public Health) chapter on the history of biological warfare, the text has five chapters regarding the Category A diseases that are (true to the title, beyond anthrax), namely, smallpox, plague, tularemia, botulism, and the viral hemorrhagic fevers. The chapters are written by some of the foremost experts of each field including representatives of the National Institutes of Health, the

Centers for Disease Control and Prevention, and UK's Defense Science and Technology Laboratory at Porton Down. The chapters for the most part contain similar sections including outbreak scenarios, a historical perspective, microbiologic considerations, natural infection with its epidemiology and diagnostic considerations, as well as specific biowarfare issues. Additionally, the chapters discuss both therapeutic and preventative measures and may include infection control, prophylactic drugs, reservoir controls, and vaccinations.

The next part of the text contains chapters dealing with many, but not all, of the Category B agents, selected for overall interest. This includes a chapter on the intentional contamination of food and water as well as ones dealing with melioidosis, epidemic typhus, and some of the biotoxins such as ricin and staphylococcal enterotoxin B. Overall, the organization of these chapters parallel that in those of the Category A diseases. With much more emphasis on the "A" diseases, the inclusion of these entities provides a good source of information for the clinician and epidemiologist.

Following the "B" list are a number of chapters that concentrate on a variety of issues that are important in any contribution in the biowarfare arena. All of these have direct applications to natural outbreaks and epidemics, and they include Public Health Infrastructure, Public Health Law, Public Health Surveillance, Mental Health Management, as well as a chapter regarding the role of the media in outbreaks written by David Brown, a physician who has written regularly for the *Washington Post*. The text ends with an overview of rapid detection of pathogens and a final chapter discussing agroterrorism, that is, biological attacks on the potentially very vulnerable food-producing systems of the world. Biowarfare aimed at flora and fauna rather than on humankind, although not as often written about, are ripe areas for further discussions and protective measures.

In several of the original versions of the "Table of Contents," several other chapters were envisioned, but as the text matured, they were not included. The editors thank those who contributed additional but unused material.

We hope that the topics contained here, as biowarfare events, remain purely didactic exercises and not issues that interject themselves into clinical medicine.

References

1. Holty, J.-E., Bravata, D. M., Liu, H., et al: A century of inhalational anthrax cases from 1900 to 2005. Ann. Intern. Med. 144, 270–280, 2006.
2. Newsom, S. W.: Pioneers in infection control: John Snow, Henry Whitehead, the Broad Street pump, and the beginnings of geographical epidemiology. J. Hosp. Infect. 64, 210–216, 2006.
3. Conly, J. M., Johnston B. L.: SARS: A tale of two epidemics. Can. J. Infect. Dis. 14, 147–149, 2003.
4. Reed, K. D., Melski, J. W., Graham, M. B., et al: The detection of monkeypox in humans in the Western Hemisphere. N. Engl. J. Med. 350, 342–350, 2004.

5. Gubler, D. J.: The continuing spread of West Nile virus in the western hemisphere. Clin. Infect. Dis. 45, 1039–1046, 2007.
6. Gorwitz, R. J.: A review of community-associated methicillin-resistant *Staphylococcus aureus* skin and soft tissue infections. Pediatr. Infect. Dis. J. 27, 1–7, 2008.
7. Tumbarello, M., Spanu, T., Sanguinetti, M., et al: Bloodstream infections caused by extended-spectrum-beta-lactamase-producing *Klebsiella pneumoniae*. Antimicrob. Agents Chemother. 50, 498–504, 2006.
8. Peiris, J. S., de Jong, M. D., Guan, Y.: Avian influenza virus(H5N1): a threat to human health. Clin. Microbiol. Rev. 20, 243–267, 2007.

Contents

1 **The History of Bioterrorism: Old Idea, New Word, Continuing Taboo** 1
Stuart Handysides

2 **Smallpox and Bioterrorism** 17
Daniel R. Lucey, Joel G. Breman and Donald A. Henderson

3 **Plague** 55
Petra C. F. Oyston and Richard W. Titball

4 **Tularemia** 77
Daniel S. Shapiro

5 **Botulism** 85
Jeremy Sobel

6 **The Viral Hemorrhagic Fevers** 107
Daniel G. Bausch and C. J. Peters

7 **Melioidosis** 145
Pooja Tolaney and Larry I. Lutwick

8 **Epidemic Typhus Fever** 159
Mohammad Mooty and Larry I. Lutwick

9 **Category B Biotoxins** 181
Larry I. Lutwick, Jeremy Gradon and Jonathan Zellen

10 **Intentional Terrorist Contamination of Food and Water** 207
Jeremy Sobel and John C. Watson

11 **Public Health Infrastructure** 219
Isaac B. Weisfuse

12 **Public Health Law and Biological Terrorism** 239
Lance Gable and James G. Hodge, Jr.

13 **Public Health Surveillance for Bioterrorism** 253
Peter N. Wenger, William Halperin and Edward Ziga

14 **Psychosocial Management of Bioterrorism Events** 279
David M. Benedek and Thomas A. Grieger

15 **The Role of the Media in Bioterrorism** 295
David Brown

16 **Rapid Detection of Bioterrorism Pathogens** 317
David Perlin

17 **Plant Pathogens as Biological Weapons Against Agriculture** 335
Forrest W. Nutter and Lawrence V. Madden

Index 365

Contributors

Daniel G. Bausch, MD, MPH&TM
Department of Tropical Medicine, Tulane School of Public Health and Tropical Medicine, New Orleans, Louisiana, dbausch@tulane.edu

David M. Benedek, MD, LTC, MC, USA
Center for the Study of Traumatic Stress, Uniformed Services University, Bethesda, Maryland, dbenedek@usuhs.mil

Joel G. Breman, MD, DTPH
Fogarty International Center, National Institutes of Health, Bethesda, Maryland

David Brown, MD
The Washington Post, Washington, District of Columbia, browndavidm@comcast.net

Lance Gable, JD, MPH
Wayne State University Law School; Center for Law and the Public's Health, Detroit, Michigan

Jeremy Gradon, MD
Sinai Hospital of Baltimore; Johns Hopkins Hospital School of Medicine, Baltimore, Maryland

Thomas A. Grieger, MD, Capt., MC, USN
Center for the Study of Traumatic Stress, Uniformed Services University, Bethesda, Maryland

William Halperin, MD, DrPH
Department of Preventive Medicine and Community Health, University of Medicine and Dentistry of New Jersey, New Jersey Medical School, Newark, New Jersey, wengerpn@umdnj.edu

Stuart Handysides, BSc, MBBS
Program for Monitoring Emerging Diseases, Hertford, England

Donald A. Henderson, MD, MPH
Center for Biosecurity, University of Pittsburgh Medical Center, Johns Hopkins Hospital School of Medicine Distinguished Service Professor, Baltimore, Maryland

James G. Hodge, Jr., JD, LLM
Center for Law and the Public's Health; Johns Hopkins Bloomberg School of Public Health, Baltimore, Maryland, jhodge@jhsph.edu

Daniel R. Lucey, MD, MPH
Biohazardous Threat Agents and Emerging Infectious Diseases, Department of Microbiology and Immunology, Georgetown University School of Medicine, Washington, District of Columbia, dlucey@columbus.rr.com

Larry I. Lutwick, MD
Veterans Affairs New York Harbor Health Care System, Brooklyn Campus; State University of New York, Downstate Medical Center, Brooklyn, New York, lutwick@isid.org

Suzanne M. Lutwick, BS, MPH
Director of Grant Development, Hackensack University Medical Center Foundation, Hackensack, New Jersey, slutwick@humed.com

Laurence V. Madden, PhD
Department of Plant Pathology, Ohio State University, Wooster, Ohio

Mohammad Mooty, MD
Infectious Diseases, Eastern Maine Medical Center, Bangor, Maine

Forrest W. Nutter, Jr., PhD
Department of Plant Pathology, Iowa State University, Ames, Iowa, fwn@iastate.edu

Petra C. F. Oyston, BSc, PhD
Defense Science and Technology Laboratory, Porton Down, Wiltshire, England

David Perlin, PhD
Public Health Research Institute, Newark, New Jersey, perlinds@umdnj.edu

C. J. Peters, MD
Departments of Pathology, and Microbiology and Immunology, Center for Tropical Diseases, University of Texas, Galveston, Texas

Daniel S. Shapiro, MD
Boston University School of Medicine; Director of Clinical Microbiology Laboratory, Lahey Clinic, Burlington, Massachusetts, daniel.s.shapiro@lahey.org

Jeremy Sobel, MD, MPH
Foodborne and Diarrheal Diseases Branch, Centers for Disease Control and Prevention, Atlanta, Georgia, qzs3@CDC.GOV

Richard W. Titball, BSc, PhD, DSc
School of Biosciences, University of Exeter, Exeter, England, R.W.Titball@exeter.ac.uk

Pooja Tolaney, MD
Infectious Diseases Clinician, Hartford, Connecticut

John C. Watson, MD, MPH
Captain, US Public Health Service, Division of Parasitic Diseases, National Center for Zoonotic, Vectorborne, and Enteric Diseases, Coordinating Center for Infectious Diseases, Centers for Disease Control and Prevention, Atlanta, Georgia

Isaac B. Weisfuse, MD, MPH
New York City Department of Health and Mental Hygiene, New York, New York, iweisfus@health.nyc.gov

Jonathan Zellen, MD
Department of Medicine, North General Hospital, New York, New York

Edward Ziga, MD, MPH
Office of Surveillance and Prevention, Communicable Diseases Division, Newark Department of Health and Human Services, Newark, New Jersey

Chapter 1
The History of Bioterrorism: Old Idea, New Word, Continuing Taboo

Stuart Handysides

1.1 Definitions

The word "bioterrorism" first appeared in a book called *Killing Winds*, by Jeanne McDermott, in 1987 [1], and took another 9 years to reach a biomedical publication [2]. It appears in only the post-2003 editions of large dictionaries in my local bookshop and the *Oxford English Dictionary* online [3]. A Medline search yielded 2,018 entries on the topic—none before 1996, only 50 before 2000, and then an exponential increase (70 in 2000, 445 in 2001, 862 in 2002, and 3,998 by November 13, 2007) [4]. The history of bioterrorism would be rather short if written to consider events only since the word was coined. From a historical perspective it will be better, I think, to consider the phenomenon itself and take a longer view. Nevertheless, the word itself needs defining.

The word "terrorism" goes back only as far as the French Revolution. "The reign of terror" was a 2-year period of mob rule and bloodshed, led by the Jacobin government of Robespierre and the so-called Committee of Public Safety that followed the September massacres of 1792. Edmund Burke was one of the first persons to use the word "terrorist" to describe agents of the Jacobin government, in 1795, and the word "terrorism" was first used, in the same context, the same year.

Robespierre, translated from the original French by J. M. Thompson, explained the need for harsh measures: "If the basis of popular government in time of peace is virtue, its basis in time of revolution is both virtue and intimidation—virtue, without which intimidation is disastrous, and intimidation, without which virtue has no power.... Intimidation is merely justice—prompt, severe and inflexible. It is therefore an emanation of virtue, and results from the application of democracy to the most pressing needs of the country" [5]. Thompson, commenting on these words, noted that intimidation was generally the weapon of tyrants. The new despotism of postrevolutionary France took this weapon out of the tyrant's hand and turned it against

S. Handysides
25 Fordwich Rise, Hertford SG14 2BW, England
e-mail: stuart_handysides@hotmail.com

L.I. Lutwick, S.M. Lutwick (eds.), *Beyond Anthrax*,
DOI: 10.1007/978-1-59745-326-4_1,

him in the name of the people, but ended up turning it against anyone who disagreed with the current "party line".

The word terrorist today is usually applied to a nongovernmental agent, an agent without state sponsorship, but this usage goes back only to the second half of the nineteenth century. The word was used in 1866 to describe the dissident Irish, and in 1883 Russian revolutionaries who were prepared to use violence received the same appellation. *Webster's New International Dictionary* (1913) defined terrorism as "a mode of governing, or opposing government, by intimidation" and a terrorist as "one who administers or coerces a government or community by intimidation" [6], thus covering the actions of established governments and those with grievances against them.

The word terrorist is often given a negative connotation, but history sometimes changes our perspective on people and events. As an example, the South African government imprisoned Nelson Mandela as a terrorist, but many saw his fight against oppression and demand for human rights and the end of apartheid as the just desires of a freedom fighter. The latter appear to have been right.

Central to the meaning of terrorism is the fear experienced by those being terrorized. The acts of violence or warfare themselves kill or injure, but the terror is experienced by those who wonder where it will end and whether they or their loved ones will be the next victims of pain, injury, or death. Perhaps, the greatest act of terrorism the world has seen was the unleashing of atomic bombs on Japan. Terror belonged not only to the survivors in Japan, but to the world in general in the following 40 years of the "Cold War" and the uncertainty of the deterrent power of mutually assured destruction.

The prefix "bio" denotes the use or threat of biological agents to terrorize. Human beings themselves are biological agents, whose fists, feet, and teeth may be used as weapons. Various large and/or fierce animals have been used to intimidate enemies—Hannibal's elephants must have been an awesome sight, and the pots of snakes hurled by his men onto the ships of King Eumenes of Pergamon spread fear and distracted his enemies [7, 8]; Nero's lions in the Coliseum were an attempt to reduce the attraction of Christianity; the Romans also catapulted bees and hornets at their enemies; and the horses of the Spanish conquistadors menaced the Incas and Aztecs [7]. The word bioterrorism is usually used, however, to describe the threat or deployment of microorganisms or the use of contagion or infection, as weapons. The *Oxford English Dictionary* defines bioterrorism as "the use of infectious agents or biologically active substances as weapons of terrorism" [3].

Does the term bioterrorism deserve to exist? Do we speak of ballistic, explosive, or chemical terrorism? Is the use of biological weaponry different from other methods of attack? Roman jurists protested when their attempt to conquer Germanic tribes was thwarted by the poisoning of wells: *armis bella non venenis geri*—war is fought with weapons, not with poisons [8]. Commanders might see their armies decimated by outbreaks of plague, typhoid, cholera, smallpox, or influenza, but these were misfortunes rather than potential tools. Why is the use of a biological weapon seen as "fighting dirty" or "not cricket"?

This chapter, on the history of bioterrorism, will take an inclusive approach. It will draw little distinction between those who practice "warfare" and those who practice "terrorism." It will also use the term bioterrorism to describe actions taken before the existence of microorganisms was discovered.

1.2 Acts of God

Several of the Biblical plagues meted out to the Egyptians when Pharaoh refused to allow the children of Israel their freedom could be regarded as bioterrorist acts [9]. In the first plague, the rivers turned to blood and the fish died and stank. The plague of frogs was unwelcome, as was their smell when they died and rotted in heaps. Plagues of lice and flies and a die-off of cattle, which spared the livestock of the Israelites, followed the plague of frogs. Pharaoh continued to take a hard line, refusing to bargain with the terrorists, and the next visitation was a plague of boils and blains on the skin of men and beasts. At this point, the Lord diversified, using hail and fire to destroy the ripening crops, but then again returned to a biological plague, employing locusts to finish off whatever the hail had left. The penultimate plague was a period of darkness, lasting 3 days. In the last plague, the firstborn of all families, human and animal, were slain in households where a prescribed sacrifice had not been made. At this point, Pharaoh hollered "'nough" and sent the Israelites on their way.

The exact nature and factual existence of the plagues have been debated. The boils have been attributed to both plague and anthrax, but it all happened a long time ago. At the very least, however, the biblical report indicates that the potential for bioterrorism had been realized when the book of Exodus was written (about 1500 BC). If the book is taken as a literal historical report, it could be argued that God, as well as creator, was also the first bioterrorist.

The Bible also describes an outbreak—possibly plague—that befell the Philistines, when they captured the Ark of the Covenant from the Israelites [8, 10].

Another early reference to possible bioterrorism is found in Homer's *Iliad*, which tells how the city of Troy came under siege of the Greeks, after the beautiful Helen (married to the Greek Menelaus) ran off with Paris, one of the sons of the Trojan king, Priam [11]. The tale, written perhaps 7–10 centuries before the birth of Christ, starts with a description of a plague on mules, dogs, and men meted out by Apollo, after his priest, Chryses, was sent away rudely by Agamemnon when he asked for the return of his daughter.

Thus, the earliest descriptions of what might be called bioterrorism were plagues attributed to the God of the Hebrews and the Greek god Apollo. Gods, unlike men, could not be fought. They had to be appeased. Pharaoh and Agamemnon capitulated.

1.3 Poisoning Water Supplies

A little later, in the fifth century BC, Hippocrates said that impurities in the air (Greek: *miasmata*) were the cause of plagues [12]. At much the same time, Thucydides noted that the people of Athens, suffering from plague (or was it measles? [13]), believed that the city's water supply had been poisoned by the Spartans. Although the Romans had declared that poisoning was not an appropriate way to wage war, they poisoned the wells of the remnants of the army of Aristonicus, who kept fighting despite being, to a large extent, defeated [8]. Many years later the Black Death spread from Constantinople to the whole of western Europe, following trade routes both on land and on sea. Jewish communities in some of the plague-affected cities were accused of well poisoning and were exterminated [12]. The practice of poisoning water supplies has continued: It occurred in the American Civil War, the Boer War, and, allegedly, in Turkish Kurdistan as recently as 1997 [8].

1.4 Ballistic Biological Weapons

The archers of Scythia, in about 400 BC, are said to have dipped their arrow tips in blood mixed with manure [8]. Other early instances of the ballistic distribution of biological weapons are arrow tips and darts from blowpipes poisoned with curare by native Amazonians and with batrachotoxin from frogs by Hawaiian islanders [8, 14]. A book published in 1777 suggested to dip "arrows in matter of smallpox and twang them at the American rebels" [8]. More recently, grenade shrapnel was contaminated with botulinum toxin in the Second World War [8].

Sometimes the missiles were rather larger. The original catapult and ballista, as used by the Romans, could hurl rocks of approximately 30 kg at and over the walls of castles [15]. Later developments, such as the trebuchet, could project missiles of 150 kg and even as much as 1,500 kg. When the rocks ran out, other objects could be used as ammunition. Gabriel de Mussis provided an eyewitness account of the siege of Caffa (now Feodosiya), on the Black Sea, from 1344 to 1346 [15]. The Genoese-occupied city held out for 3 years. Suddenly, the besieging Tartars and Saracens fell victim to plague: "the humors coagulated in the groins, they developed a subsequent putrid fever and died." Mountains of cadavers were "placed on their hurling machines and thrown into the city of Caffa ... soon all the air was infected and the water poisoned, corrupt and putrefied, and such a great odor increased." The Genoese took to their ships and fled, taking plague with them to Italy, Sicily, and Sardinia. It has been argued that the fleas responsible for transmission of plague would have left the dead to occupy living hosts and the cadaver missiles, therefore, may not have carried the vectors into the city [14]. But how dead were the dead, and how quickly would the fleas have fled?

Other similar incidents have been documented. A few years earlier, in 1340, dead horses and other animals were hurled mechanically at the castle of Thun L'Eveque in northern France. The reporter of this incident, Jean Froissart, wrote, "the stink and the air were so abominable . . . they could not long endure" [16]. Less successful was the siege of Carolstein, or Karlstein, in Bohemia in 1422. Despite a barrage of soldiers' bodies and 2,000 cartloads of excrement, and an outbreak of fever attributed to the stench, the siege was abandoned after 5 months [8, 15–17]. The Hippocratic idea of miasma as the means by which illness was transmitted was still commonly held at the time. A rain of mutilated, rotting corpses within the city walls might well have induced terror of contagion as well as spreading disease.

1.5 Fomites

It appears that the development of gunpowder and the ways of using it occupied the minds of militarists for the next few hundred years [8]. In the early eighteenth century, almost a 100 years before Edward Jenner showed that inoculation with cowpox offered protection against smallpox, the practice of variolation—inoculation with fluid from smallpox pustules—was recognized as a means of protecting against severe infection with smallpox [8]. Variolation had a mortality rate of 2–3%, one-tenth that of natural infection, and became popular. It offered the protection needed by an aggressor to contemplate the potential of using an infectious disease as a weapon.

British forces in North America, whether through natural infection or through variolation, probably had more immunity to smallpox than the Native Americans. In a well-documented incident from the Pontiac Rebellion in 1763, Captain Ecuyer (under the command of General Jeffrey Amherst) gave blankets and a handkerchief from the smallpox hospital at Fort Pitt to Delaware Indians, with the hope that they would "have the desired effect" [18]. An epidemic of smallpox among the Native American tribes in the area followed, although it is not clear whether it was the blankets or other contacts with colonists that introduced the virus into the Native American population [14]. The intention to harm was clear, and letters expressing genocidal intent have been preserved [18]. The attempt was made, however, in a way intended to cause harm without, necessarily, intimidation. Both British and American troops were variolated during the American War of Independence [8], and the British are said to have used smallpox against the Americans in both Quebec and Boston [16]. Fomites are said to have been used by "land speculators and corrupt agents of the Brazilian Indian Protective Service" to spread smallpox among native American tribes of the Amazonian basin between 1957 and 1965 [16].

1.6 Living Human Carriers

The traditional image of people with leprosy is of their being herded into colonies, being cut off from their healthy fellows, and having to carry a bell and ring it to warn people of their arrival and enable them to get out of the way [13, 19]. The potential for transmission was clearly known: Spaniards are said to have spiked French wine with blood from people with leprosy in 1495. The potential for using infectious people to spread disease was at least discussed in the American War of Independence. A letter from General Alexander Leslie to General Cornwallis in 1781 talks of distributing a cohort of 700 Negroes suffering from smallpox in the rebel plantations [8].

1.7 Economic Sabotage Through Biological Weapons

The work of Robert Koch and Louis Pasteur in the 1870s identified specific infectious agents as the causes of contagion rather than the "bad air" hypothesis that had held since the days of Hippocrates [13]. Bacteria could be grown in a laboratory and, presumably, released among or dispatched to your enemies. Germany tried it out in the First World War. The targets were not humans, however, but animals, which perhaps reflects persistence of the Roman sensitivity about the rules of engagement. The attacks were made, in general, on nonaligned countries that were supplying Germany's enemies with animals for transport and food [14]. Romanian sheep to be exported to Russia, mules from Mesopotamia, horses from the United States destined for the allied forces, livestock from Argentina, and reindeer and horses from Norway were all attacked. The organisms used were *Bacillus anthracis* and *Pseudomonas mallei*, the pathogens associated with anthrax and glanders, respectively. Several methods were used: injections using needles that had been dipped in cultures, infected solutions poured onto feed, and capillary tubes embedded in sugar lumps [16]. The effectiveness of the campaign is not clear [16], but the intention was plain. In Mesopotamia, 4,500 mules were inoculated, and in Argentina over 200 mules died after infection with *B. anthracis* and *P. mallei* [14].

1.8 Biological Warfare and Terrorism by Established Powers Since the Geneva Protocol

Although biological weapons had not been used against humans in the First World War, their potential use and the need to control them were recognized in the 1925 Geneva Protocol for the Prohibition of Asphyxiating, Poisonous or Other Gases, and of Bacteriological Methods of Warfare [14]. The treaty banned the use of biological weapons, but did not outlaw research, production, or possession, and made no provision for inspection [14]. Several countries that had ratified the protocol set up basic research programs; Britain, France, and the Soviet Union declared that they were bound only so long as their enemies did not use chemical or biological weapons [20]; the United States refused to ratify the protocol until 1975 [14].

1.8.1 Japan

Japan, like the United States, did not ratify the protocol in 1925. Japan conducted large-scale research from 1932 to 1945 using human subjects, mainly in the occupied Chinese province of Manchuria [14, 16]. Led by Shiro Ishii, the main focus of activity was the "Epidemic Prevention and Water Supply Unit" designated Unit 731, near the town of Ping Fan [14, 16, 21]. Over 10,000 people (political prisoners, local people, and prisoners of war) died as a result of experimental infection and subsequent vivisection. Several infectious agents were tried: *B. anthracis*, *Neisseria meningitidis*, *Shigella* sp., *Vibrio cholerae*, and *Yersinia pestis* [14]. Experiments also employed typhoid, paratyphoid, and glanders [21].

Field attacks on military and civilian targets in China followed the early Unit 731 experiments. Starting in 1939, saboteurs contaminated wells with intestinal pathogens; distributed infected food; dropped biodegradable bombs that contained live plague-infected rats and fleas, which exploded to let the creatures fall safely to the ground; and dropped anthrax-infected birds and feathers [16, 21]. Hundreds of thousands of Chinese (also Russians and Koreans) in at least 11 cities are believed to have been killed in these attacks [16, 21]. Japanese troops were themselves not immune: 1,700 are estimated to have died from enteric diseases (mainly cholera) among about 10,000 casualties of biological warfare [14, 16].

Some of the officers from Unit 731 were captured by Soviet troops and served sentences of hard labor for war crimes [14, 16]. The leaders of the bioweapons program, having been captured by Western forces in Tokyo, were granted immunity from war crimes prosecution in return for full disclosure about the program [16, 21]. Whether this was done in order to use the "treasure trove" of the results of these barbaric experiments for Western bioweapons programs [21] or whether it represented an altruistic intention to prevent the (distrusted) Soviet Union from acquiring the information [16] will probably never be known.

1.8.2 Germany

Germany made little use of biological weaponry in the Second World War; apparently Hitler prohibited their development [14]. Some research was carried out in concentration camps, where prisoners were infected forcibly with rickettsiae, hepatitis A virus, and malaria in experiments on pathogenesis and vaccine and drug testing [14]. One of the Germans' last acts of the war was the pollution with sewage of a large reservoir in Bohemia [14]. Evidence recently came to light that the Nazis sabotaged hydraulic pumps in southern Italy that were used to drain the Pontine Marshes [22]. Mosquitoes, and malaria, had flourished in the marshes between the decline of the Roman Empire, when irrigation and drainage became neglected, and the start of restoration of drainage in the eighteenth century, which was completed by Mussolini in the 1930s [13]. With the pumps out of action, seawater again flooded the area, the mosquitoes returned, and a large outbreak of malaria followed. A national malaria eradication program was set up in 1947, using insecticide (DDT) spraying and environmental sanitation measures, as a result of which transmission ceased [23].

1.8.3 Allied Forces

Both Britain and the United States researched bioweaponry during the Second World War. The Scottish island of Gruinard, which was bombed experimentally with weaponized anthrax spores, remained contaminated with viable spores until 1986, when it was decontaminated with formaldehyde and seawater [14]. The US offensive biological weapons program started in 1942, and 5,000 bombs filled with *B. anthracis* spores were produced at a pilot plant at Camp Detrick, Maryland [14]. A production plant at Terre Haute, Indiana, and its surroundings were shown to be contaminated, which precluded large-scale production [14].

It was alleged that an outbreak of tularemia that arose among German troops in 1942, and then spread to Russian troops in the Volga basin, was due to Soviet biowarfare [16]. The outbreak is said to have affected 10,000 people, and 70% of the early cases were pneumonic, an unusual frequency for a disease most often transmitted by insect bite or exposure to infected animals or their remains [24]. Further analyses of the outbreak have concluded that there is insufficient evidence to say whether the Soviet Union was prepared to use bioweaponry in 1942 and that the outbreak may have been natural [16].

The fear of biological warfare was a motivation for the development of communicable disease surveillance institutions. Examples include the Emergency Public Health Laboratory Service, later without the "Emergency" and now part of the Health Protection Agency in England and Wales [25], and the Centers for Disease Control and Prevention in the United States [26].

1.8.4 Postwar Stockpiling, Psychology, and Propaganda

The Cold War is generally thought of as a nuclear standoff, but its period included various wars and other military conflicts—Korea, Vietnam, Suez,

Cuba, and the Middle East. There were continuing battles worldwide for hearts and minds; both the east and the west attempted to claim the moral high ground and discredit the opposing side. Allegations about the development and use of biological weapons were a way of bringing shame upon the enemy and of spreading distrust. They contributed to the pervading fear, or terror, about what would happen if a major war were to break out again.

The US program of research, development, and production of biological weapons was extensive and is said to have built on information obtained from secret debriefings of Shiro Ishii and other Japanese scientists [14, 16, 21]. The American experiments utilized animals, military and civilian volunteers, and both active biological agents and supposedly harmless organisms. Several lethal and incapacitating agents and anticrop agents were weaponized and stockpiled [14]. The "harmless" simulants were aerosolized and dropped surreptitiously over cities such as New York and San Francisco to assess their dispersibility [14].

Both North Korea and China alleged that the United States dropped various fomites and live insects contaminated with infective agents over their countries in 1952 [14, 16]. The concerned countries argued about which body would be impartial and competent to investigate. An International Scientific Commission investigated the issue, but relied on evidence supplied by the Chinese, rather than collecting its own [16]. A subsequent investigation concluded that the evidence was fabricated [16], but publicity at the time reduced international goodwill toward the United States [14].

Further allegations were made over the next 20–30 years. America was said to have infected turkeys in Cuba with Newcastle disease, to have introduced African swine fever to Cuba, and to have released the insect *Thrips palmi* from an aircraft flying over the country's air space [16]. The United States was also accused of testing plague weapons on Canadian Eskimos, conducting an attack on Colombian and Bolivian peasants, releasing dengue in Cuba, and planning to initiate a cholera epidemic in China [14].

For their part, the Americans alleged that the Soviet-backed Vietnamese troops had used mycotoxins ("yellow rain"—plant-based toxins that inhibit protein synthesis) in Laos, Cambodia, and Afghanistan [14, 16]. No evidence for the claim was found. Further allegations of the use of glanders in Afghanistan by Soviet troops were also not substantiated [16].

Over 10,000 human cases of anthrax, including 182 deaths, occurred in the black-held Tribal Trust Lands in Rhodesia (now Zimbabwe), during its War of Independence in 1979–1980. Allegations that this outbreak was begun deliberately have not been substantiated, and the outbreak is believed to have arisen because the preventive vaccination program in the area had broken down [16].

All these stories seem to have provided useful propaganda in their time, but seem to have been backed by little evidence when investigated thoroughly. Interested parties made the allegations and refutations. Were investigators, however independent and disinterested, privy to full and unbiased data? Could they, necessarily, have known if information was being withheld or "spun"? Outbreaks of infection can arise without military help, which makes it hard to investigate suspected biological warfare or terrorism.

Biological "friendly fire" is no easier to identify. Covert drops of *Serratia marcescens* over San Francisco in 1951 were followed by an outbreak of urinary tract infections caused by *S. marcescens* at Stanford University Hospital [27]. The army convened an investigation of the possible link, but the organism continued to be used as a simulant until 1968 [14]. The public became aware of these experiments in 1976 when an article in the *Washington Post* brought them to light [14]. A subsequent investigation of *S. marcescens* outbreaks by the Centers for Disease Control and Prevention showed that they were caused by strains different from those used by the military [14]. The US Army published data on occupational infections among workers at Fort Detrick, to demonstrate the attention paid to the safety of workers there [14].

Just as the Americans said little about their biological weapons experiments in the 1950s, similarly little is known in the public domain about what was happening elsewhere. The British chemical and biological defense establishment at Porton Down in Wiltshire was famous for common cold experiments, but National Service Volunteers (sworn to secrecy) were exposed to far more sinister substances. A verdict of "misadventure" was returned when serviceman Ronald Maddison died there in 1953 after the nerve gas sarin was dripped onto his arm [28]. After a long campaign the inquest was reopened and in 2004 the verdict was changed to "unlawful killing" [29].

These incidents occurred long ago and were hidden from the public eye for many years. The two world wars were still close enough for people to remember fighting against external enemies. The Cold War had continued to focus attention on "them" rather than on "us." Nevertheless, concern grew in the late 1950s and the 1960s that, perhaps, good and bad were not always clearly demarcated on national lines and that those in authority did not always know best. Further, if we were all going to die in a nuclear holocaust, there was nothing to be lost by protesting about the way things were and by trying to change them.

1.9 Biological and Toxins Weapons Convention, 1972

The next step toward control was the Biological and Toxins Weapons Convention (formally the Convention on the Prohibition of the Development, Production and Stockpiling of Bacteriological [Biological] and Toxin Weapons and on Their Destruction [BWC]), which was opened for signature in 1972 and came into effect in 1975 [14, 20]. It has been signed by 140 nations. The 1925 Geneva Protocol had failed to prevent the proliferation of biological weapons and concern had grown that biological weapons were indiscriminate and unpredictable, and their effects uncontrollable. Several nations—the United States, Canada, Sweden, the Warsaw Pact countries, and the United

Kingdom—announced proposals in 1969 along the lines of the subsequent treaty's title [14, 20]. Ratification of the treaty required a signatory nation to destroy stocks of biological agents, delivery systems, and equipment within 9 months.

Despite the scope of the BWC, it does not include provisions for implementation or verification [20]. It is known that the Soviet Union violated the treaty and that a large outbreak of inhalational anthrax in Sverdlovsk resulted from an accident at a military biological weapons facility [14, 20]. At least one successful assassination was performed using ricin, a toxin derived from castor beans, sealed into a tiny pellet and shot from a modified umbrella [14]. Another signatory, Iraq, was said to have an offensive biological weapons program at the time of the first Persian Gulf War in 1991 [20]. A defector reported that missiles, bombs, and aircraft spray tanks were prepared with botulinum toxin, aflatoxin, and anthrax spores, and research had been carried out on *Clostridium perfringens*, rotavirus, echovirus 71, and camelpox [20]. Weapons inspectors of the United Nations Special Commission have never found them [20, 30].

1.10 Non-state-Sponsored Bioterrorism

The essence of terrorism is fear, and the fear that extremist factions—whether political, religious, or psychopathic—will perpetrate bioterrorist acts has been around for over 30 years [31]. The threat has been taken more seriously since the Aum Shrinrikyo cult released sarin gas into the Tokyo subway in 1995, killing 11 people and injuring over 5,000 [32]. The cult was alleged to be researching the use of botulinum toxin and *Coxiella burnetii* (the bacterium responsible for Q fever) [14], trying to obtain Ebola virus [14], and is known to have sprayed a suspension of a vaccine strain of *B. anthracis* from its headquarters building in Tokyo in 1993 [32].

The sarin attack in 1995 was big enough to prompt the realization that chemical and biological weapons were not only in the hands of nations (with a lot to lose if they used them) but also available to other groups with various motives, who might be prepared to use them whatever the consequences. A distinction was drawn between traditional terrorists, whose aims might well be shared by a proportion of the public even if they did not endorse their methods, and a new breed of wanton destroyers whose target was society in general [2].

Biological weapons were said to be cheap to produce and the raw materials easy to acquire, they were not detected by metal detectors and x-rays, and those who used them could be far away by the time the target population felt their effects [2, 33]. It was said, however, that the United States itself had only two laboratories designated Biosafety Level 4, which were equipped to handle the most dangerous pathogens [2]. This suggests that such resources would not be readily available for the would-be bioterrorist. The technical expertise was said to be available from scientists and technicians previously employed in such countries as the Soviet Union and South Africa and now (so the thesis implied) in the marketplace [31]. The disadvantages of biological weapons—that they were indiscriminate and unpredictable, and their effects uncontrollable [14]—seemed to be forgotten.

Despite their attractions, and the fear they have generated, biological weapons seem to have been little used. The database of the Monterey Institute's Center for Nonproliferation Studies identified 66 criminal and 55 terrorist incidents in which biological agents were used between 1960 and 1999 [31]. Among these, eight criminal attacks caused casualties (29 deaths and 31 injuries), and only one terrorist attack—salmonella used by members of a religious commune to contaminate restaurant salad bars—was associated with casualties (751; no deaths) [31, 34]. Case studies collected by the Monterey Institute between 1970 and 1998, other than those already mentioned, included plots hatched by anti-imperialist, ecoterrorist, Marxist, right-wing anti-government, and white supremacist groups and individuals [31]. Two of the cases appear to have been hoaxes; several expressed persecutory or apocalyptic visions and were led by charismatic figures [31].

A series of hoax letters were sent and telephone calls were made in the United States between October and December 1998 [35, 36]. Letters sent to health clinics and a private business were said to contain anthrax, and telephone threats said that ventilation systems of public and private businesses had been contaminated with anthrax [35, 36]. The incidents prompted emergency responses, with decontamination and chemoprophylaxis of sites and of those who might have been exposed and examination of samples from the allegedly contaminated letters and the ventilation systems. Security and public health strategists drew up plans for how best to respond to such events [35].

The real thing followed in 2001, early in October, just as the United States was reeling from the attacks of September 11 [37]. The country's first case of inhalational anthrax in 25 years was confirmed in Florida and—over the next 6 weeks—a total of 22 cases of anthrax (11 inhalational, 5 of which were fatal) were identified in seven states plus the District of Columbia [37]. *B. anthracis* was isolated from powder in four envelopes; 20 of the patients were either mail handlers or had links to the workplaces where contaminated mail was processed or sent [37].

Who mailed the contaminated envelopes from New Jersey, and why, is not known. Speculation was rife: Was it the work of Al-Qaida, the organization responsible for the September 11 attacks, or could the bioterrorist attacks have been made by a party who wished to prompt and justify what became known as the "war on terror"? Terror was certainly achieved, and a massive industry for the surveillance of diseases that might represent future attacks, civil defense, and the protection of public health swiftly evolved [38–43]. Ciprofloxacin (an antibiotic active against anthrax) was stockpiled, and mass vaccination against smallpox, a virus infection that the World Health Organization had declared eradicated over 20 years earlier, began (and ended "because few people volunteered for it") [44].

1.11 Continuing Bioterror?

The loss of life from bioterrorism in the past 50 years has been infinitesimal in comparison with that caused by conventional terrorism, warfare, homicide, and road accidents. It is miniscule compared with the loss of life associated with the Japanese experiments on bioweaponry in the 1930s and 1940s. The threat of biological weapons has not required enormous loss of life to spread fear, however, or to divert time, effort, and money into responding to the perceived threat. Why, in an era when suicide attacks occur almost daily, do terrorists rarely take advantage of biological weapons?

Perhaps, the idea that they themselves may die from disease is more fearsome or less honorable than the prospect of dying swiftly from a bomb. Perhaps, they fear falling into the hands of their enemy and giving way to interrogation while weakened by disease. Perhaps, the adverse publicity for the terrorist's cause, brought about by scenes of innocent victims disfigured by open sores, choking, vomiting, convulsing, and expiring, acts as a deterrent.

We can only hope that the taboo retains its power. Whether biological weapons of mass destruction will be unleashed and whether the infrastructure will cope with them remains to be seen.

Acknowledgments My thanks are due to the following people for their advice on sources and helpful discussions about the drafting of this chapter: Julia Heptonstall, Harry Leonard, Larry Madoff, and David Woolliscroft.

References

1. McDermott, J. *Killing Winds*. New York: Arbor House Pub Co, 1987.
2. Stephenson, J. Confronting a biological Armageddon: experts tackle prospect of bioterrorism. *JAMA* 1996; 276: 349–351.
3. *Oxford English Dictionary* online. <http://www.oed.com/> accessed 14 November 2003.
4. *Medline*. <http://www.ncbi.nlm.nih.gov/sites/entrez/> accessed 13 November 2007.
5. Thompson, JM. *Robespierre*. Oxford: Blackwell, 1988 (reprint from 1935 edition).
6. Harris, WT (editor in chief). *Webster's New International Dictionary*. London: Bell, 1913.
7. Loefler, I. Bioterrorism. *BMJ* 2003; 327: 817.
8. *A Brief History of Chemical and Biological Weapons: Ancient Times to The 19th Century*. <http://www.cbwinfo.com/History/History.html/> accessed 30 September 2003.
9. *The Bible* (King James version): Exodus chapters 8–12.
10. *The Bible* (King James version): I Samuel chapters 4–6.
11. Homer. *The Iliad* (translated by E. V. Rieu). Harmondsworth: Penguin, 1950.
12. Leven, K-H. Poisoners and "plague-smearers". *Lancet* 354(Suppl.) SIV53, 1999.
13. Thomas, H. *An Unfinished History of the World*. London: Pan, 1981, 137–147, 562–573.

14. Christopher, GW, Cieslak, J, Pavlin, JA, Eitzen EM Jr. Biological warfare: a historical perspective. *JAMA* 1997; 278: 412–417.
15. Derbes, VJ. De Mussis and the Great Plague of 1348. *JAMA* 1966; 196: 179–182.
16. Wheelis, M. A short history of biological warfare and weapons. In: Chevrier MI, Chomiczewski K, Dando MR, Garrigue H, Granasztoi G, Pearson GS (eds.). *The Implementation of Legally Binding Measures to Strengthen the Biological and Toxin Weapons Convention.*Dordrecht: Springer, 2004.
17. *History of Biowarfare.* <http://www.pbs.org/wgbh/nova/bioterror/hist_nf.html/> accessed 18 July 2003.
18. d'Errico, P. *Jeffrey Amherst and Smallpox Blankets.* <http://www.nativeweb.org/pages/legal/amherst/lord_jeff.html/> accessed 18 July 2003.
19. Handysides, S. All the history that you can remember. *Commun Dis Public Health* 1999; 2: 230–232. <http://www.hpa.org.uk/cdph/issues/CDPHvol2/no4/editorials.pdf/> accessed 25 November 2003.
20. Kadlec, RP, Zelicoff, AP, Vrtis, AM. Biological weapons control: prospects and implications for the future. *JAMA* 1997; 278: 351–356.
21. Hill, A. The day the earth died. *Observer* 2003; 20 August <http://observer.guardian.co.uk/print/0,4616329–110648,00.html/> accessed 13 November 2007.
22. *BBC.* Document: mosquito wars. 8 September 2003. <http://www.bbc.co.uk/radio4/history/document.shtml/> accessed 26 November 2003.
23. Sabatinella, G, Majori, G. Malaria surveillance in Italy: 1986–1996 analysis and 1997 provisional data. *Eurosurveillance* 1998; 3: 38–40. <http://www.eurosurveillance.org/em/v03n04/0304-223.asp/> accessed 26 November 2003.
24. Benenson, AS. (editor). *Control of Communicable Diseases Manual* (16th edition). Washington DC: American Public Health Association, 1995.
25. Williams, REO. *Microbiology for the Public Health.* London, UK: PHLS, 1985.
26. Centers for Disease Control and Prevention. History of CDC. *MMWR Morb Mortal Wkly Rep*1996; 45: 526–530. <http://www.cdc.gov/mmwr/PDF/wk/mm4525.pdf/> accessed 1 November 2003.
27. Wheat, RP, Zuckerman, A, Rantz LA. Infection due to chromobacteria. *Arch Intern Med* 1951; 88: 461–466.
28. *Wellcome Trust.* Death of a serviceman. <http://www.wellcome.ac.uk/doc_WTX023670.html/> accessed 13 November 2007.
29. Shukman D. MoD pays out over nerve gas death. *BBC News online.* 2006; 25 May. <http://news.bbc.co.uk/2/hi/uk_news/england/5018084.stm/> accessed 13 November 2007.
30. Anonymous. Weapons: a question of trust. *Observer* 2003; 1 June. <http://observer.guardian.co.uk/iraq/story/0,12239,968036,00.html/> accessed 25 November 2003.
31. Tucker, JB. Historical trends related to bioterrorism: an empirical analysis. *Emerg Infect Dis* 1999; 5: 498–504.
32. Keim, P, Smith, KL, Keys, C, et al. Molecular Investigation of the Aum Shinrikyo Anthrax Release in Kameido, Japan. *J Clin Microbiol* 2001; 39: 4566–4567. <http://jcm.asm.org/cgi/content/full/39/12/4566/> accessed 15 November 2003.
33. Henderson, DA. Weapons for the future. *Lancet* 2000; 354(Suppl.): SIV64.
34. Török, TJ, Tauxe, RV, Wise, RP, et al. A large community outbreak of salmonellosis caused by intentional contamination of restaurant salad bars. *JAMA* 1997; 278: 389–395.
35. Centers for Disease Control and Prevention. Bioterrorism alleging use of anthrax and interim guidelines for management—US. *MMWR Morb Mortal Wkly Rep* 1999; 48: 69–74.
36. Bales, ME, Dannenberg, AL, Brachman, PS, et al. Epidemiologic response to anthrax outbreaks: field investigations, 1950–2001. *Emerg Infect Dis* 2002; 8: 1163–1174.
37. Jernigan, DB, Raghunathan, PL, Bell, BP, et al. Investigation of bioterrorism-related anthrax, United States, 2001: epidemiologic findings. *Emerg Infect Dis* 2002; 8: 1019–1028.

38. Hoffman, RE. Preparing for a bioterrorist attack: legal and administrative strategies. *Emerg Infect Dis* 2003; 9: 241–245.
39. Dworkin, MS, Xinfang, M, Golash, RG. Fear of bioterrorism and implications for public health preparedness. *Emerg Infect Dis* 2003; 9: 503–505.
40. Ashford, DA. Planning against biological terrorism: lessons from outbreak investigations. *Emerg Infect Dis* 2003; 9: 515–519.
41. Kaplan, EH, Patton, CA, Fitzgerald, WP, Wein, LM. Detecting bioterror attacks by screening blood donors: a best-case analysis. *Emerg Infect Dis* 2003; 9: 909–914.
42. M'ikanatha, NM, Southwell, B, Lautenbach, E. Automated laboratory reporting of infectious diseases in a climate of bioterrorism. *Emerg Infect Dis* 2003; 9: 1053–1057.
43. Buehler JW, Berkelman, RL, Hartley, DM, Peters CJ. Syndromic surveillance and bioterrorism-related epidemics. *Emerg Infect Dis* 2003; 9: 1197–1204.
44. ProMED-mail. Smallpox vaccination adverse events—USA (11): few. ProMED-mail 2003; 20 June: 20030620.1519 <promed@promedmail.org>accessed 26 November 2003.

Chapter 2
Smallpox and Bioterrorism

Daniel R. Lucey, Joel G. Breman, and Donald A. Henderson

2.1 Introduction

This chapter will focus on information regarding smallpox and smallpox vaccination since 2001, notably, the persisting threat of smallpox as a bioterrorist agent, international preparedness for a smallpox outbreak, vaccine adverse event issues including myopericarditis, second- and third-generation smallpox vaccines, HIV/AIDS issues, similarities with other microbial threats such as monkeypox and SARS, and an example of hospital and city smallpox preparedness efforts beginning in late 2001. Recent reviews by us and others, including the Centers for Disease Control and Prevention (CDC) and the World Health Organization (WHO), have addressed the history, clinical features, pathogenesis, prevention, diagnosis, and management of smallpox [1–7]. In addition, reference is also made to classic comprehensive texts on smallpox from 1962, 1972, and 1988 [8–10].

After the terrorist airplane hijacking attacks of September 11, 2001, and the subsequent anthrax bioterrorism attacks, additional international efforts were undertaken to reassess the threat of smallpox being reintroduced into the human population a quarter century after its eradication. These efforts, including those of the WHO, were focused on recognition of the clinical aspects of smallpox, the public health response, smallpox vaccination, and the need for expanded smallpox vaccine stockpiles [11–20].

In the United States, the CDC and the Department of Defense (DoD) initiated extensive educational training regarding smallpox and smallpox vaccination [21–29]. According to CDC [30], between January 2003, the beginning of the civilian vaccination program, and October 31, 2004, at least 39,597 civilians were vaccinated against smallpox. The civilian program declined by the summer of 2003, temporally linked with three events that began in March 2003: These were the unexpected finding of myopericarditis in a small

D.R. Lucey
Georgetown University School of Medicine, NE 317, Medical-Dental Building, 3900 Reservoir Road, Washington, DC 20057-1411, USA
e-mail: DRL23@georgetown.edu

L.I. Lutwick, S.M. Lutwick (eds.), *Beyond Anthrax*,
DOI: 10.1007/978-1-59745-326-4_2, © Springer Science+Business Media, LLC 2008

percentage of vaccinees, a growing appreciation of the risks of vaccination, and the apparent absence of biological weapons in Iraq, as confirmed subsequent to invasion. In the DoD, between December 13, 2002, and October 14, 2004, over 656,000 smallpox vaccinations were administered [24] (www.smallpox.army.mil/event/SPSafetySum.asp). Unlike the civilian program, the DoD smallpox vaccination program has continued without pause, and in fact, expanded in the latter half of 2004. On June 28, 2004, a memorandum from the Pentagon by the Deputy Secretary of Defense directed the expansion of the vaccination programs in the military for both smallpox and anthrax. Expansion of vaccination included "all uniformed DoD personnel serving in the Central Command Area of Responsibility," which includes central Asia, parts of east Africa, and the Korean peninsula areas considered at special risk for military personnel [31] (www.smallpox.army.mil/resources/policies.asp).

2.2 Smallpox: A Persisting Bioterrorist Threat

The primary source threat of smallpox being reintroduced into the world was the former Soviet Union because of its alleged former massive program to weaponize smallpox. As reported by Alibek [32], the former deputy director of this Soviet effort, after the WHO announced in 1980 that smallpox had been eradicated [33], the Kremlin provided the resources and planning to produce and store up to 20 tons of smallpox per year. This alleged illegal and secret smallpox production effort, involving tens of thousands of persons over multiple years, was cited again in October 2003 at an international smallpox vaccine meeting in Geneva [34] by Henderson. According to Alibek, this viral production facility was located at Zagorsk, now known as Sergiyev Posad, located less than an hour northwest of Moscow [32]. This is still a top-secret facility under the Russian Ministry of Defense, according to Henderson, and it is unknown whether smallpox is still present in this facility [35].

There are only two facilities that are approved by the WHO for storage of variola virus and for limited research: the CDC and the State Research Center of Virology and Biotechnology (VECTOR) in Koltsovo, Novosibirsk, Siberia [35]. Increased laboratory research on smallpox at these two locations since 2001, including monkey and other animal model studies and efforts to develop antiviral drugs and attenuated vaccines against smallpox, inevitably carry an intrinsic risk of an accidental laboratory-associated infection. A laboratory-associated variola virus infection would trigger international public concern such as the one that occurred with SARS coronavirus infection in lab workers in Singapore, Taipei, and Beijing in late 2003 and 2004 [36].

In addition, there is concern that some workers in the former Soviet smallpox weapons program have left Russia, and may have taken variola virus with them and shared their expertise on smallpox with other nations or organizations [34, 35]. Such linkages could serve as a means whereby smallpox could be reintroduced into a now largely unvaccinated and susceptible human population. In an attempt to decrease the risk of smallpox and other biological weapons, the United States and European nations are reported to be devoting $90 million each year to assist Russia to employ approximately 6,000 former bioweapons scientists and to secure better its large bioweapons complex. One example of these funding initiatives is the planned construction in 2005 of new and more secure laboratories to study high-risk pathogens, although not smallpox, in Kazakhstan [37].

Prior to the 2003 war with Iraq, the *Washington Post* reported in a front-page article on November 5, 2002, that unnamed sources in the US government suggested that Iraq and North Korea, as well as the United States and Russia, possessed the variola virus [38]. No specific information was provided. On February 5, 2003, the US Secretary of State Colin Powell, in his detailed presentation at the United National Security Council regarding specific concerns about Iraqi weapons of mass destruction, mentioned smallpox only once, in referring to Saddam Hussein: "And he also has the wherewithal to develop smallpox" [39].

Even though the war with Iraq did not reveal any smallpox stockpiles or weapons of mass destruction, concern persists regarding the possible use of smallpox as a bioterrorist weapon. In the summer of 2003, Richard Danzig, former secretary of the US Navy and a biodefense expert, argued that aerosolized smallpox and aerosolized anthrax are two of the four major catastrophic bioterrorism threats for which the United States needs to prepare better [40]. He discussed specific measures and made recommendations for dealing with an emergency of 200,000 smallpox-infected persons. These difficult issues include rapid detection of the aerosol smallpox attack and rapid vaccination of large numbers of persons within a 4-day (96 h) window after infection, the period when vaccination can prevent or decrease the severity of clinical illness. Similarly, Alibek and Charles Bailey, bioweapons experts from the former Soviet Union and the United States, respectively, have recently emphasized the threat of an aerosolized attack with a bioterrorism weapon [41].

In the summer of 2004, the CDC and Federal partners began the planning and implementation with Departments of Health in multiple US cities, including the Washington, DC, National Capital Region of the new "Cities Readiness Initiative (CRI)." The specific funding and rationale for the CRI, listed on the CDC website in June 2004, is to enhance readiness in at least 20 US cities and their surrounding regions for a catastrophic event, such as an aerosol release of a bioterrorist agent over or within one or more cities [42].

Multiple organizations continue to create and critique computer models of smallpox outbreaks [43–47]. A recent review article on smallpox modeling by Ferguson and colleagues discussed the benefits and drawbacks of different types of smallpox vaccination policy options in controlling a smallpox attack [43]. These options included quarantine/isolation, movement restrictions, containment by "ring" vaccination, targeted vaccination, mass vaccination, and prophylactic vaccination.

In 2004, Dr. Alibek published a paper [48] on smallpox as a disease and as a weapon, in which he reviewed in detail specific aspects of the former Soviet Union's program to weaponize smallpox such as field testing at Vozrozhdenie island until the late 1970 s and production and testing using large reactors (up to 630 L) during the 1980 s. He also presented information on methods that might be used to release smallpox virus as a bioterrorist weapon, such as the use of mechanical devices to generate an aerosol, explosive devices, contamination of food or various articles, or release within a subway to generate an aerosol by evaporation of a liquid smallpox formulation or a dry powder.

2.2.1 Genetic and Immunologic Scenarios

Alibek concludes his paper with a discussion of genetically modified variola virus, designed to enhance its effectiveness as a weapon of mass destruction. This scenario builds on the work published from Australia in 2001 involving mousepox (ectromelia) with a gene inserted for interleukin (IL)-4 [49]. The IL-4 cytokine weakens the cell-mediated immune response against viruses such as orthopoxviruses, by inhibiting cytotoxic T-cells and interferon (IFN)-γ production. Clinically, the mice infected with this IL-4-modified mousepox had increased mortality and significantly decreased protection against mousepox by prior vaccination [49].

Similar laboratory work with variola virus, such as inserting the gene for IL-4 or related cytokines such as IL-13, has not been performed or approved by WHO for future experiments, given the risk that the findings with mousepox-IL-4 might be similar to that with variola-IL-4. However, IL-4-modified vaccinia virus has been studied recently in a mouse model. In these experiments, reported in 2004 by NIH researchers, an otherwise fatal challenge with vaccinia virus that had been modified to express murine IL-4 could be prevented by prior immunization with the non-replicating, attenuated vaccinia virus, Modified Vaccinia Ankara (MVA) [50]. This was an important finding because vaccinia virus, with or without the expression of IL-4, can infect humans (as well as mice), whereas mousepox virus does not infect humans.

Additional research has applied the immunologic model [51, 52] of type 1 cytokines (Th1) such as IFN-γ and type 2 cytokines (Th2) such as IL-4 to mousepox and vaccinia; such studies in mice and inferences from human conditions such as atopic dermatitis, immunocompromising diseases, and pregnancy could lead to a rationale for novel immunologic therapies for orthopoxviruses including vaccinia and variola.

In a paper published in 2004 from Australia [53], mousepox (ectromelia) infection of virus-resistant mice (C57BL/6) resulted in IFN-γ production and a strong cytotoxic T-cell cellular immune response. In contrast, mousepox infection of susceptible mice (BALB/c and A/J) resulted in little or no IFN-γ, but instead resulted in production of IL-4. Deletion of the IL-4 gene did not change the disease in the susceptible mice, but loss of IFN-γ function in the resistant mice lead to 100% mortality. Similar earlier studies [54] from Australia and Japan found that mousepox-susceptible mice (BALB/c) were made less susceptible when "STAT-6" (signal transducer and activator of transcription), the intracellular signaling molecule for IL-4, was deleted.

A common theme in these studies is that a strong Th1 response that is exemplified by IFN-γ is needed to prevent or decrease mousepox disease. Since the Th1 IFN-γ and the type 2 cytokine IL-4 are cross-inhibitory [51, 52], the impairment of IFN-γ may be at least as important as the enhancement of IL-4. A strong cellular immune response (controlled by type 1 or Th1 cytokines) may be more critical than a predominant antibody immune response (controlled by type 2 or Th2 cytokines); this is particularly true when response is directly associated with a weak cell-mediated immune response as evidenced by impaired IFN-γ and cytotoxic T-cell production. In the early 1990 s, IFN-γ itself had been reported to have antiviral activity against vaccinia [55–57].

In extending the type 1/type 2 cytokine model to humans, the situation is often less clear cut than in mice [51, 52]. There are data to support the view that atopic dermatitis, immunocompromising diseases, such as HIV/AIDS and some malignancies, and even normal human pregnancy are characterized by a relative decrease in the normal ratio of IFN-γ (type 1 cytokine) to IL-4 (type 2 cytokine) [52, 58–62]. These conditions have been associated with a relative decrease in cell-mediated immune responses. In addition, they are all associated with an increased risk of adverse events due to smallpox vaccination with vaccinia.

These observations on the importance of IFN-γ for the control of orthopoxviruses could generate the hypothesis that subcutaneous IFN-γ, already FDA licensed since 1990 for chronic granulomatous disease and specific medical conditions [63], could be beneficial to control some life-threatening adverse effects of smallpox vaccination including progressive vaccinia. Specifically, for the rare cases of progressive vaccinia that do not respond to Vaccinia Immune Globulin (VIG), and for which surgical therapy (resection) is being considered, along with VIG, subcutaneous IFN-γ could be administered under an investigational new drug (IND) protocol, if one were available. If successful in such a clinical setting, IFN-γ use would avoid surgical resection.

2.3 The Two Viruses: Vaccinia virus (Smallpox Vaccine) and Variola virus (Smallpox)

Vaccinia virus is the virus found in smallpox vaccine, while variola virus is the causative agent of smallpox; they are two distinct viruses. Table 2.1 compares these two related orthopoxviruses, their routes of transmission, virus–immune system interactions, and potential therapy. Vaccinia virus never causes smallpox. Vaccinia virus is not spread via respiratory droplets, and therefore no

Table 2.1 Comparison of vaccinia virus and variola virus

Vaccinia virus: smallpox vaccine	Variola virus: smallpox disease
VACCINIA : the vaccine virus	VARIOLA: the disease virus
Definitions	
Vaccinia: The virus in the smallpox vaccine	Variola: The virus that causes smallpox disease
Vaccinia does not cause smallpox	Variola is not used in smallpox vaccines
Distinct from cowpox (L. "vacca," cow)	Two forms: variola major and variola minor
Transmission	
Vaccinia is spread only by direct contact	Variola is usually spread by direct contact, occasionally in bedding or clothes
Vaccinia is not spread through the air	Variola is spread through the air by droplet aerosols
Virus–immunity interactions	
Vaccinia induces immunity against variola	Variola major is often (30%) fatal if unvaccinated
Immunocompromised persons can develop more severe vaccine reactions, e.g., "progressive" or "necrotic" vaccinia	Immunocompromised and pregnant persons may have more severe smallpox and present with atypical skin lesions: "Hemorrhagic", or "flat" smallpox (both with >90% mortality).
Therapy	
Vaccinia Immune Globulin (VIG) is effective for some, not all, serious vaccine reactions.	Vaccination within 3–4 days can protect against disease [166]. VIG is not used against variola.
No FDA-licensed antiviral drugs.	No FDA-licensed antiviral drugs
Cidofovir may be tested as an antiviral on an investigational new drug (IND) basis.	Cidofovir may be tested as an antiviral on an investigational new drug (IND) basis.

respiratory precautions are needed for persons vaccinated with vaccinia. Some serious vaccination reactions can be treated with VIG, whereas smallpox disease due to variola virus is not responsive to VIG. An intravenous formulation of VIG has replaced the older intramuscular formulation (IM) [64–66] after approval by the FDA on February 18, 2005 (www.fda.gov/cber/products/ vigivdyn021805.htm) [64–66]. There are no FDA-licensed antiviral drugs to prevent or treat illness due to either vaccinia virus or variola virus. Table 2.2 lists 10 ways that smallpox vaccine differs from other FDA-licensed vaccines, including routine use of a bifurcated needle (Fig. 2.1), and that a successful vaccination (a "take") is documentable on the skin by day 6–8 (Fig. 2.2).

Variola virus can be transmitted in multiple ways: By far, the most common is via respiratory droplets, but transmission by fomites such as clothing or bed linens, has occurred [1]. Transmission as an aerosol, involving droplet nuclei, is rare but occasionally has been documented such as in a hospital in Meschede, Germany [67].

The incubation period of variola virus is 7–17 (mean = 12) days, after which a febrile prodrome begins with headache, backache, nausea, and prostration

Table 2.2 Ten (10) ways that smallpox vaccine differs from other vaccines

1. Rationale for use: to protect against a disease eradicated over 25 years ago.
2. One virus (vaccinia) protects against disease due to a second virus (variola).
3. Contraindications (absent smallpox exposure) include any history of eczema.
4. A "bifurcated" needle is routinely used for vaccination.
5. Either 3 (naïve) or 15 (revaccinee) intradermal jabs of the needle are recommended.
6. A trace of blood must be seen after last intradermal jab, or vaccination is repeated.
7. A successful vaccination (a "take") is documentable on the skin by day 6–8.
8. The vaccine site is infectious to self and "contacts" until the scabs are fully formed: $\sim$3 weeks.
9. Least safe FDA-licensed vaccine: 15 life-threatening reactions, and one or two deaths, per million primary vaccinations.
10. Some, but not all, serious vaccine reactions can be treated with Vaccinia Immune Globulin (VIG).

(Table 2.3) [1, 9, 68]. Some have speculated that the incubation period may be shorter if a highly virulent and high-dose exposure to smallpox is accomplished by an aerosol release as a bioweapon [48]. After 1–4 days of the febrile prodrome, a rash begins in the oral mucosa and then in the skin; typically the rash is concentrated centrifugally, including the face, palms, and soles. Infectivity prior to the clear-cut onset of rash is rare, and the highest degree of infectivity occurs once the rash is present [1].

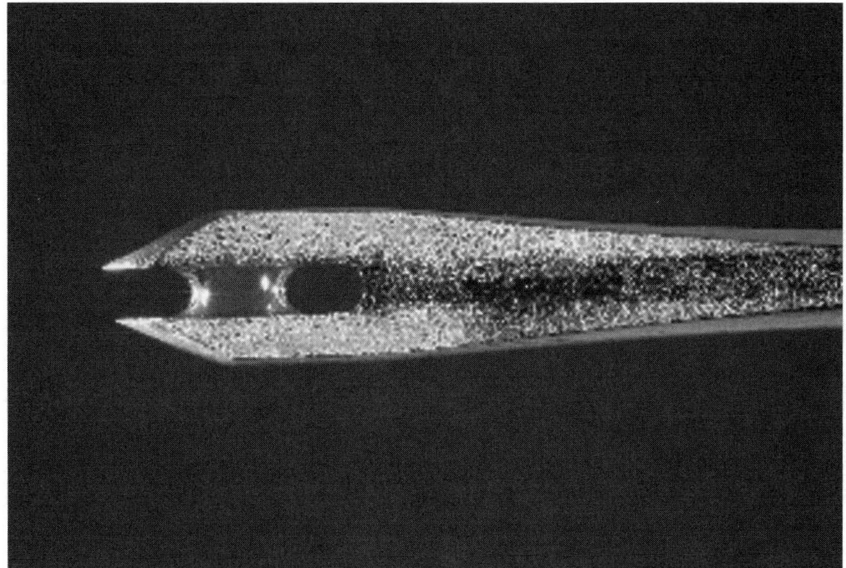

Fig. 2.1 Bifurcated needle with smallpox vaccine liquid (CDC)

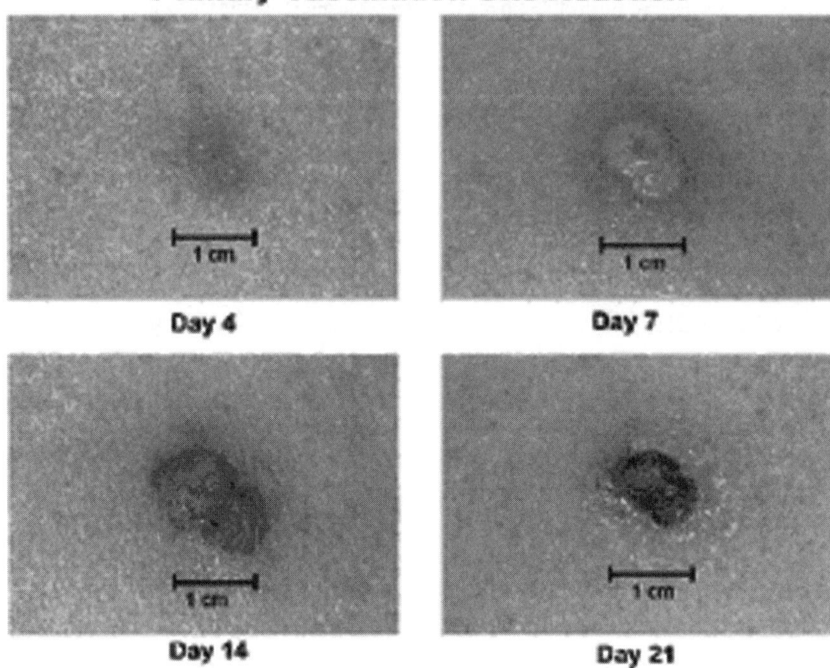

Fig. 2.2 Time course of typical skin reactions to smallpox vaccination in a vaccinia-naïve person (CDC)

Table 2.3 Major and minor criteria for the diagnosis of smallpox

Major criteria (3)

1. **Febrile prodrome:** occurs 1–4 days before rash. Fever >101F and at least one of the following: prostration, headache, backache, chills, vomiting, or severe abdominal pain.
2. **Classic smallpox lesions:** deep-seated, firm-hard, round well-circumscribed vesicles or pustules as they evolve lesions may become umbilicated or confluent.
3. **Lesions in the same stage of development:** on any one part of the body lesions are all in the same stage, e.g., all vesicles or all pustules at the same time.

Minor criteria (5)

1. Centrifugal distribution with greatest concentration of lesions on face and distal extremities.
2. First lesions on the oral mucosa/palate, face, or forearms.
3. Patient appears toxic or moribund.
4. Slow evolution of lesions evolving from macules to papules to pustules over several days.
5. Lesions on the palms and soles.

"High," "Moderate," and Low" risk of smallpox defined using these major and minor criteria

"High" Risk: all three major criteria

"Moderate" Risk: Febrile prodrome and either one other major criteria or 4–5 minor criteria.

"Low" Risk: either no febrile prodrome or febrile prodrome and <4 minor criteria.

Reference [21] http://www.bt.cdc.gov/agent/smallpox/diagnosis/pdf/spox-poster-full.pdf.

2.4 Myopericarditis and other adverse events after vaccination: 2002–2004

Prior to 2003, cases of myocarditis and/or pericarditis after smallpox vaccination were seldom reported in the United States, but were reported from Europe, especially Scandinavia, and from Australia [69–76]. One possible explanation was the use of a different vaccinia strain in the United States (New York City Board of Health strain) from those used in Europe and Australia. In a study of military conscripts from Finland [76], all of whom were routinely vaccinated against smallpox, an incidence of symptomatic myocarditis after the smallpox vaccination was approximately 1:10,000. This figure was based on 12 cases of myocarditis occurring 8–14 days after vaccination, without any other etiology for the myocarditis being found on investigation.

In the United States, the initial reports of myopericarditis after smallpox vaccination appeared in March 2003 and triggered immediate investigation by the CDC and the DoD [27, 77–80]. While investigations were ongoing to assess causality, new safeguards were implemented to avoid vaccination in persons with a history of either cardiac disease or stroke, or in those in whom three or more risk factors were present (Table 2.4). These traditional risk factors for heart disease included high blood pressure, elevated cholesterol, diabetes, smoking, and a positive family history of heart disease before the age of 50 years [27].

As of October 14, 2004, the DoD had diagnosed 82 cases of myopericarditis in over 656,000 vaccinees (about 1:8,000), most of whom were primary vaccinees. Out of 39,213 vaccinees, the CDC identified 5 probable and 16 suspected cases of myopericarditis after smallpox vaccination [81]. The DoD published

Table 2.4 CDC updated (November 15, 2003) smallpox guidelines for "Smallpox Pre-Vaccination Information Packet: Contents and Instructions." "Smallpox Vaccination Patient Medical History and Consent Form." Heart Problems

1. Have you ever been diagnosed by a doctor as having a heart condition with or without symptoms such as a previous myocardial infarction (heart attack), angina (chest pain caused by a lack of blood flow to the heart), congestive heart failure, or cardiomyopathy?
2. Have you ever had a stroke or transient ischemic attack (a "mini-stroke" that produces stroke-like symptoms but no lasting damage)?
3. Do you have chest pain or shortness of breath when you exert yourself (such as when you walk up stairs)?
4. Do you have any other heart condition for which you are under the care of a doctor?
5. Do you have three or more of the following risk factors?
   a. You have been told by a doctor that you have high blood pressure.
   b. You have been told by a doctor that you have high blood cholesterol.
   c. You have been told by a doctor that you have diabetes or high blood sugar.
   d. You have a first-degree relative (for example, mother, father, brother, or sister) who had a heart condition before the age of 50).
   e. You smoke cigarettes now.

their initial findings in June 2003 [82] and in two updated articles [83, 84] in 2004 as well as on the DoD website dedicated to their smallpox vaccination program (www.smallpox.army.mil/event/SPSafetySum.asp). A causal relationship has been accepted for the myopericarditis, in part because it is more common in the DoD after primary vaccination than revaccination, because of its occurrence within 7–14 days after vaccination, and because of the absence of other etiologies. The DoD reported in 2004 a statistically significant association between developing myopericarditis and being male and white. Among primary vaccinees there was a significantly increased risk of myopericardits within 30 days after smallpox vaccination, with an observed incidence of 16.11/100,000. In contrast, the DoD found no increased risk of myopericarditis in revaccinees [83]. No deaths have occurred, and the prognosis has been good for a full recovery after vaccine-associated myopericarditis. The DoD reported that 64 of the initial 67 patients (96%) had normalization of their functional status, echocardiography, EKG, and graded exercise testing at a mean of 32 weeks' follow-up. Atypical, but non-limiting, persistent chest discomfort was reported by 8 of the 67 patients (13%) [84].

No causal relationship has been found for myocardial infarction or other ischemic events after smallpox vaccination [24, 85]. Likewise, a retrospective analysis of cardiac deaths after the 1947 mass vaccination program of approximately 6.4 million persons in New York City revealed no evidence of an increase in cardiac deaths [86].

Among other adverse events following vaccination, the DoD reported as of October 14, 2004, that one death may have been attributable to smallpox vaccination, although the results are inconclusive, according to two independent civilian physician panels. This patient was a 22-year-old reservist who received five vaccines, including smallpox vaccine, at the same time and developed a lupus-like illness prior to her death 33 days after the five vaccinations [84] (www.smallpox.mil/event/panelreport.asp). Six other deaths after vaccination were judged to be clearly unrelated to vaccination. Sixteen other cases of "ischemic heart disease" such as angina or myocardial infarction occurred within 6 weeks after smallpox vaccination in the 656,000 vaccinees, but these cases were judged to be "similar to what normally occurs among unvaccinated military personnel of similar age" [86, October 14, 2003, summary at www.smallpox.mil/event/panelreport.asp]. Forty cases of generalized vaccinia were reported, and most were treated as outpatients; 50 cases of contact vaccinia were found, nearly all between spouses and adult intimate contacts outside the workplace [24]. More importantly, no cases of vaccinia transmission occurred between the 27,700 vaccinated health-care workers (HCWs) and patients or co-workers. Neither progressive vaccinia nor eczema vaccinatum cases were observed in military or civilian vaccinees (www.smallpox.army.mil/event/SPSafetySum.asp). Similarly, there were no episodes of vaccinia transmission from a civilian health-care worker to a patient or a co-worker.

2.5 HIV/AIDS and Smallpox Vaccination

In 2004, the DoD reported that 10 of the initial 438,000 patients who received smallpox vaccination since December 2002 also had undiagnosed infection with the human immunodeficiency virus (HIV) [88]. All 10 persons had a normal major reaction to the vaccination and normal healing. More importantly, however, none of these persons had AIDS-defining CD4-cell counts (<250 cells/ul), opportunistic infections, or malignancies. Their CD4 counts ranged from 286 to 751 cells/ul. In addition, 7 of 10 patients had previously been vaccinated against smallpox.

Only one patient with HIV infection has been reported to have had a serious, but nonfatal, adverse event after receiving the standard smallpox vaccination [89]. This occurred in 1984 in the US Army, prior to the availability of HIV antibody testing. At that time, smallpox vaccination was still routinely administered in the military due to concern about the potential use of smallpox virus as a bioweapon. Soon after smallpox vaccination, the first for this 19-year-old army recruit, the patient presented with AIDS-defining cryptococcal meningitis, and oral candidiasis. His CD4 T-cell count was <25 cells/ul. Four weeks after vaccination, while hospitalized for meningitis, a 3 cm × 4 cm ulcer developed at the vaccination site, and then over the next 3 days, 80–100 pustular lesions appeared on the posterior legs and buttocks. These lesions also ulcerated, and vaccinia virus was cultured from the lesions. After 12 weekly intramuscular treatments with VIG, the skin lesions completely resolved. When this case report was published in 1987, the accompanying editorial by Halsey and Henderson [90] commented that several hundred HIV-infected military recruits must have received multiple immunizations, including vaccinia, without complications prior to the mandatory HIV-antibody testing and exclusion of HIV-positive recruits.

Although no other instances of complications of smallpox vaccination in patients with HIV infection have been reported, the use of recombinant vaccinia to express HIV proteins as an investigational form of cell immunotherapy did raise concerns about vaccinia virus potentially contributing to the deaths of three patients with AIDS and CD4 T-cell counts <50 cells/ul in a Phase I trial in Paris in 1989–1990 [91, 92]. According to Zagury, earlier clinical trials at the Cliniques Universitaires, Kinshasa, Democratic Republic of the Congo, and Paris had not shown similar toxicities [93]. This particular HIV cell immunotherapy, using paraformaldehyde inactivation and recombinant vaccinia to express HIV proteins in autologous EBV-transformed B-cells, was reviewed in 1991 and the decision was made to discontinue its use [92, 93].

Since 2001, concerns regarding complications of smallpox vaccination and smallpox infection in persons with immunocompromised conditions, such as HIV/AIDS or transplantations [94], have been discussed by Bartlett and others [95–97]. Issues regarding HIV/AIDS and smallpox and smallpox vaccination were presented at the 2002 International AIDS conference in Barcelona, Spain

[98]. In the event of a smallpox attack and possible exposure, the possibility of rapid testing for HIV infection has been considered as a possible screening tool. However, the critical point is that if a person has been exposed to smallpox, there are no contraindications to vaccination with vaccinia, including HIV infection.

One such rapid test for HIV antibody using fingerstick specimens, called OraQuick Rapid HIV-1 antibody test, was approved by the FDA on November 7, 2002 [99, 100]. The FDA later approved the OraQuick test for use with routine whole blood venipuncture samples in September 2003. The FDA revised the time during which the results of the test would be interpreted to between 20 and 40 min.

How would the ongoing global HIV/AIDS pandemic impact the global public health response if smallpox was to reenter the human population as a bioterrorist weapon? The potential public health, societal, and economic implications in terms of trying to contain and control smallpox in this setting, especially in parts of the world with the highest prevalence of HIV infection, such as sub-Saharan Africa and India have been debated. Some [101] have viewed with alarm the potential for dual infections with HIV and variola, or vaccinia, but there are others who doubt that this would pose an insuperable problem.

Safer smallpox vaccines are needed. Third-generation smallpox vaccines, using attenuated vaccinia viruses such as MVA or the LC16m8 strain used in a smallpox vaccine that was licensed in Japan in 1975, are being reevaluated as options for immunocompromised patients in the event of a smallpox attack. An immunocompromised animal model has been studied in which rhesus macaques are infected with simian immunodeficiency virus (SIV) or a SIV/HIV hybrid virus. They are vaccinated with an attenuated, replication-deficient vaccinia and/or with the standard non-attenuated first-generation Dryvax vaccine. Giving the attenuated vaccinia vaccine first, followed by Dryvax, decreases the adverse events seen with Dryvax alone [102].

Given the global susceptibility to smallpox since its eradication 25 years ago and subsequent cessation of routine vaccination, the threat of smallpox being reintroduced as an act of bioterrorism makes the insufficient amount of smallpox vaccine in most nations of the world today particularly concerning. For these and other reasons, it is evident why destruction of all stocks of smallpox virus has been called for and its use as a bioterror weapon has been characterized as a "crime against humanity" as one of several recommended international measures to prevent the return of smallpox [68, 103].

2.6 Hemorrhagic Smallpox

The rare and highly fatal (92–100%) form of smallpox known as "hemorrhagic smallpox" deserves specific consideration. Due to the striking and rapidly progressive clinical illness, some have speculated that terrorists would attempt a smallpox attack that will cause a high incidence of hemorrhagic smallpox [104, 105], if such a strain of variola were able to be identified. At this time no strain of variola has been reported that reproducibly causes hemorrhagic smallpox.

The "early" form of hemorrhagic smallpox was found by Rao in his 1964 report of 100 such patients to have a much shortened time (mean of 5.95 days) from the onset of the smallpox febrile prodrome until death [106]. If an aerosol attack with smallpox occurs in which tens or thousands of persons are infected, some of the index cases may be patients with early hemorrhagic smallpox. Recognition of this rare (~1%) manifestation of smallpox would be critical to trigger an immediate public health response to such a smallpox outbreak.

A monkey model of hemorrhagic smallpox has been developed at the CDC by the US Army researchers [107–109]. High-dose intravenous challenge with variola virus caused a hemorrhagic form of smallpox with a monocyte-associated viremia. Analysis of the immune response in these animals suggested marked impairment of both the tumor necrosis factor alpha (TNF-α) response and the expression of the transcription factor NF-kB, in these animals [109]. Cidofovir did not confer any prophylactic protection in this hemorrhagic smallpox model—a finding that the authors attributed to the overwhelming nature of the hemorrhagic smallpox with 100% lethality and a mean time to death of 4 days [108]. The high-level viremia with variola associated with hemorrhagic smallpox in the above-mentioned monkey models is reminiscent of the findings published in 1969 by a team of researchers from India, England, and the United States working in Madras, India, that patients with hemorrhagic smallpox also had high-level viremia with variola [110].

As an example of concern regarding hemorrhagic smallpox as a clue to weaponization of the virus, in late 2001, information was made public in a Russian newspaper and to the West regarding a previously unreported smallpox outbreak involving 10 patients in Aralsk, Kazakhstan, in the former Soviet Union in 1971 [111]. The fact that 3 of the 10 patients were diagnosed with hemorrhagic smallpox was raised as a possible clue by one investigator that a more virulent smallpox virus was being developed and tested at that time near Aralsk, on Vozrozhdeniye island in the Aral Sea, by the Soviet military [111]. Henderson doubted this interpretation, pointing out that the one person who was ostensibly infected by the aerosol actually had a mild case. All other cases resulted from secondary transmission, and the three who subsequently manifested hemorrhagic smallpox did not transmit infection to others. This would be consistent with Rao's thesis that the cause of hemorrhagic smallpox relates to host response rather than to the intrinsic character of the virus strain [8, 112].

Rao has reported the largest series of hemorrhagic smallpox cases [8, 106]. Although earlier clinicians, such as Osler in his 1892 textbook of Medicine, had recognized two types of hemorrhagic smallpox, a rapidly fatal "black smallpox" and a later pustular form [113], the most detailed description of the clinical and epidemiological aspects of the disease has been given by Rao. In 1964, he published a paper describing in detail 240 hemorrhagic cases seen between

1959 and 1963, representing 2.3% of 10,857 total smallpox cases [106]. In his 1972 smallpox monograph [8], Rao reviewed 200 patients with hemorrhagic smallpox beginning in 1961 (and thus partially overlapping with his earlier series from 1959 to 1963), for a total of 385 cases of hemorrhagic smallpox out of approximately 30,000 total smallpox cases he had seen over 30 years of his work in India. Rao reported that, of these 385 cases of hemorrhagic smallpox, not even one transmitted hemorrhagic smallpox to another person, suggesting that it was the host response rather than the virus strain that was the critical variable.[8].

This observation by Rao is also used to counter the argument advanced by Sarkar and Mitra in 1967 that hemorrhagic smallpox patients have a more virulent virus than patients with confluent or discrete smallpox. Working in Calcutta, they isolated variola virus from 75 patients, comparing 25 with hemorrhagic smallpox, 25 with confluent smallpox, and 25 with discrete smallpox [114]. They used four methods to assess virulence: at least 50% mortality in the chick embryo, at least 50% mortality in infant mice, the histopathology of pocks on the chorioallantoic membrane (CAM), and at least 1,000 pock-forming units (PFU) per gram of liver in an infected chick embryo. These four methods were used, in part, because there were no standard methods to assay virulence of the variola virus. A positive result leading to being classified as more virulent was found in all four assays in 48% of hemorrhagic smallpox cases, compared with 36% of confluent cases, and 0% of discrete-type smallpox cases. A virological mechanism for these findings has never been reported, but one methodological difference, albeit of uncertain significance, is that the variola virus from all 25 hemorrhagic smallpox cases was isolated from venous blood, whereas 49/50 confluent and discrete cases were isolated from vesicular or pustular fluid. These studies from 1967 have not been replicated or restudied.

Salient clinical points from Rao's 240 hemorrhagic smallpox patients [106] distinguish the "early" and "late" form of hemorrhagic smallpox. The "early" form (100 of 240 patients) presented with fever and severe prodromal symptoms including excruciating backache and severe headache with hemorrhages into the mucous membranes and skin, which was described as having a "velvety touch and colour." Death occurred in 100% of these patients on average 5.95 days later. Classic smallpox skin lesions never developed, an important point because the current CDC algorithm for evaluating a rash would likely miss a patient with early hemorrhagic smallpox because of the lack of an acute, generalized vesicular or pustular rash, which is one of the major criteria in the CDC algorithm [21] (Table 2.3). Potentially diagnostic clues to even atypical forms of smallpox would still be recognized at autopsy [115, 116].

Rao's description of "late" hemorrhagic smallpox, based on the remaining 140 of the total 240 hemorrhagic smallpox patients, starts with the febrile prodrome that may or may not be severe, but with a rash actually developing to a papulovesicular stage [106]. The average time to death, which occurred in 92% of the 140 cases, was 10.2 days, considerably longer than the 5.95 days found in the early hemorrhagic smallpox form. In both early and late forms, pregnant women were especially vulnerable to hemorrhagic smallpox. This was most striking with the early form in which 44 of the 100 patients (44%) were pregnant women, compared with 14 of the 140 patients (10%) with the late form.

In both early and late forms, death occurred despite past successful vaccination, at least a few of which were recent. However, the vaccines used in India during Rao's studies were of variable quality, and an apparent vaccination scar could be caused by trauma to the skin when a rotary lancet was used even when the smallpox vaccine was impotent. An illustrated historical review of devices and tools used to administer smallpox vaccines was provided by Baxby in 2002 [117]. This visually striking review emphasizes that the bifurcated needle (Fig. 2.1), successfully used during the smallpox global eradication program, became available only in the late 1960 s.

Increased hormone levels associated with pregnancy were considered by Rao and other researchers to contribute to the predisposition and high case fatality rate of pregnant women for hemorrhagic smallpox [118]. In 1963, Rao and colleagues in India reported on their extensive clinical experience with smallpox and pregnancy, totaling 244 pregnant women. They also compared in detail 94 consecutive pregnant women admitted over a 12-month period from 1961 to 1962 with a comparison group of non-pregnant women and men. Their multiple findings included that the highest risk of premature termination of pregnancy occurred if the woman was infected with variola in the very early or very late months of pregnancy. The incidence of hemorrhagic smallpox was much higher in pregnant women than in non-pregnant women or in men. The specific manifestation of hemorrhagic smallpox was reported to be lowest in the first trimester, then increasing to a peak in the sixth month, declining in the seventh and eighth month, but rising again at the end of pregnancy.

In his 1972 monograph, Rao summarized results of his experiments, published in 1968 in the Indian Journal of Medical Research [119], using a monkey model to define the pathogenesis of smallpox in pregnancy and in immunocompromised hosts, for example, by administering corticosteroids (cortisone) prior to infection with variola [8]. He concluded: "Thus cortisone has been shown to enhance the disease of variola in monkeys. Adequate doses of cortisone before and after variolation produced a fatal form of smallpox, associated with internal as well as external hemorrhages. Pregnant monkey and cortisonised monkey reacted to smallpox infection in the same way as a pregnant woman to smallpox. The mechanism by which cortisone enhances the disease is still vague."

The monkeys used in these experimental variola infection studies were Indian bonnet monkeys (*Macacus radiata*), 2–4 kg in weight, and caught in and around Madras. Only one of these monkeys was pregnant. A fourth egg passage variola virus suspension derived from vesicular fluid from a patient with smallpox was used to infect these monkeys by variolation on the abdomen, using a tuberculin syringe and injecting the variola suspension intradermally. A total of 30 monkeys were variolated, 16 of whom also received varying doses of cortisone before and after infection, while 14 others received a placebo rather than cortisone. Twelve of sixteen (75%) of the cortisoned animals died of smallpox, whereas 0/14 of the control monkeys died. All 16 of the cortisonized monkeys developed varying degrees of generalized smallpox rash, as did 13/14 control animals albeit less extensive. Comparing the time course of viremia in both groups showed that higher percentage of cortisonized animals were viremic on days 4, 6, and 8 after infection. Autopsies of the 12 cortisonized monkeys that died revealed macroscopic petechial hemorrhages in the lungs and gastrointestinal mucosal membranes. Variola was found in the viscera of multiple cortisonized animals at autopsy, but no virus was found in the single control animal sacrificed. The pregnant monkey did not receive cortisone, aborted on the sixth day after variolation and died on the twelfth day with extensive hemorrhages in the lung and intestinal mucous membranes at autopsy.

For unknown reasons, few other viral infections, with the exception of Lassa Fever virus and hepatitis E [120], have such an increased case fatality rate in pregnant women as does smallpox. Whether the immunologic paradigm described during pregnancy of increased type 2 cytokines such as IL-4 and decreased type 1 cytokines such as IFN-γ plays an etiologic role in hemorrhagic smallpox is uncertain [59–62]. Interestingly, progesterone, a hormone elevated during pregnancy, has been reported to increase IL-4 production from T-cells, including those not normally producing this cytokine [62]. A speculative analogy to pregnancy and increased risk of severe smallpox exists in the recent experiments with mousepox engineered to express IL-4 and inhibit cytotoxic T-cells that produce IFN-γ, causing more virulent disease and overcoming the protective effect of prior mousepox vaccination.

2.7 International Preparedness for Smallpox

In October 2001, the director of the WHO, Dr. Gro Harlem Brundtland, stated [121]: “I want to emphasize that should an outbreak of smallpox be detected in any country, this should be considered an international emergency. WHO will help countries to pool available resources so as to contain the disease as rapidly and effectively as possible.”

The WHO has continued to provide international support to efforts related to smallpox detection and vaccination, including the provision of educational resources on its website and the sharing of results of annually sanctioned research on variola virus in Russia and the United States. Worldwide, the WHO provides support to surveillance networks for smallpox and other outbreaks via their Global Outbreak Alert and Response Network (GOARN). Preparations for a possible smallpox virus release and other potential bioterrorist events were initiated by a number of nations. These planning efforts involved the WHO, US scientists, public health officials, politicians, regulatory officials, and others.

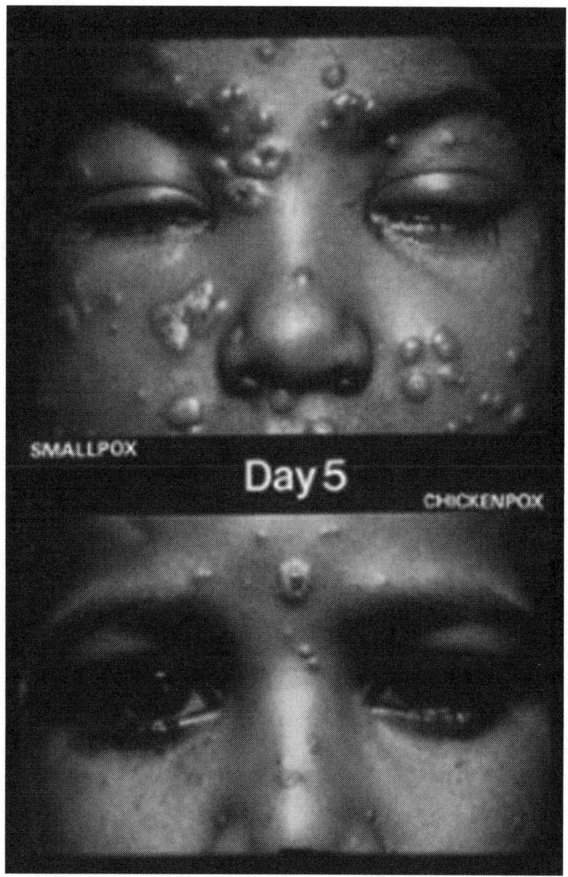

Fig. 2.3 Smallpox skin lesions (WHO): day 5 of smallpox vs. chickenpox

The WHO has provided regular updates on smallpox and smallpox vaccination since 2001. These updates include addressing smallpox as a global public health emergency if even one case occurs [11–13], posting on their website photographs of smallpox and smallpox vaccination responses, including comparisons with chickenpox (Fig. 2.3), updating in 2004 the WHO 1970 review of the risks posed by biological weapons [5], and posting annually the laboratory research on variola virus in Russia and the United States. Such work has included the pathogenesis of variola infections, serological assays, PCR-based diagnostic assays, animal model development, studies of new vaccines, and antiviral drugs including the tyrosine kinase inhibitors such as the anti-leukemia drug "Gleevac" (5, 13 and www.who.int/csr/disease/smallpox/research/en/).

Israel was the first nation to begin smallpox vaccination following the anthrax attacks of September–October 2001 in the United States. An initial phase of vaccination was carried out between September 2002 and January 2003 when 17,000 first responders, including HCWs, were vaccinated using the Lister strain of vaccinia [122]. A study of a subset of these vaccinees, all of whom had been previously vaccinated, showed that only 96/158 (61%) of these vaccinees had a successful clinical take, but this was understandable because vaccine titers were much lower than international standards..

On September 5–6, 2002, a multination (G7+) Global Health Security Initiative (GHSI) workshop was held at the Paul Ehrlich Institute in Langen, Germany, on "Best practices in vaccine production for smallpox and other potential pathogens" [10]. National and regional information on current and projected smallpox vaccines and antiviral drugs was presented by scientists from Japan, the Pan American Health Organization, the European Union, Germany, France, Belgium, the United States, the WHO, and others. The US Food and Drug Administration (FDA) regulatory requirements for licensure of smallpox vaccines were presented [123].

On September 8–10, 2003, an international command post exercise named "Global Mercury," involving a scenario with multiple "terrorists" who were inoculated with smallpox and traveled to different parts of the world was conducted. Canada, Mexico, Japan, Italy, Germany, France, the UK, the United States, the European Commission, and the WHO were involved with this real-time exercise, details of which were posted on the Health Canada website (www.hc-sc.gc.ca/english/media/issues/global_mercury_summary.html). Six recommendations resulted from this exercise. One of the most important was the recognition of the need to strengthen already existing national smallpox response plans by "greater elaboration of their international components." It was also found that all forms of communications were to maintain in an adequate real-time manner during the exercise across multiple continents and nations. Better communications infrastructure, improved information management processes, and trained public health personnel were needed [14, 15].

In October 2003, an international conference was held in Geneva on past smallpox weapons development, current threats, and smallpox vaccination issues. Copies of slide presentations were posted online at www.smallpoxbiosecurity.org and partly in a special supplement of the International Journal of Infectious Diseases [124].

In November 2003, at a symposium on smallpox and smallpox vaccination held in Hong Kong, sponsored by the Health Department of Hong Kong, one of us (DL) presented both pre-event and post-event smallpox vaccination scenario discussions. Lessons learned from the US smallpox vaccination program were also presented. The smallpox preparedness program in Hong Kong had already been initiated prior to the onset of the SARS epidemic in February 2003. Issues regarding sharing of smallpox vaccine if needed to help control an international outbreak were also discussed.

As of December 2003, the UK had posted on its Department of Health website (www.dh.gov.uk) its updated smallpox plan [125]. This is a valuable reference document, with 17 appendices and a large amount of detail regarding the common and critical public health issues that would occur anywhere in the world once a smallpox outbreak had occurred. Particularly helpful are highly specific algorithms for how to manage initial suspected smallpox cases depending on where they are first located. Separate algorithms are given if the suspected case is at home, in the emergency department ("Accident and Emergency"), on a general hospital ward, in a surgery clinic, in an intensive care unit, in an infectious disease unit, or in a port health control unit.

Additionally, detailed recommendations are provided for vaccination strategies at each level of alert, for example, if smallpox is reported outside the UK (alert level 2) or in the UK (alert level 3). Notably, the UK plan includes a specific smallpox outbreak alert level for when a large-scale outbreak occurs that is not contained by "ring" vaccination (alert level 4). Whereas "surveillance and containment" (sometimes referred to as "ring" vaccination) is recommended by the UK for alert levels 2 and 3, as it is done by the WHO, and the CDC mass vaccination is to be considered for alert level 4, depending on the circumstances and the risk/benefit analyses at that time.

In January 14, 2005, a smallpox tabletop exercise named "Atlantic Storm" was carried out, as described online at www.upmc-biosecurity.org. In this hypothetical scenario, terrorists released smallpox virus in six target areas via a commercially available dry powder dispenser hidden in a backpack. The targets included crowded public sites in Frankfurt, Istanbul, Rotterdam, Warsaw, Los Angeles, and New York City [17–21].

Two observations from this Atlantic Storm exercise deserve particular notice: (1) With respect to the availability of vaccine, only 40 of more than 200 nations now have any stocks of smallpox vaccine, and no country has more vaccine than what it believes it would need for its own citizens. The total global stockpiles of vaccine amount to about 750 million doses (about 10–12% relative to the global population); the WHO stockpile consists of only 2.5 million doses; there are only five vaccine production laboratories and, under emergency conditions, output would not be much more than 40 million doses per month. At present, there is, in place, no mechanism for deciding on priorities for global allocation of vaccine in case of an emergency. (2) There is, at present, no forum wherein different countries, in case of an emergency, could work to effect common policies with respect to restrictions on travel, harmonization of national policies, and mobilization of non-health resources.

In sum, the need to work collaboratively on an international basis, including discussion of sharing smallpox vaccine supplies, prior to a smallpox outbreak, is critical to prepare best for what could rapidly become a global public health emergency.

2.8 The Centers for Disease Control and Prevention: Smallpox algorithm for generalized vesicular or pustular rash

After the events of 2001, the CDC developed an algorithm to evaluate suspected patients with smallpox, focusing on patients with fever followed by a generalized vesicular or pustular rash [21]. During 30 months (from January 2002 until

June 2004), the CDC was consulted on 43 patients with suspected smallpox as part of this algorithm [126]. Major and minor criteria were developed (Table 2.3), and "high," "medium," and "low" risk patients identified. To decrease the number of false-positive laboratory tests for variola virus, only persons classified by this algorithm as "high-risk" for smallpox underwent testing for variola. Any "high-risk" case was not to undergo laboratory testing for another disease until laboratory testing was completed for variola virus. According to this algorithm, all patients with a generalized vesicular or pustular rash and fever were immediately placed on airborne and contact precautions, and the infection control team was notified.

The CDC investigators reported that, during the 30-month period, none of the 43 cases of suspected smallpox met the criteria for "high-risk"; eight were classified as "moderate-risk"; and 35 as "low-risk". Despite not being classified as "high-risk," one patient did have variola testing performed and the result was negative; the final diagnosis was HSV-2. The most common diagnosis was varicella. Of the eight "moderate-risk" cases, five were due to varicella, one due to a drug reaction, one due to erythema multiforme, and one due to eczema. On seven occasions, hospital or emergency department closures or diversions occurred. Use of the algorithm facilitated the prompt reversal of these closures and diversions.

The CDC authors added an important caveat to this algorithm, that it "is not designed to detect the most severe and atypical forms of smallpox – that is, flat-type or hemorrhagic type." A color poster and online version of this CDC smallpox algorithm, with rapid interactive individual patient classification options, is available via the CDC website at: www.bt.cdc.gov/agent/smallpox/diagnosis/pdf/spox-poster-full.pdf.

The CDC website on smallpox, www.bt.cdc.gov/agent/smallpox/index.asp, contains extensive information on smallpox, smallpox vaccination, contact tracing, quarantine and isolation, criteria for a "contagious" facility where smallpox patients could be hospitalized or otherwise cohorted for care, VIG, cidofovir, and multiple other related issues. Several hundred photographs illustrating key points about smallpox and smallpox vaccination are available (e.g., Figs. 2.1 and 2.2) at www.bt.cdc.gov/agent/smallpox/smallpox-images/.

The CDC has sought outside guidance from the Institute of Medicine (IOM) on smallpox vaccine–related issues. Reports of at least six meetings have been submitted to the CDC director by The Institute of Medicine Committee on Smallpox Vaccination Program Implementation. Each of the six IOM reports can be found online at www.iom.edu/report.asp?id = 21243.

The committee recommendations and assessments have traced a course from focusing on smallpox and smallpox vaccination, including active surveillance for adverse events, to recommending that smallpox preparedness be incorporated into a more general "all-hazards" emergency preparedness program. The committee has emphasized that smallpox vaccination is only one aspect of preparedness for smallpox and that detailed preparedness plans for smallpox and other public health emergencies should be written, critiqued, and assessed via training exercises [127].

2.9 Smallpox Vaccines 2004: First, Second, and Third Generations

Smallpox vaccine development can be divided into three generations of vaccines. The first generation vaccines are those that use vaccinia virus grown on the skin of a calf and subsequently purified after harvest. In the United States, through 2007, this vaccine was a lyophilized (freeze-dried) preparation produced by Wyeth–Ayerst that was reconstituted before use [128]. This has been replaced by a second-generation vaccine, ACAM 2000 (see below) [129].

Another first-generation smallpox vaccine, available in the United States, was stored frozen, rather than lyophilized, and approximately 80 million doses were provided to the US government by Aventis Pasteur. Dilution studies in 340 vaccinia-naïve adults using 1:5 and 1:10 dilutions of this vaccine showed equivalent vaccination take rates with this vaccine (undiluted: 100%; 1:5 dilution: 98.2%; and 1:10 dilution: 100%) [130]. Under field conditions, lower take rates would be expected; thus, the vaccine is recommended for use at a 1:5 dilution at most and only under emergency circumstances.

So-called second-generation smallpox vaccines are grown in tissue cell cultures. The vaccinia virus strains are plaque purified strains derived from those used in preparation of the animal lymph vaccines; the frequency of adverse events is expected to be comparable. At least two different tissue cell culture vaccines of this type entered clinical trials. These are ACAM 2000 grown in African green monkey kidney ("Vero" cells) made by Acambis in partnership with Baxter and a chick embryo cell-culture smallpox vaccine made by Bavarian Nordic, a Danish company. The ACAM 2000 vaccine uses a vaccinia virus derived from the New York City Board of Health seed strain [131, 132]; Bavarian Nordic uses a Lister-derived vaccinia strain. On September 1, 2007, the FDA announced licensure of this second-generation smallpox vaccine, ACAM 2000, including a medication guide (www.fda.gov/cber/products/acam2000qa.htm). This six-page medication guide includes information regarding possible side effects of the vaccine, what are the medical conditions that predispose to some of these side effects, how to care for the vaccination site, and what to avoid after getting vaccinated. As of 2007, Acambis has produced and supplied to the US stockpile some 200 million doses of their new vaccine.

Initial Phase I clinical trials of ACAM 2000 demonstrated comparable safety and immunogenicity with the Dryvax first-generation vaccine. In 2004, during the larger Phase III trials required for licensure, patients with myopericarditis were diagnosed, both in the Dryvax comparator-control vaccine recipients and in the tissue culture vaccine recipients. The symptoms were mild and transient, and no sequelae were detected.

Third-generation smallpox vaccines include those made from attenuated vaccinia virus strains, such as MVA and LC16m8, and more recently, DNA-based vaccines [133–135], using only selected DNA segments of the vaccinia virus, rather than the entire virus [133]. The central concept behind the third-generation vaccines is to increase the safety profile by using attenuated vaccinia viruses or DNA-based vaccines rather than non-attenuated live, replicating vaccinia virus as are used in the first- and second-generation vaccines. The DNA subunit vaccine approach reported in 2004 by Hooper et al. demonstrated that rhesus macaques monkeys were protected from severe disease when a normally lethal challenge with monkeypox virus was administered [135].

MVA is a non-replicating attenuated vaccinia strain. It was developed in Germany in the 1960 s and 1970 s to be used prior to vaccinating with the traditional Lister lymph vaccine strain in expectation that MVA might protect against vaccine complications caused by the Lister strain. It has not been tested for efficacy during a smallpox outbreak. Immunocompetent monkeys given either two doses of MVA or one dose of MVA followed by one dose of Dryvax [136] have been successfully protected against intravenous infection with monkeypox, an orthopoxvirus closely related to smallpox. The precise vaccine-associated correlates of protection are unknown [137–140], but these authors found that antibody binding and neutralization titers, as well as vaccinia-virus-specific IFN-γ producing T-cells, were equivalent or higher in the immunized monkeys compared with those who received a single dose of the standard lymph vaccine (Dryvax) [136].

Extending the lethal monkeypox virus challenge to immunocompromised monkeys, specifically macaques infected with the AIDS-causing SIV, failed to show vaccine protection if the animals had become severely immunodeficient (CD4+ T-cell counts <300 cells/ul) [141].

On June 4, 2007, the US government announced purchase of approximately 20 million doses of MVA to stockpile in the event of a smallpox bioterrorist attack. Using a two-dose regimen, this stockpile would be sufficient to vaccinate the estimated 10 million immunocompromised people in the USA (www.hhs.gov/news/press/2007pres/06/pr20070604a.html).

Another attenuated vaccinia virus third-generation vaccine, LC16m8, is a smallpox vaccine developed in Japan by repeated low-temperature tissue cell culture passage of Lister strain vaccinia; it was licensed for use in Japan in 1975. The vaccine is a replicating strain, cultured in primary rabbit kidney cell cultures. It has been administered to more than 50,000 Japanese children and produces a smaller primary vaccination lesion and fewer secondary symptoms and signs than Dryvax (www.who.int/entity/csr/disease/smallpox/lance_gordon.pdf).

2.10 Vaccinia Immune Globulin and Antiviral Drug Development

VIG is being produced and tested as an intravenous formulation rather than the intramuscular form that has been traditionally used. In 2004, a study using IV-VIG showed that, compared with the IM product, IV-VIG is very safe and well tolerated, yielding higher peak levels sooner than the 3–7 days seen after administration of lyophilized IM-VIG. A liquid form of IV-VIG was found to have a comparable adverse reaction rate to the lyophilized formulation [64]. The FDA licensed an intravenous formulation of VIG ("VIGIV" by DynPort Vaccine Company LLC) in February 2005.

In an historical review of VIG use and efficacy, Hopkins and Lane found that there have been no randomized controlled trials of VIG prior to FDA licensure [65]. Thus, recommendations for use of VIG are based on observational data. VIG is believed to prevent or decrease vaccinia complications in persons at increased risk, such as those with eczema or atopic dermatitis. In studies performed in Dutch military recruits, ~50,000 of whom received VIG before smallpox vaccination using a European strain of vaccinia, compared with the same number receiving a placebo before vaccination, only three recruits developed encephalitis in the group receiving VIG compared to 14 controls. The significance of this observation is puzzling as it has been believed that the pathogenesis of post-vaccinal encephalitis is an auto-immune response rather than the result of vaccinia infection of the brain.

No antiviral drug has yet been licensed by the FDA for the prevention or treatment of smallpox, monkeypox, or vaccinia virus disease. In June 2003, the IOM convened a committee to review and discuss the possibilities for the development of smallpox of an antiviral smallpox drug. Several new candidate antiviral drugs and strategies were reviewed, and seven recommendations with regard to future initiatives were made. These included the expansion of broad international collaborations, centralized resources, pharmaceutical company engagement, the training of a new cohort of investigators, and the formation of a high-level oversight panel, much like the AIDS Vaccine Research Working Group that would report to the directors of the NIH, CDC, and other federal agencies [142].

The antiviral drug, cidofovir, has been extensively studied for its possible uses in treatment or prevention of orthopoxvirus infection as well as other DNA viruses. The drug is licensed by the FDA only for the treatment of cytomegalovirus (CMV) in immunocompromised patients with HIV/AIDS. Recent literature on cidofovir for poxvirus infection, including investigational oral formulations, has been published by Bray and colleagues [143–145]. The possible role of cidofovir in prophylaxis is limited as it prevents infection in experimental animals (and presumably man) only if given at the time of actual infection or before. Since vaccination itself serves to protect even when given several days after infection, cidofovir offers no advantage. It has not been shown to have any effect in animal studies after infection is established. The current IV form of cidofovir is highly toxic, including renal toxicity. Renal shut down has occurred after the administration of only a single dose, and an oral formulation is under development.

2.11 Smallpox Preparedness in Hospitals and Public Health Partners

To illustrate one hospital's effort to implement a smallpox response plan, an example is given from Washington Hospital Center, the largest (909 bed) hospital in Washington, DC, where one of us (DRL) has worked, in partnership with the DC Department of Health. By noon of September 11, 2001, a 30-min education program about the major bioterrorism agents, including anthrax, plague, and smallpox, had begun in the Department of Medicine, including trainees and senior physicians. This effort was directed by Infectious Diseases and Infection Control Services and by late September 2001, included many other disciplines. Photographic and written information regarding the clinical recognition and diagnosis of smallpox, issues related to smallpox vaccine and bifurcated needle access limitations, and infection control issues to prevent transmission of variola were discussed. By September 21, thousands of N-95 respirators had been stockpiled with thousands of bottled doses of doxycycline for management of potential bacterial bioterrorism threats. On October 1, the interim biodefense plans were discussed in a meeting with the director of the DC Department of Health and President of the DC Hospital Association. A multidimensional educational program about bioterrorism, including smallpox, was initiated throughout the hospital in September and accelerated in October and November after the anthrax attacks.

By December 2001, an initial protocol for the management of patients with suspected or confirmed smallpox was completed by the Infection Control and Infectious Diseases services in coordination with the multidisciplinary bioterrorism preparedness task force working closely with the Department of Emergency Medicine. Information on the potential off-label use of the antiviral drug cidofovir for therapy of variola or vaccinia viruses was obtained and a protocol submitted to the hospital Institutional Review Board (IRB) for its use against smallpox or severe vaccinia reactions not resolved with VIG [146]. In addition, Medicine Grand Rounds was given on smallpox and vaccinia vaccination.

Beginning in January 2002, a series of 17 monthly bioterrorism 2-h continuing medical education (CME) public forums began for regional hospitals, clinics, and public health officials. These presentations were offered across the DC and surrounding areas of Virginia and Maryland within the National Capital Region. The subsequent monthly meetings included discussions on smallpox and smallpox vaccination and included smallpox experts from the NIH and Johns Hopkins University. These monthly meetings included hands-on opportunities to use the bifurcated needle on an artificial skin-covered deltoid teaching device by June 2002.

These hands-on training sessions were combined with a standardized powerpoint slide presentation and expanded to health-care settings across the region, including private clinics, hospitals, and the Medical Society of DC. Smallpox vaccination information and plans were shared between DC hospitals via the

DC Hospital Association Infectious Disease and Infection Control Committee. These hospitals included three DC-regional military medical facilities as well the civilian hospitals in DC. The smallpox vaccination training slides were posted on a biodefense website, www.bepast.org, along with related information and frequently asked questions (FAQs).

As partners in this effort, the DC Department of Health began to co-sponsor the training exercises and to issue "smallpox immunization technician" certification cards to over 300 persons completing these hands-on educational sessions. The Department of Health initiated a written record of contact information for recipients of these training certificates, anticipating that in the event of a smallpox emergency these persons could volunteer to assist the Department of Health with vaccination efforts.

The nursing director and senior nurses within the hospital were trained in these same hands-on sessions, and copies of the training slides were provided for "train-the-trainer" exercises with other nurses. Similarly, senior members of the largest DC-regional Visiting Nurse Association (VNA) joined in the training on vaccination issues and how to use the bifurcated needle if they were needed for large-scale hospital or community-based smallpox vaccinations.

Bifurcated needle hands-on training exercises were also coordinated with colleagues in nearby areas of northern Virginia and Maryland starting in September 2002. These sessions included both the respective health departments and clinicians and emergency response volunteers. From this experience, we learned of one superb example of a large community-based "Bioterrorism Medical Action Team (B-MATS)" [147]. Initiated by a senior pediatrician, Dr. Daniel Keim, and his colleagues in Fairfax County, Virginia, and then integrated into, and expanded by, the Fairfax Department of Health, this B-MATS organization began with a focus on being able to administer smallpox vaccinations to everyone in the county on a round-the-clock basis. Thousands of volunteers were organized into teams of 75–80 people, only few of whom were physicians. Specific community facilities that were well known to each neighborhood in Fairfax County were identified as mass vaccination sites. Volunteers were recruited who were not full-time hospital employees to avoid any potential conflict of duties in the event of a major emergency. While the focus of these teams was initially on smallpox mass vaccination, the B-MATS concept was enlarged to include any type of bioterrorism. Details of the Fairfax County B-MATS are posted on their website at www.fairfaxcounty.gov/service/hd/actsurv_clinic.htm.

An illustrated teaching guide for the prevention, diagnosis, and management of the six CDC Category A bioterrorism agents, including smallpox, was created using the acronym "BE Past" for these six agents (botulism, ebola-viral hemorrhagic fevers, plague, anthrax, smallpox, and tularemia) in June 2002. This poster guide was disseminated throughout the hospital, and thousands were provided to regional and national hospitals, clinics, public health facilities, and fire/EMS stations, were posted on the website (www.bepast.org), and shared with colleagues in Italy, Hong Kong, China, Thailand, and the Czech Republic.

By December 2002, a separate nine-page illustrated community guide to smallpox and smallpox vaccine was co-authored with the DC Department of Health. This guide was subsequently distributed in the District of Columbia by the Department of Health. The guide was posted on their health department website [148] and translated into Spanish, Mandarin Chinese, and several additional languages.

In early March 2003, four persons volunteered to be the first to be vaccinated against smallpox by the Washington, DC, Department of Health. Two of the vaccinees, a DC health department pediatrican and a hospital infectious disease physician (DL), then worked with colleagues at Washington Hospital Center and the health department to immunize 40 HCWs on March 20. The following month, a 270-person multidisciplinary smallpox tabletop exercise was organized by the Washington Hospital Center for the DC National Capital Region. Issues ranging from clinical recognition of a smallpox outbreak to communication mechanisms across the region to vaccination plans and implementation were discussed. By 2004, however, only 105 non-military persons had been vaccinated by the DC Department of Health.

2.11.1 Vaccination Coverage

Reasons for the near-complete cessation of smallpox vaccination included the following: a lack of adequate liability and compensation protection in place at the time the vaccination program began [149] (Table 2.5); potentially mandated time away from clinical work ("furlough") until the vaccination scab fell off; perceived health risk of transmitting vaccinia to colleagues or patients; health

Table 2.5 Compensation coverage for smallpox (Vaccinia) vaccine injuries*

Injury or condition in vaccine recipient or in a contact of the recipient.
1. Significant local skin reaction
2. Stevens–Johnson syndrome
3. Inadvertent inoculation
4. Generalized vaccinia
5. Eczema vaccinatum
6. Progressive vaccinia
7. Postvaccinial encephalopathy, encephalitis, or encephalomyelitis
8. Fetal vaccinia
9. Secondary infection
10. Anaphylaxis or anaphylactic shock
11. Vaccinial myocarditis, pericarditis, or myopericarditis
12. Death resulting from an injury referred to above in which the injury arose within the defined time frame.

*Above table and detailed definitions of each vaccine injury listed online at the Health Resources and Services Administration (HRSA) at www.hrsa.gov/smallpoxinjury/table.htm and in the Federal Register [149].

concerns of the candidate vaccinees; insufficient definition of the threat of smallpox being used as a bioterrorism weapon [167]; hospital legal concerns; competing obligations; priorities and resources by departments of health; unanticipated myopericarditis cases (nonfatal); the small number of cardiac deaths that were temporally, but not causally, linked to smallpox vaccination and the media coverage given to them; lack of weapons of mass destruction being found in Iraq after the March 2003 invasion; and the lack of additional terrorism attacks during 2002–2004.

To prepare for a potential bioterrorism agent such as smallpox is also to prepare for an emerging disease such as SARS (for similarities see Table 2.6) [36, 150, 151], or pandemic influenza [152], or another new respiratory infectious disease in terms of similarities in transmission, needed personal protective equipment (PPE), hospital preparedness, and public health responses. Accordingly, over the course of 5 months starting at the end of 2003, the Washington Hospital Center undertook a formal fit-testing program for N-95 respirators that successfully trained over 6,000 clinical and non-clinical workers in the appropriate use of these respirators. This better prepared the hospital to care for patients with a spectrum of droplet or aerosol-transmitted respiratory diseases, including smallpox, viral hemorrhagic fevers, pneumonic plague, and recently emerging diseases such as SARS, avian or pandemic influenza, Nipah virus, and traditional threats such as tuberculosis and measles. Similar to the smallpox hospital outbreak in Meschede, Germany [67], the SARS coronavirus was reported to be transmitted on at least some occasions via droplet

Table 2.6 Similarities between smallpox and SARS

1. Viral etiology: orthopoxvirus (smallpox) vs coronavirus (SARS)
2. No antiviral therapy or prophylactic drug proven effective.
3. Transmission by close contact face-to-face contact, including by respiratory droplets.
4. Transmission sometimes by airborne aerosol: (e.g., smallpox outbreak in a hospital in Meschede, Germany 1970 and SARS in Amoy Gardens apartments, Hong Kong, 2003).
5. Health care workers, family, and other close contacts at high risk or infection.
6. Infection control recommendations include: standard, contact, droplet, and airborne.
7. Personal protective equipment recommended by CDC includes: fit-tested N-95 (or higher) respirator, eye protection, gowns, and gloves.
8. Patients should wear a surgical mask to decrease transmission risk.
9. Patient isolation, contact tracing, and quarantine-monitoring of contacts.
10. Hospitals would actively screen persons entering hospitals for the disease and restrict entrance of visitors to non-essential personnel.
11. Require a "surge" in medical and public health response personnel and facilities.
12. Safeguards would be implemented by blood banks to prevent transfusion-related viral transmission.
13. Significant, and perhaps catastrophic, economic burden to affected nations.
14. On the list of mandated reportable diseases in the USA.
15. Would involve potential limitations on travel and gathering of large numbers of people.
16. Would require a coordinated global response, with the WHO, CDC, and National and Health Departments.

nuclei as an aerosol such as in the Amoy Gardens residential complex outbreak in 2003 [153].

At the city-wide level, while working at the DC Department of Health in the spring of 2004, one of us (DL) initiated the purchase and stockpiling of a large number of N-95 respirators (435,000) and surgical masks (2.5 million). Because of the experience of other nations hard hit by the SARS epidemic, acute shortages of N-95 respirators and surgical masks must be anticipated. These would need to be available immediately following the release of smallpox, certain hemorrhagic fevers, pandemic influenza, SARS, or other bioterrorist or emerging pathogens.

To prepare for smallpox is to prepare for many of the other public health threats that we face today and will face in the future. The integration of smallpox preparedness measures into broader public health preparedness locally, regionally, and nationally is one of the primary recommendations from the Committee on Smallpox Vaccination Program Implementation of the IOM of the National Academy of Science [127]. Explicit comparisons between smallpox, pandemic influenza, and SARS are made in the August 28, 2004, US draft pandemic influenza plan [152].

Preparing optimally for smallpox in the United States requires preparing on a global basis to prevent the return of smallpox. Whereas an intensified global program was required to eradicate smallpox from the human population in the 1960 s and 1970 s, today and in our future an intensified long-term global program of watchfulness and preparation for response is required to prevent smallpox from being reestablished as an endemic disease.

2.12 Monkeypox: An Emerging Disease in the United States in 2003 and in Sudan in 2005

In 2003, an outbreak of monkeypox occurred for the first time in the United States [154, 155]. The outbreak component involving humans began in May and was confirmed by laboratory testing at the CDC by early June 2003. Monkeypox, known in animals since 1958 and in humans since 1970, is an orthopoxvirus related to variola and vaccinia viruses. Monkeypox had never previously been reported outside of Africa. There, secondary attack rates were low and did not extend beyond four generations, making it a disease of low epidemic potential. Two clades had been found, one West African and one Congolese. Unlike smallpox, monkeypox is a zoonosis. As in Africa, the US outbreak in 2003 was linked to infected animals.

In general, clinical manifestations of monkeypox, including fever and the sequential appearance and resolution of the skin lesions, as well as the incubation period, are similar to smallpox. One specific finding that distinguishes monkeypox from smallpox is lymphadenopathy, especially in the cervical and inguinal regions, in patients with monkeypox [156]. Chickenpox (VZV) is another disease that should routinely be considered in the differential diagnosis of monkeypox. Indeed, in 2007 Rimoin and colleagues from the United States, the Democratic Republic of the Congo (DRC), and the WHO reported in a laboratory study of 136 patients from the DRC with suspected monkeypox, 51 (37.5%) were confirmed to have monkeypox, whereas 61 (45%) had Varicella-Zoster Virus (VZV) and one had infection with both viruses [157].

The potential for monkeypox to be an emerging disease problem was discussed by Breman in 2000 and is related to the increasing contact of humans with animals in endemic areas and the waning of vaccinia-induced immunity [158]. In addition to the US outbreak in 2003, Inger Damon at the CDC and colleagues from the WHO and Medecins sans Frontiers (MSF) reported in 2006 laboratory confirmation of monkeypox virus for the first time in Sudan. They identified monkeypox virus isolated in November 2005 from the mother of a young child in southern Sudan, both of whom had clinically suspected monkeypox. Genetic sequencing of this isolate was most consistent with the clade from the Congo basin. Epidemiologic studies in Sudan by the MSF revealed "small clusters of self-limited disease compatible with monkeypox had occurred that were not widely spread within the community. No deaths were reported among patients with suspected cases" [159].

The endemic natural host for monkeypox is not known with certainty, but serologic evidence of orthopoxvirus infections, presumably due to monkeypox, has been found in some rodents in Africa, including the Gambian giant pouch rat and the rope squirrel. The first outbreak in the United States was traced to imported wild rodents from Accra, Ghana, West Africa, that arrived in Texas on April 9, 2003. Subsequent testing of these animals by the CDC revealed PCR, and virus isolation demonstrated that at least one Gambian giant rat, three dormice, and two rope squirrels were positive for monkeypox. Some of the Gambian giant rats were housed with prairie dogs at an Illinois pet distributor [160]. These prairie dogs were found to be susceptible to monkeypox, and close contact between humans and infected pets, including prairie dogs, resulted in monkeypox infection of at least 37 persons. Initial studies of the pathogenesis of monkeypox in the North American prairie dog were published in 2004 [161].

Most of these 37 laboratory-confirmed infections in the United States were mild, manifest as fever and a rash with a limited number of lesions. Patients were confirmed with monkeypox in Illinois, Indiana, Kansas, Missouri, and Wisconsin. Occupational exposure to prairie dog–associated monkeypox infection in veterinary facilities in Wisconsin was reported in detail [162]. On June 11, 2003, a combined order from the CDC and the FDA prohibited the importation of African rodents and the sale or transport in the United States of six genera of African rodents and of US prairie dogs [160]. All patients had had direct exposure to infected animals; no evidence of person-to-person transmission occurred [163]. One-third of the patients had a known history of at least one smallpox vaccination in the distant past.

None of the patients died. Two children became seriously ill, but eventually recovered. One child had respiratory difficulty with marked cervical adenopathy and pharyngeal lesions, but did not require mechanical ventilation. Severe encephalitis occurred in one previously healthy 6-year-old whose family purchased one of the monkeypox-infected prairie dogs [164]. Two adults in this same family had mild monkeypox disease. One of these adults who had been vaccinated as a child had minimal symptoms and very few skin lesions. All three members of the family had one or more skin lesions on the palms. The child with encephalitis also had cervical lymphadenopathy, an uncommon finding with smallpox. She developed seizures and was placed on a ventilator. Her cerebrospinal fluid was IgM positive for orthopoxvirus, while PCR and culture of the CSF were negative. Eventually, she made a full recovery. As with smallpox and vaccinia-associated encephalitis, neither VIG nor cidofovir are recommended in the treatment of monkeypox encephalitis. Neither agent was given to this patient.

On June 12, 2003, the CDC issued interim guidance regarding use of smallpox vaccine, VIG, and the antiviral drug cidofovir for prevention and therapy of monkeypox during this outbreak [165]. Regarding smallpox vaccination (vaccinia virus), it was known from studies in Africa to confer protection (≥85%) against monkeypox when given before exposure to monkeypox. Unlike smallpox disease [166], no data exist on the efficacy of giving smallpox vaccine after exposure to monkeypox, in terms of preventing or decreasing the severity of illness although it is believed that it would be effective. Accordingly, the CDC offered guidance for use of smallpox vaccination in different groups at risk for exposure to monkeypox.

HCWs caring for proven or suspected cases of monkeypox, and veterinarians exposed to animals (such as prairie dogs) with monkeypox, were advised to receive the smallpox vaccine within 4 days of initial exposure and to consider vaccination up to 2 weeks after the most recent exposure. CDC also advised that even previously vaccinated HCWs workers should continue to use PPE including a fit-tested N-95 respirator and should follow airborne, contact, and standard infection control precautions. HCWs who could be assigned to care for patients with monkeypox in the future were advised to receive smallpox vaccine and to have a confirmed take before caring for such patients. If this had not been done, then vaccination just before caring for these patients was indicated.

Similar to smallpox, vaccination of close contacts of monkeypox patients was addressed by CDC. The same working definition for close contact was applied to monkeypox as has been used for smallpox.

Some, but not all, medical contraindications to smallpox vaccination were maintained even for persons with close or intimate contact with a symptomatic, laboratory-confirmed case of monkeypox within the prior 2 weeks. Persons with T-cell immunodeficiencies were advised not to be vaccinated, including AIDS-defining CD4 T-cell counts, solid or bone marrow transplant recipients, or other persons receiving high-dose immunosuppressive medications, hematologic malignancies, or congenital T-cell defects. Otherwise, neither pregnancy, nor age or a history of active eczema were to be considered contraindications to smallpox vaccination.

VIG was not recommended for either prophylaxis or treatment of monkeypox patients because no data existed on its role in either setting. Consideration of cidofovir was only to be given as a last resort in the clinical setting of a life-threatening monkeypox infection, and not for prophylaxis.

The pathologic findings and clinical presentation of monkeypox were reported in two of the prairie dogs infected during this outbreak in the United States [161]. Evidence of viral replication was found in both the lungs, where a necrotizing bronchopneumonia was found, and in ulcerative lesions of the tongue. The potential for transmission of monkeypox from both mucocutaneous exposures and from the respiratory route is evident. Given the susceptibility of the prairie dog to severe monkeypox disease, this animal could serve as a model for further research into antiviral drug and new vaccine development against monkeypox [161]. There is no evidence to date that monkeypox has become endemic in US animals such as the prairie dog, as occurred with *Yersinia pestis* (plague) after emerging in California in the early 1900 s following its spread from China (Guangdong Province to Hong Kong [167]) to San Francisco.

References

1. Breman JG, Henderson DA. Diagnosis and management of smallpox. N Engl J Med 2002;346:1300–1308.
2. Albert M, Lucey DR, Breman JG. Preparedness for a bioterrorism attack with smallpox. In: *Hospital Epidemiology and Infection Control*, 3rd edition. Mayhall, CG, editor. 2004:1965–1978. Lippincott, Williams & Wilkins, Philadelphia.
3. Rotz LD, Cono J, DamonI. *Smallpox and Bioterrorism. Principles and Practices of Infectious Diseases*, 6th edition 2005. Mandell GL, Benett JE, Dolin R, editors. 2005. Elsevier, Inc., Philadelphia.
4. Henderson DA, Inglesby TV, Bartlett JG, et al. Smallpox as a biological weapon. Medical and Public Health Management. J Am Med Assoc 1999;281:2127–2137.
5. WHO. Public health response to biological and chemical weapons: WHO guidance (2004). www.who.int/csr/delibepidemics/biochemguide/en/index.html
6. Henderson DA, Moss B. Smallpox and Vaccinia (chapter 6). In: *Vaccines*, 3rd edition. Stanley Plotkin, Walter Orentstein, editors. 1999:74–97. W.B. Saunders Company, Philadelphia.
7. Cono J, Casey CG, Bell, DM. Centers for disease control and prevention. Smallpox vaccination and adverse reactions: guidance for clinicians. MMWR Recomm Rep 2003;52:1–28.
8. Dixon CW. *Smallpox* (512 pages). 1962. Little, Brown, and Company, Boston.
9. Rao AR. *Smallpox* (220 pages). 1972. Kothari Book Depot, Bombay.
10. Fenner F, Henderson DA, Arita I, et al. Smallpox and its eradication. (1460 pages). In: *History of International Public Health*. No. 6. 1988. World Health Organization, Geneva.
11. WHO. *G7+ Global Health Security Initiative (GHSI) Workshop* (5–6 September 2002). "Best practices in vaccine production for smallpox and other potential pathogens". Paul-Ehrlich-Institut, Langen, Germany. www.who.int/csr/disease/smallpox/preparedness/en/print.html
12. WHO. *Smallpox. Historical Significance*. www.who.int.mediacentre/factsheets/smallpox/en/print.html

13. WHO. *Preparedness in the Event of a Smallpox Outbreak*. www.who.int/csr/disease/smallpox/preparedness/en/print.html
14. Health Canada website. www.hc-sc.gc.ca/english/media/issues/global_mercury_summary.html
15. Vedantam S. WHO assails wealthy nations on bioterror. Coordination of defenses poor in simulation; U.S. support for agency questioned. Washington Post. 5 November 2003:A08.
16. Lucey D, Sum M. *Hong Kong Department of Health. Symposium on Smallpox Vaccination*. 1 November 2003. Wanchai, Hong Kong.
17. Drogin B. Smallpox exercise poses big question: Is anyone ready? Los Angeles Times, 17 January 2005.
18. Mintz J. Bioterrorism war game shows lack of readiness. Washington Post, 15 Jan 2005, A12.
19. De Vreij H. *Atlantic Storm. On a Tabletop*. Radio Netherlands. www.wereldomroep.nl
20. *Center for Biosecurity-University of Pittsburgh Medical Center. Atlantic Storm Scenario Assumptions*. 14 January 2005. www.upmc-biosecurity.org
21. *Centers for Disease Control and Prevention. Evaluating Patients for Smallpox*. http://www.bt.cdc.gov/agent/smallpox/diagnosis/pdf/spox-poster-full.pdf.
22. *Centers for Disease Control and Prevention. Smallpox Response Plan and Guidelines. Annex 3: Smallpox Vaccination Clinic Guide*. http://www.bt.cdc.gov/agent/smallpox/response-plan/index.asp.
23. *Centers for Disease Control and Prevention. Smallpox Response Plan and Guidelines. Draft Guide A: Smallpox Surveillance and Case Reporting; Contact Identification, Tracing, Vaccination, and Surveillance; and Epidemiologic Investigation*. http://www.bt.cdc.gov/agent/smallpox/response-plan/index.asp.
24. *Department of Defense Smallpox Vaccination Website*. www.smallpox.army.mil/event/SPSafetySum.asp
25. Damon I, Li Y, Kline R, et al. (2002). Variola virus and smallpox: past, present, or future tense? From Centers for Disease Control and Prevention Web site: http://ftp.cdc.gov/pub/infectious diseases/iceid/2002/pdf/regnery.pdf
26. *Centers for Disease Control and Prevention. Smallpox Fact Sheet: People Who Should Not Get the Smallpox Vaccine*. http://www.bt.cdc.gov/agent/smallpox/vaccination/contraindications-public.asp.
27. *Centers for Disease Control and Prevention. Interim Smallpox Fact Sheet: Smallpox Vaccine and Heart Problems*. http://www.bt.cdc.gov/agent/smallpox/vaccination/heartproblems.asp.
28. Grabenstein JD, Winkenwerder W. US military smallpox vaccination program experience. JAMA 2003;289:3278–3282.
29. LeDuc JW, Damon I, Meegan JM, et al. Smallpox research activities: U.S. interagency collaboration, 2001. Emerging Infect Dis 2002;8:743–745.
30. CDC. *Smallpox Vaccination Program Status State by State* (as of 31 August 2004). www.cdc.gov/od/ocmedia/spvaccin.htm
31. *Department of Defense*. www.smallpox.army.mil/resources/policies.asp
32. Alibek K. Biohazard. 1999. Delta, New York.
33. Breman JG, Arita I. The confirmation and maintenance of smallpox eradication. N Engl J Med 1980;303:1263–1273.
34. http://www.smallpoxbiosecurity.org, Geneva 21–22 October 2003.
35. Henderson DA, Borio L. Bioterrorism: An Overview. In: *Principles and Practice of Infectious Diseases* 2004, 6th Edition. Mandell GL, Bennett JE, Dolin R, editors. Elsevier Co., Philadelphia.
36. WHO. *SARS Lab Outbreaks. WHO Guidelines for the Global Surveillance of Severe Acute Respiratory Syndrome (SARS)*. Updated recommendations, October 2004.
37. Malakoff D. Biosecurity goes global. Science 2004;305:1706–1707.

38. Gellman B. 4 Nations thought to possess smallpox. Iraq, N. Korea named, two officials say. Washington Post 2002;Nov 5:A1.
39. Powell C. Publication of presentation to the United Nations Security Council on February 5, 2003. Washington Post 6 February 2003.
40. Danzig R. *Catastrophic Bioterrorism-What is to be Done*? *August* 2003. *Center for Technology and National Security Policy*. National Defense University, Washington DC.
41. Alibek K, Bailey C. Bioshield or Biogap? Biosec and Bioterr Biodef Strat Pract Sci 2004;2(2):132–133.
42. CDC. *Cities Readiness Initiative*. June 14, 2004. http://www.bt.cdc.gov/cri/
43. Ferguson NM, Keeling MJ, Edmunds WJ, et al. Planning for smallpox outbreaks. Nature 2003;425:681–685.
44. Bozzette SA, Boer R, Bhatnagar V, et al. A model for a smallpox vaccination policy. N Engl J Med 2003;348:416–425.
45. Massoudi MS, Barker L, Schwartz B. Effectiveness of postexposure vaccination for the prevention of smallpox: results of a Delphi analysis. J Infect Dis 2003;188:973–976.
46. Kaplan EH, Craft DL, Wein LM. Emergency response to a smallpox attack: the case for mass vaccination. Proc Natl Acad Sci 2002;99:10935–10940.
47. Bauch CT, Galvani AP, Earn DJD. Group interest versus self-interest in smallpox vaccination policy. Proc Natl Acad Sci 2003;100:10564–10567.
48. Alibek K. Smallpox: a disease and a weapon. Intl J Infect Dis 2004;852:S3–S8.
49. Jackson RJ, Ramsay AJ, Christensen CD, Beaton S, Hall DF, Ramshaw IA. Expression of mouse interleukin-4 by a recombinant ectromelia virus suppresses cytolytic lymphocyte responses and overcomes genetic resistance to mousepox. J Virol 2001;75:1205–1210.
50. McCurdy LH, Rutigliano JA, Johnson TR, Chen M, Graham BS. Modified vaccinia virus Ankara immunization protects against lethal challenge with recombinant vaccinia virus expressing murine interleukin-4. J Virol 2004;78(22):12471–12479.
51. Mosmann T, Cherwinski H, Bond M, Giedlin M, Coffmann R. Two types of murine helper T cell clones. 1 Definition according to profiles of lymphokine activities and secreted proteins. J Immunol 1986;136:2348–2357.
52. Lucey DR., Clerici M, Shearer G. Type 1 and type 2 cytokine dysregulation in human infectious, neoplastic, and inflammatory diseases. Clin Microbiol Reviews 1996;9(4):532–562.
53. Chaudri G, Panchanathan V, Buller RML, et al. Polarized type 1 cytokine response and cell-mediated immunity determine genetic resistance to mousepox. Proc Nal Acad Sci 2004;101(24):9057–9062.
54. Mahalingam S, Karupiah G, Takeda k, Akira S, Matthaei KI, Foster PS. Enhanced resistance in STAT-6 deficient mice to infection with ectromelia virus. Proc Natl Acad Sci 2001;98(12):6812–6817.
55. Karupiah G, Xie QW, Buller RM, Nathan C, Duarte C, MacMicking JD. Inhibition of viral replication by interferon-gamma-induced nitric oxide synthase. Science 1993;261:1445–1448.
56. Harris N, Nuller RM, Karupiah G. Gamma-interferon-induced, nitric-oxide-mediated inhibition of vaccinia virus replication. J Virol 1995;69:910–915.
57. Ruby J, Ramshaw I. The antiviral activity of immune CD8+ T-cells is dependent on interferon-gamma. Lymphokine Cytokine Res 1991;10:353–358.
58. Engler RJM,Kenner J, Leung DYM. Smallpox vaccination: risk consideration for patients with atopic dermatitis. J Allergy Clin Immunol 2002;110:357–365.
59. Jones CA, Williams KA, Finlay-Jones J, Hart PH. Interleukin 4 production by human amnion epithelial cells and regulation of its activity by glycosamnoglycan binding. Biol Reprod 1995;52:839–847.
60. Lin H, Mosmann T, Guilbert L, Tuntipopipat S, Wegmann T. Synthesis of T helper-2 type cytokines at the maternal fetal interface. J Immunol 1993;151:4562–4573.

61. Wegman T, Lin H, Guibert L, Mosmann T. Bidirectional cytokine interactions in the maternal-fetal relationship: is successful pregnancy a Th2 phenomenon? Immunol Today 1993;14:353.
62. Piccinni M, Guidizi M, Biagiotti R, et al. Progesterone favors the development of human T helper cells producing Th2-type cytokines and promotes both IL-4 production and membrane CD30 expression in established Th1 cell clones. J Immunol 1995;155:128–133.
63. Interferon-gamma. www.biopharma.com/sample_entries/184.html
64. Hopkins RJ, Kramer WG, Blackwelder WC, et al. Safety and pharmacokinetic evaluation of intravenous vaccinia immune globulin in healthy volunteers. Clin Infect Dis 2004;39:759–766.
65. Hopkins RJ, Lane JM. Clinical efficacy of intramuscular vaccinia immune globulin: a literature review. Clin Infect Dis 2004;39:819–826.
66. Bray M. Editorial commentary: Henry Kempe and the birth of Vaccinia Immune Globulin. Clin Infect Dis 2004;39:767–769.
67. Wehrle PF, Posch J, Richter KH, et al. An airborne outbreak of smallpox in a German hospital and its significance with respect to other recent outbreaks in Europe. Bull World Health Organ 1970;43:669–679.
68. Breman JG, Henderson DA. Poxvirus dilemmas – monkeypox, smallpox, and biologic terrorism. N Engl J Med 1998;339:556–559.
69. Matthews AW, Griffiths ID. Post-vaccinial pericarditis and myocarditis. Brit Heart J 1974;36:1043–1045.
70. Helle E-P, Koskenvuo K, Heikkila J, Pikkarainen J, Weckstrom P. Myocardial complications of immunizations. Ann Clin Research 1978;10:280–287.
71. Feery BJ. Adverse reactions after smallpox vaccination. Med J Australia 1977;2:180–183.
72. Finlay-Jones LR. Fatal myocarditis after vaccination against smallpox. N Engl J Med 1964;270:41–42.
73. Moschos A, Papaioannou AC, Nicolopoulos D, Anagnostakis D. Cardiac complications after vaccination for smallpox. Helv Paediatr Acta 1976;31:257–260.
74. Mead J. Serum transaminase and elcetrocardiographic findings after smallpox vaccination: Case report. J Am Geriatr Soc 1966;14(7):754–756.
75. Bengtsson E, Holmgren A, Nystrom B. Circulatory studies in patients with abnormal ECG in the course of postvaccinial complications. Acta Med Scand Suppl 1966;464:113–126.
76. Karjalainen J, Heikkila J, Nieminen MS, et al. Etiology of mild acute infectious myocarditis. Acta Med Scand 1983;213:65–73.
77. CDC. Update: cardiac and other adverse events following civilian smallpox vaccination. United States, 2003. MMWR Morb Mortal Wkly Rep 2003;52:639–642.
78. Couzin J. Panel urges caution over heart problems. Science 2003;300:2013–2014.
79. *Centers for Disease Control and Prevention. Smallpox Fact Sheet: Adverse Reactions Following Smallpox Vaccination.* http://www.bt.cdc.gov/agent/smallpox/vaccination/reactions-vacc-clinic.asp.
80. Chen RT, Lane MJ. Myocarditis: the unexpected return of smallpox vaccine adverse events. Lancet 2003;362:1345–1346.
81. CDC. Update: Adverse events following civilian smallpox vaccination—United States, 2003. MMWR 2004;53(5):106–107.
82. Halsell JS, Riddle JR, Atwood JE, et al. Myopericarditis following smallpox vaccination among vaccinia naive US military personnel. JAMA 2003;289:3283–3289.
83. Arness MK, Eckart RE, Love SS, et al. Myopericarditis following smallpox vaccination. Am J Epidemiol 2004;160:642–651.
84. Eckart RE, Love SS, Atwood JE, et al. Incidence and follow-up of inflammatory cardiac complications after smallpox vaccination. J Am Coll Cardiol 2004;44:201–205.
85. CDC. Update: Adverse events following smallpox vaccination—United States, 2003. MMWR 2003;52(13):278–282.

86. DoD. http://www.smallpox.mil/event/panelreport.asp.
87. CDC. Cardiac deaths after a mass smallpox vaccination campaign – New York City, 1947. MMWR 2003;52(9):933–936.
88. Tasker SA, Schnepf GA, Lim M, et al. Unintended smallpox vaccination of HIV-1-infected individuals in the United States military. Clin Infect Dis 2004;38:1320–1322.
89. Redfield R, Wright DC, James WD, Jones TS, Brown C, Burke DS. Disseminated vaccinia in a military recruit with human immunodeficiency virus (HIV) disease. N Engl J Med 1987;316:673–676.
90. Halsey NA, Henderson DA. HIV infection and immunization against other agents. N Engl J Med 1987;316:683–685.
91. Guillaume JC, Saiag P, Wechsler J, Lescs MC, Roujeau JC. Vaccinia from recombinant virus expressing HIV genes. Lancet 1991;337:1034–1035.
92. Picard O, Lebas J, Imbert JC, Bigel P, Zagury D. Complication of intramuscular/subcutaneous immune therapy in severely immune-compromised individuals. J AIDS 1991;4(6):641–643.
93. Zagury D. Anti-HIV cellular immunotherapy in AIDS. Lancet 1991;338:694–695.
94. Dropulic LK, Rubin RH, Bartlett JG. Smallpox vaccination and the patient with an organ transplant. Clin Infect Dis 2003;36:786–788.
95. Bartlett J, Borio L, Radonovich L, et al. Smallpox vaccination in 2003: key information for clinicians. Clin Infect Dis 2003;36:883–902.
96. Bartlett JG. Smallpox vaccination and patients with human immunodeficiency virus infection of acquired immunodeficiency syndrome. Clin Infect Dis 2003;36:468–471.
97. Amorosa VK, Isaacs SN. Separate worlds set to collide:smallpox, vaccinia virus vaccination, and human immunodeficiency virus and acquired immunodeficiency syndrome. Clin Infect Dis 2003;37:426–432.
98. Shoham S, Lucey DR. *Smallpox and HIV/AIDS: Patient and Public Health Preparedness. XIVth International Conference on HIV/AIDS*. 7–12 July 2002. Barcelona, Spain.
99. *OraQuick Rapid HIV-1 Antibody Test Package Insert*. www.orasure.com
100. CDC. Approval of a new rapid test for HIV antibody. MMWR 2002;51(46):1051–1052.
101. Heymann DL. Smallpox containment updated: considerations for the 21st century. Intl J Infect Dis 2004;852:S15–S20.
102. Edghill-Smith Y, Venzon D, Karpova T, et al. Modeling a safer smallpox vaccine regimen, for human immunodeficiency virus type 1-infected patients, in immunocompromised macaques. J Infect Dis 2003;188:1181–1191.
103. Breman JG, Arita I, Fenner F. Preventing the return of smallpox. N Engl J Med 2003;348:463–466.
104. Zanders JP. Addressing the concerns about smallpox. Intl J Infect Dis 2004;852:S9–S14.
105. Lucey DR. *Hemorrhagic Smallpox: Initial Clue to a Smallpox Attack*? Washington Newsletter 15 November 2004. www.bepast.org
106. Rao AR. Hemorrhagic smallpox: A study of 240 cases. J Indian Med Assoc 1964 (Sept 1);43(5):225–229.
107. Jahrling PB, Hensley LE, Martinez MJ, et al. Exploring the potential of variola virus infection of cynomolgous macaques as a model for human smallpox. Proc Natl Acad Sci 2004;101:15196–15200.
108. Huggins JW, Zwiers SH, Baker RO, Hensley LE, Larsen T, Martinez MJ, Jahrling PB. Cidofovir treatment of variola (smallpox) in the hemorrhagic smallpox primate model and the IV monkeypox primate model. WHO website.www.who.int/csr/disease/smallpox/smallpox/cidofovirtreatment/en/print.html.
109. Rubins KH, Hensley LE, Jahrling PB, et al. The host response to smallpox: analysis of the gene expression program in peripheral blood cells in a nonhuman primate model. Proc Natl Acad Sci 2004;101:15190–15195.
110. Downie AW, Fedson DS, Vincent LS, Rao AR, Kempe CH. Hemorrhagic smallpox. J Hyg (Camb) 1969;67:619–629.

111. Tucker JB, Zilinskas RA. *The 1971 Smallpox Epidemic in Aralsk, Kazakhstan, and the Soviet Biological Warfare Program*. July 2002. Monterey Institute of International Studies, Monterey.
112. Henderson DA. Commentary on Dr. Alan Zelicoff's epidemiological analysis of the Aralsk outbreak (No. 3). Crit Rev Microbiol 2003;29(2):169–170.
113. Osler W. *The Principles and Practice of Medicine*. 1892:46–60. D. Appleton and Company, New York. Smallpox.
114. Sarkar JK, Mitra AC. Virulence of variola virus isolated from smallpox cases of varying severity. Indian J Med Res 1967;55:13–20.
115. CDC. Medical Examiners, coroners, and biologic terrorism. MMWR 2004;53/No.RR-8:1–36.
116. Martin DB. The cause of death in smallpox: an examination of the pathology record. Mil Med 2002;167:546–551.
117. Baxby D. Smallpox vaccination techniques; from knives and forks to needles and pins. Vaccine 2002;20:2140–2149.
118. Rao AR, Prahlad I, Swaminathan M, Lakshmi A. Pregnancy and smallpox. J Indian Med Assoc 2003;40(8):353–363.
119. Rao AR, Sukumar, MS, Kamalakshi S, et al. Experimental variola in monkeys. Part 1. Studies on disease enhancing property of cortisone in smallpox: a preliminary report. (1968). Ind J Med Res 1968;56:12, 18655–18665.
120. Kumar A, Beniwal M, Kar P, Sharma JB, Murphy NS. Hepatitis E in pregnancy. Int J Gynaecol Obstet 2004 (June);85(3):240–244.
121. Brundtland, Gro Harlem. October 2001. www.who.int/inf-pr-2001/en/state2001-16.html.
122. Orr N, Forman M, Marcus H, et al. Clinical and immune responses after revaccination of Israeli adults with the Lister strain of vaccinia virus. J Infect Dis 2004;190:1295–1302.
123. Midthun K. *Smallpox – Regulatory Requirements for Historical and New Smallpox Vaccines. G7+ Workshop*. Langen, Germany. 5–6 September 2002. www.fda.gov/cber/smplx/smplxreg.htm
124. Gouvras G. Policies in place throughout the world: action by the European Union. Intl J Infect Dis 2004;852:S21–S30.
125. *United Kingdom Smallpox Plan Update December 2003*. www.dh.gov.uk/PublicationsAndStatistics/Publications/PublicationsPolicyAndGuidance/PublicationsPolicyAndGuidanceArticle/fs/en?CONTENT_ID = 4070830&chk = XRWF7m
126. Seward JF, Galil K, Damon I, et al. Development and experience with an algorithm to evaluate suspected smallpox cases in the United States, 2002–2004. Clin Infect Dis 2004;39:1477–1483.
127. Baciu A, Anason AP, Stratton K, Strom B. (editors). *The Smallpox Vaccination Program. Public Health in an Age of Terrorism. Institute of Medicine*. 2005:1–370. The National Academies Press, Washington, D.C.
128. *Dryvax Package Insert*. www.fda.gov/cber/label/smalwye102502LB.htm
129. Artenstein A, Johnson C, Marbury T, et al. A novel, cell culture-derived smallpox vaccine in vaccinia-naïve adults. Vaccine 2005 (May);23:3301–3309.
130. Talbot TR, Stapleton JT, Brady RC, et al. Vaccination success rate and reaction profile with diluted and undiluted smallpox vaccine. JAMA 2004;292(10):1205–1212.
131. Monath TP, Caldwell JR, Mundt W, et al. ACAM 2000 clonal Vero cell culture vaccinia (New York Board of Health strain) – a second generation smallpox vaccine for biological defense. Intl J Infect Dis 2004;852:S31–S44.
132. Weltzin R, Liu J, Pugachev KV, et al. Clonal vaccinia virus grown in cell culture as a new smallpox vaccine. Nat Med 2003;9(9):1125–1130.
133. Hooper JW, Custer DM, Thompson E. Four-gene combination DNA vaccine protects mice against a lethal vaccinia virus challenge and elicits appropriate antibody responses in nonhuman primates. Virology 2003;306:181–195.

134. Enserink M. Smallpox vaccines: looking beyond the next generation. Science 2004;304:809.
135. Hooper JW, et al. Smallpox DNA vaccine protects nonhuman primates against lethal monkeypox. J Virol 2004;78.9:4433–4443.
136. Earl PL, Americo JL, Wyatt LS, et al. Immunogenicity of a highly attenuated MVA smallpox vaccine and protection against smallpox. Nature 2004;428:182–185.
137. Ennis FA, Cruz J, Demkowicz WE, et al. Primary induction of human CD8 + cytotoxic T lymphocytes and interferon-gamma-producing T cells after smallpox vaccination. J Infect Dis 2002;185:1657–1659.
138. Belyakov IM, Earl P Dzutsev A, et al. Shared modes of protection gainst poxvirus infection by attenuated and conventional smallpox vaccine viruses. Proc Natl Acad Sci 2003;100:9458–9463.
139. Hammarlund E, Lewis MW, Hansen SG, et al. Duration of antiviral immunity after smallpox vaccination. Nat Med 2003;9(9):1131–1137.
140. Kennedy JS, Frey S, Yan L, et al. Induction of human T cell-mediated immune responses after primary and secondary smallpox vaccination. J Infect Dis 2004;190:1286–1294.
141. Edghill-Smith Y, Bray M, Whitehouse CA, et al. Smallpox vaccine does not protect macaques with AIDS from a lethal monkeypox virus challenge. J Infect Dis 2005;191:372–381.
142. Harrison SC, Alberts B, Ehrenfield E, et al. Discovery of antivirals against smallpox. Proc Natl Acad Sci 2004;online July 12.
143. Smee DF, Bailey KW, Sidwell RW. Treatment of lethal vaccinia virus respiratory infections in mice with cidofovir. Antivir Chem Chemother 2001;12:71–76.
144. Bray M, Martinez M, Smee DF, et al. Cidofovir protects mice against lethal aerosol or intranasal cowpox virus challenge. J Infect Dis 2000;181:10–19.
145. Bray M. Pathogenesis and potential antiviral therapy of complications of smallpox vaccination. Antiviral Res 2003;58:101–114.
146. Wilck M, Dass, K, Shoham S, Moore J, Lucey DR. *Smallpox Vaccination: Use of Cidofovir for Severe Complications*. American College of Physicians (ACP) Associates Annual Meeting, Washington DC, 11 May 2002.
147. Bioterrorism–Medical Action Team ("B-MATS"). www.fairfaxcounty.gov/service/hd/actsurv_clinic.htm
148. Richardson M, Lucey D, Berry K, Coleman B. *Washington DC Department of Health Community Guide on Smallpox and Smallpox Vaccination.* http://bioterrorism.doh.dc.gov/biot/frames.asp?doc = /biot/lib/biot/pdf/smallpox_9_panel.pdf
149. Health Resources and Services Administration. Department of Health and Human Services. Smallpox vaccine injury compensation program: smallpox (Vaccinia) vaccine injury table. Fed Regist 2003;68(166):(August 27):51492–51499.
150. Saijo M, Ami Y, Suzaki Y, et al. LC16m8, a highly attenuated vaccinia virus vaccine lacking expression of the membrane protein B5R, protects monkeys from monkeypox. J Virol 2006;80:5179–5188.
151. Lucey DR, Perl T, Karchmer T, et al. *SARS Lessons Learned for the USA from IDSA Physicians Who Worked in Toronto. Late-Breaker Abstract.* 9–12 October 2003. Annual Meeting of the Infectious Disease Society of America, San Diego.
152. USA Draft Pandemic Influenza Plan (26 August 2004). Annex 12. Synergies and Differences in Preparedness and Response for Influenza and Other Infectious Disease Threats. http://www.hhs.gov/nvpo/pandemicplan/
153. Ignatius TSY, Li Y, Wong TW, et al. Evidence of airborne transmission of the severe acute respiratory syndrome virus. N Engl J Med 2004;350:1731–1739.
154. Reed KD, Melski JW, Graham MB, et al. The detection of monkeypox in the Western Hemisphere. N Engl J Med 2004;350:342–350.

155. Update: multistate outbreak of monkeypox – Illinois, Indiana, Kansas, Missouri, Ohio, and Wisconsin, 2003. MMWR Morb Mortal Wkly Rep 2003;52:642–646.
156. Nalca A, Rimoin A, Bavari S, Whitehouse C. Reemergence of monkeypox: prevalence, diagnostics, and countermeasures. Clin Infect Dis 2005;41:1765–1771.
157. Rimoin A, Kisalu N, Kebela-Ilunga B, et al. Endemic human monkepox, Democratic Republic of Congo, 2001–2004. Emerg Infect Dis 2007 (June);13(7). http://www.cdc.gov/EID/content/13/6/934.htm
158. Breman JG. Monkeypox: an emerging infection for humans? In: *Emerging Infections*. Scheld WM, Craig WA, Hughes JM (editors). 2000;45–67. ASM Press, Washington D.C.
159. Damon I, Roth C, Chowdhary V. Discovery of monkeypox I Sudan. N Engl J Med 2006;355(9):962–963.
160. CDC. Multistate outbreak of monkeypox – Illinois, Indiana, Kansas, Missouri, Ohio, and Wisconsin, 2003. MMWR. Morb Mortal Wkly Rep 2003;52:616–618.
161. Guarner J, Johnson BJ, Paddock CD, et al. Monkeypox transmission and pathogenesis in prairie dogs. Emerg Infect Dis J 2004;10:426–431.
162. Croft D. Sotir M, Kazmierczak J, et al. Occupational risks during a monkeypox outbreak, Wisconsin, 2003. Emerg Infect Dis 2007; (August). http://www.cdc.gov/EID/content/13/8/1150.htm
163. CDC. Update: Multistate outbreak of monkeypox – Illinois, Indiana, Missouri, Ohio, and Wisconsin, 2003. MMWR Morb Mortal Wkly Rep 2003;52:642–646 (11 July).
164. Sejvar JL, Chowdary Y, Schomogyi M, et al. Human monkeypox infection: a family cluster in the Midwestern United States. J Infect Dis 2004;190:1833–1840.
165. CDC. Interim guidance for use of smallpox vaccine, cidofovir, and vaccinia immune globulin (VIG) for prevention and treatment in the setting of outbreak of monkeypox infections. 12 June 2003:1–6. www.cdc.gov/ncidod/monkeypox
166. Sommer A. The 1972 smallpox outbreak in Khulna municipality, Bangladesh. II. Effectiveness of surveillance and containment in urban epidemic control. Am J Epidemiol 1974;99(4):303–313.
167. Solomon T. The Hong Kong plague of 1894 and the discovery of the cause of plague. Hong Kong Museum of Medical Sciences, 2 Caine Lane, Mid-Levels, Hong Kong. Museum visited 2 November 2003 (DL).
168. Lucey DR. Surveillance and Management of SARS in the Emergency Department. www.BePast.org March 19, 2003. (Accessed on July 3, 2008).

Chapter 3
Plague

Petra C.F. Oyston and Richard W. Titball

3.1 Outbreak Scenarios

3.1.1 India 2002 – Spread in an Endemic Area

A hunter spent a night in the jungle areas of the Himalayas, probably dismissing the fleabite on his leg as innocuous. Falling ill several days later, he was admitted to a local hospital with severe chest pain, difficulty in breathing, and a cough with bloody sputum [1]. He died soon after admission to hospital. Five relatives, who had paid their last respects to the patient, developed pneumonic plague and died [1].

While this is a true report of a recent case of plague in India, this is also the type of event that might have been the start of the Indian epidemic in 1994. Although some controversy still remains over the identity of the pathogen that was responsible for the outbreak of disease in Surat, in west central India, a general consensus exists that a significant proportion of these cases were indeed plague [2–4]. The outbreak is believed to have started with an individual who had contracted bubonic plague in the Beed district and traveled to Surat in August of 1994 [2]. Coincidentally, there had been major earthquakes in that area of India, resulting in people abandoning their homes [2]. Grain and other foodstuffs left in these abandoned houses became a source of food for rodents, the zoonotic reservoir for plague, whose numbers increased rapidly.

From the Surat index case of plague, events unfolded, which had consequences worldwide. By 24 September, more than 300 suspected cases of pneumonic plague were reported in the Surat area, with 36 deaths [5]. Hundreds of thousands fled from Surat to the major cities of Bombay, Calcutta, and New Delhi [5]. The actual incidence of disease is uncertain because confirmatory tests were not available. The reports of pneumonic plague, however, sparked a frenzy of press reporting, which in turn fanned a great degree of public concern.

R.W. Titball
School of Biosciences, Geoffrey Pope Building, University of Exeter, EX4 4QD, U.K
e-mail: R.W.Titball@Exeter.ac.uk

L.I. Lutwick, S.M. Lutwick (eds.), *Beyond Anthrax*,
DOI: 10.1007/978-1-59745-326-4_3, © Springer Science+Business Media, LLC 2008

This outbreak provides a valuable indication of the types of problems that might be associated with a biowarfare attack with *Yersinia pestis* [6], due in no small part to mass panic induced by reports of plague. During the Surat outbreak and against a background of fear of the disease spreading, some countries closed their borders to travelers from India [5]. Others introduced strict control procedures. In the USA, travelers who arrived from India were given a plague alert notice and requested to notify the public health authorities if they developed a febrile illness within 7 days of arriving in the USA [5]. Those who arrived with a febrile illness were examined and quarantined if plague was suspected. This outbreak of plague had a marked impact on the economy of India, with losses totaling $1.7 billion [7]. Hotel bookings fell by as much as 60%, and one airline alone lost $1 million each week during the outbreak [7].

3.1.2 New York City 2002 – Importation to a Nonendemic Area

On 7 November 2002 [8], a 53-year-old man, while staying at a midtown hotel in New York City, sought medical attention for fever and fatigue with left-sided inguinal pain and swelling for 2 days. He and his wife, who was also ill, had arrived in the city from Santa Fe County, New Mexico, 4 days earlier.

The husband, the sicker of the two, was found to have a temperature of 40.2°C, a blood pressure of 78/50, painful left groin lymphadenopathy, and lower extremity cyanosis. One blood culture yielded Gram-negative bacilli with bipolar staining and, within a day of admission, was identified as *Y. pestis* by both direct fluorescent antibody staining and PCR. He was treated in an intensive care unit with multiple antimicrobials and activated protein C and survived with diagnoses of bubonic and septicemic plague associated with adult respiratory distress syndrome, disseminated intravascular coagulation, acute renal failure requiring hemodialysis, mechanical ventilation, and bilateral foot amputations.

The wife had fever to 39°C and right inguinal lymphadenopathy. Both blood cultures and lymph node aspiration were nondiagnostic, and she was treated for plague. Paired acute and convalescent serum samples revealed a fourfold rise to antibody against *Y. pestis* F1 antigen. Subsequently, flea pools from areas around the couple's home revealed *Y. pestis*, which was found to be indistinguishable from the husband's isolate by pulsed field gel electrophoresis.

It was quickly recognized that the couple had *Y. pestis* infection and that the infection was likely to have been acquired in New Mexico, not in New York (the latter a nonendemic area). No evidence for bioterrorism was found. Although there was no clear secondary plague pneumonia proven, the possibility of such spread was present. This had occurred in the USA in the early part of the twentieth century as exemplified by a northern California cluster of pneumonic plague in the fall of 1919 [9].

3.2 The Organism

3.2.1 History of Plague

Plague has been suggested to have caused the death of 200 million people through history [10]. The toll of deaths from this disease had a significant impact on shaping the European civilization in the Middle Ages [11, 12]. Cycles of plague have swept across the world in three documented pandemics. The first pandemic is known as the Justinian Plague (AD 541–544). The plague arrived in Egypt from Ethiopia, and then spread through North Africa, Europe, Arabia, and Central and Southern Asia. Subsequent epidemics spread in 8–12-year cycles, often repeatedly infecting the same areas.

The second pandemic started in the fourteenth century, spreading from the steppes of Central Asia westward along trade routes. The plague arrived in Europe following the first documented use of plague as a biological weapon [13]. During a siege of Kaffa, corpses of plague victims were catapulted into the city. As plague broke out in the city, the besieged merchants fled on ships back to Genoa, taking the infection with them. The plague then spread northwards in Europe, killing an estimated 40% of the population and earning it the name of Black Death.

The third pandemic appears to have originated in the Chinese province of Yunnan in 1855, spreading due to war and troop movements to the southern coast, reaching Hong Kong in 1894. Maritime routes facilitated the global spread of infection. The Americas were infected for the first time, resulting in stable enzootic foci on every major continent except Australia. The vestigial remnants of the third pandemic persist to the present day, although the number of cases is much reduced, largely due to effective public health measures and the introduction of antimicrobial agents.

3.2.2 Yersinia pestis

Plague is caused by the bacterial pathogen *Y. pestis,* a Gram-negative nonmotile, non-spore-forming bacillus. It is capable of growth between 4 and 40°C, but grows optimally at 28–30°C. Growth is somewhat slow, requiring 48 h on enriched media for colony formation. The organism exhibits a range of auxotrophies [14, 15]. Interestingly, although the mutation of the aromatic amino acid biosynthetic pathway has been shown to be attenuating for many pathogenic bacteria, an *aroA* mutant of *Y. pestis* retained virulence for mice [16].

Y. pestis is very closely related to the enteropathogen *Yersinia pseudotuberculosis*. It has been proposed that *Y. pestis* is a clone evolving from *Y. pseudotuberculosis* serotype O:1b 1,500–20,000 years ago [17]. Comparing these species, extensive genome rearrangements and reductive evolution through gene loss appeared to be more important than acquisition of new genes in the evolution of the plague bacillus [18].

Three biovars are recognized, separated by their ability to ferment glycerol and reduce nitrate. Strains belonging to all of the biovars (Antiqua, Medievalis, and Orientalis) are virulent, and it has been suggested that each bivor is associated with one of the three pandemics. Nowadays, biovar Antiqua strains can be isolated from human cases of plague in Africa, and these strains may be descended from the bacteria that caused the first pandemic. Biovar Medievalis strains are isolated in central Asia and may be related to the bacteria of the second pandemic. Orientalis strains are widespread and appear to be the cause of the third pandemic [19].

Complete genome sequences are available for several strains of *Y. pestis*, including a biovar Orientalis strain (strain CO92) [20] and a biovar Medievalis strain (strain KIM) [21]. The genome of strain CO92 consists of a 4.56 megabase chromosome and three plasmids. These plasmids are designated pFra/pMT1, pYV/pCD1, and pPst/pPCP [22–24], and carry many of the known virulence factors of *Y. pestis*. The genome possesses a large number of insertion sequences and appears to have undergone frequent intragenomic recombinations. Indeed, recombination appears to be an ongoing process even in the present day [20]. While the organism has acquired additional genes during its adaptation from enteric pathogen to a systemic, insect-vectored pathogen, it also contains many pseudogenes in pathways no longer essential in its new niche. *Y. pestis* appears to have passed through an evolutionary bottleneck, and in this relatively isolated niche, it is unable to restore the array of pseudogenes it possesses. It is thus probably at an evolutionary dead end.

3.2.3 Virulence Factors

Many of the known virulence factors of *Y. pestis* were identified as far back as the 1950s, although for many, their role was not elucidated until recently. For example, V antigen was recognized as a protein essential for virulence in the mid-1950s [15]. Expression of V antigen coincides with resistance to phagocytosis by polymorphonuclear leukocytes and multiplication in monocytes, and V antigen is only expressed at 37°C. It was only recently that V antigen was shown to belong to the paradigm type III secretion system carried on plasmid pCD1 [25], and even now the full role of V antigen has not been elucidated [26].

Upon contact with a macrophage, the type III secretion system injects Yop effectors into the host cell. The effectors assist the bacteria to resist phagocytosis by disrupting the macrophage cytoskeleton, downregulating the inflammatory response and inducing apoptosis [27, 28]. More recently, a second type III secretion system has been shown to be present on the chromosome of *Y. pestis* [20]. The role of this second system is not yet known.

Many bacterial pathogens express a capsule, which is required for virulence, by conferring serum resistance. *Y. pestis* produces a protein capsule composed of F1 antigen and encoded by the *caf* operon. The F1 antigen is expressed only at 37°C and is exported to the cell surface where fibrillar structures are formed [29]. Natural mutants of *Y. pestis* unable to produce the F1 capsule exist and are more susceptible to phagocytosis by macrophages [30], but they remain virulent [31]. However, the time to death is delayed in comparison with wild-type strains. Therefore, *Y. pestis* is unusual in that the capsule is a relatively minor virulence factor for this pathogen.

A further example of the divergence in the role between the virulence factors of *Y. pestis* and other Gram-negative pathogens is the somatic O antigen of the lipopolysaccharide. Many Gram-negative bacilli protect their surface from the lytic activity of complement by the expression of the O antigen. Inactivation of the O antigen results in attenuation, including in *Y. pseudotuberculosis* [32]. *Y. pestis*, however, does not produce an O antigen as the biosynthetic operon has been inactivated by multiple mutations [33, 34]. The basis for serum resistance in the absence of an O antigen is not known, although it may be in part due to surface proteases such as Pla cleaving complement components [35]. Expression of a heterologous O antigen in *Y. pestis* had no effect on virulence or alteration in other surface-dependent phenotypes such as resistance to cationic antimicrobial peptides, serum, or polymyxin [36].

The plague bacillus encounters many diverse environments in transmission from flea to mammal as well as at various stages during infection of the mammal. The organism must therefore regulate expression of its genes differentially for survival in these niches. Temperature is an important signal in regulation of gene expression by *Y. pestis*. The transcription and secretion of Yops (the effectors of the pCD1 type III secretion operon) as well as of the F1 antigen only occur at 37°C. The pH within the macrophage phagolysosome is acidic. The pH6 antigen is expressed only at acidic pH and at 37°C. On release from the macrophage, therefore, the organism expresses pH6 antigen, which appears to bind to lipoproteins in plasma and on the surface of macrophages [37]. Although thought to be an adhesion, pH6 antigen seems to promote resistance to phagocytosis [38]. Mutants unable to produce functional pH6 antigen correctly are attenuated [39].

The ability of the plague bacillus to survive in macrophages is critical to the early stages of infection. *Y. pestis* possesses a PhoPQ two-component response regulatory system that has been shown to play a role in virulence in other Gram-negative bacteria, including *Salmonella enterica* serovar Typhimurium. In this latter organism, PhoPQ has been shown to be essential for survival within macrophages and for virulence in mice [40]. Inactivation of the *phoP* gene of *Y. pestis* resulted in a change in the expression of more than 20 proteins [41]. The identity of these regulated proteins is not known at present but appears to include those responsible for modification of lipo-oligosaccharide [42]. The *phoP* mutant was more susceptible to macrophage killing and less virulent in the mouse model [41], but the impact of the mutation was not as marked as had been observed for *Salmonella*. This may reflect the intracellular lifestyle of the *Salmonella* organism versus the predominantly extracellular location of *Y. pestis*.

3.3 Natural Infection

3.3.1 Epidemiology

Plague is one of three epidemic diseases notifiable to the World Health Organization. Infection circulates in sylvatic foci of rodent populations, transmitted between animals by the bite of infected fleas. Humans are accidental hosts, with most infections occurring following the bite of an infected flea which has been in close contact with the reservoir rodent. In hunters, infection can result from the handling and skinning of animals that have been suffering from plague. Domestic animals such as cats are also susceptible to plague and can transmit the infection to humans by aerosol during close contact [43].

The distribution of human plague coincides with the distribution of sylvatic plague (Fig. 3.1). Figure 3.2 shows the records of the worldwide reported incidence of disease since 1954. During the years 1954–1997, plague was reported in 38 countries, with 80,613 cases and 6587 deaths [44]. More than half of the cases were reported from Asia, followed by Africa and the Americas. The peak incidence occurred during the period 1967–1974, which corresponded to the conflict in Vietnam.

It is assumed that the number of cases of plague is significantly under-reported for many parts of the world. In the USA, where reporting may be closer to the number of cases, 247 cases were reported from 1980–1997 with a

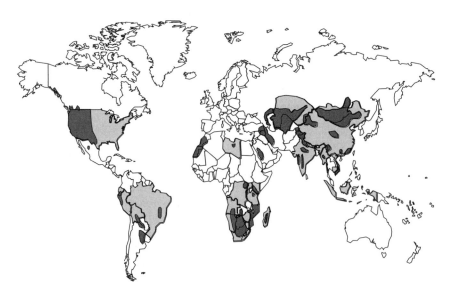

Fig. 3.1 Geographical distribution of natural plague foci in rodent population, 1997 (reproduced with permission from the World Health Organization). All regions reporting plague are shown in gray. Regions where plague is endemic are shown in dark gray

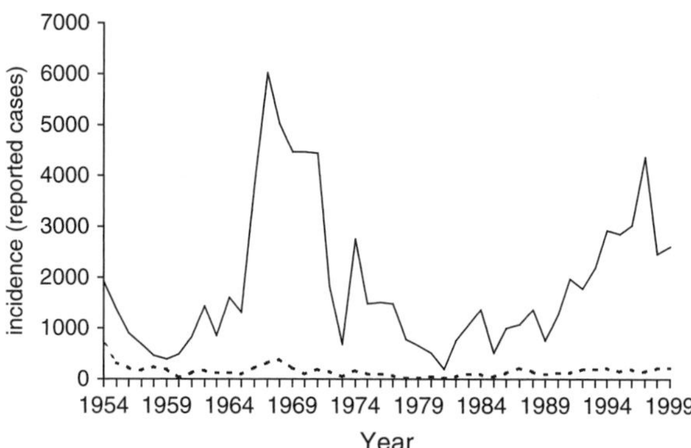

Fig. 3.2 Worldwide incidence of plague, 1954–1999. (Data from the World Health Organization, the Centers for Disease Control and Prevention, and country sources). Total reported cases of plague are shown as the solid line. Deaths from plague are shown as the dashed line

case fatality rate of 15%. Human cases occur most often in two regions: the southwestern region includes northeastern Arizona, southern Colorado, southern Utah, and New Mexico, and the Pacific region includes California, southern Oregon, and western Nevada. The US cases occur primarily (93%) during the months between April and November, with a peak incidence in July [45]. Rapid urbanization has resulted in increasing number of people living near active plague foci and increased peridomestic transmission, and infection by domestic cats have become significant sources of plague.

3.3.2 Life Cycle of Plague

Naturally occurring plague is primarily a zoonotic disease affecting rodents. A range of other mammals are susceptible to infection, but play no role in the long-term survival of the organism. The susceptibility of different animal species varies. Humans are considered to be highly susceptible, while rodents, which form the enzootic hosts, are more resistant. Transmission between rodents is by infected fleas, and the cyclic infection of rodent and flea is essential for the maintenance of plague in nature.

Fleas become infected upon feeding on the blood of a rodent itself suffering from bacteremic infection. The bacteria are restricted to the alimentary tract of the flea where they multiply in the midgut. The bacteria form large brown clumps that extend throughout the midgut, esophagus, and proventriculus, a valve-like chamber situated between the esophagus and the midgut. The clumps increase in mass over a few days until the proventriculus is blocked. The "blocked" flea then feeds on blood, but the meal is unable to pass into the stomach. The flea continues to attempt to feed, but as it futilely sucks blood from the host, the blood meal mixes with bacteria from the foregut and is regurgitated into the mammal. As many as 24,000 bacilli may be transmitted in a single attempted feeding [46].

Blockage of the flea, and thus efficient transmission of bacteria, has been shown to be dependent on the *Y. pestis* hemin storage locus (*hms*) [47]. Although originally identified as being responsible for binding and storage of hemin (and Congo Red) in the outer membrane, the *hms* (+) phenotype appears to be required for the hydrophobic surface properties of the bacteria. *Y. pestis hms* mutants are hydrophilic and not autoaggregating in aqueous environments. The mutants are unable to colonize the proventriculus and produce blockage, although they do colonize the midgut and produce the large pigmented masses. Proventriculus blockage is temperature dependent, with temperature $\geq$30°C preventing the obstruction. The effect is not due to differences in *hms* protein expression but rather due to posttranslational stability [48]. Since one *hms* protein possesses enzyme activity similar to enzymes vital to the production of polysaccharides for biofilms, it is possible that biofilm, rather than the *hms* proteins directly, is responsible for the blockage [48].

The introduced phagocytosed plague bacilli are carried to the local lymph nodes draining the site where they multiply. In humans, the resulting swollen, tender, inflamed lymph node is termed a bubo. A bubo, by definition, is a swelling caused by an inflamed, tender lymph node usually in the groin. The bacteria lyse the phagocytic cells, enter the bloodstream, and are taken up by cells in the liver and spleen. Multiplication in these organs can result in populations of 10^6 bacteria per gram of tissue [14]. Bacteria appear in increasing numbers in the bloodstream until death, probably related to diffuse endovascular injury and endotoxic shock. The bacilli are seeded through the bloodstream throughout the body, most importantly on a transmission basis, possibly causing metastatic (secondary) plague pneumonia and the generation of infectious aerosols.

Flea-vectored transmission depends on a significant septicemia developing in the infected mammal. The Oriental rat flea *Xenopsylla cheopis* is considered the classic vector with the highest transmission efficiency of fleas studied. Analysis has shown that transmission by fleas is inherently variable, as about half of fleas ingested a high-grade bacteremia blood meal are able to clear the organisms and less than half of those colonized develop proventriculus blockage [49]. Cat fleas (*Ctenocephalides felis*) and human fleas (*Pulex irritans*) appear to be poor vectors [46, 50]. Although transmission to humans is usually through the bite of an infected animal flea, human-to-human transmission vectored by fleas is, therefore, considered rare.

Human epidemic spread primarily occurs when a plague victim develops secondary pneumonia. The infectious respiratory aerosols generated from the pneumonic infection allow the development of primary pneumonic plague cases, which are of concern in public health. A cluster of fulminating pneumonia with hemoptysis should bring up the possibility of pneumonic plague. This epidemic has been of natural causes but may be biowarfare related, particularly relevant when occurring in a non-plague endemic area.

3.4 Diagnosis

3.4.1 Clinical Presentation

Y. pestis infection occurs principally in three clinical forms in humans: bubonic, septicemic, and pneumonic. Bubonic plague is the classical form of the disease, representing 85–90% of clinical presentations. Individuals present with fever, chills, headache, and the painful bubo, arising as a result of a bite from an infected flea or by contamination of an open skin lesion. Local bacterial proliferation is sometimes evident (4–10% of cases) as an abscess or ulcer at the site of infection [45].

Symptoms of fever and malaise develop 2–6 days after exposure. The bubo generally occurs in the groin lymph nodes (90%), more commonly in the femoral area than in the inguinal area. Axillary and cervical lymph nodes may be involved reflective of the location of the flea bite. Usually heralded by very severe pain within 6–8 h after the onset of constitutional symptoms, the bubo becomes evident within 24 h. It has been said [45] that the bubo may be so tender that semicomatose patients will posture in a way as to attempt to decrease pressure on the swelling. Sometimes, the bubo may not be evident in the first few days of symptoms. Furthermore, involvement of deeper lymph nodes may not be visible. In these cases, abdominal pain suggestive of appendicitis, colitis, enteritis, or cholecystitis may be described. In such cases, tenderness upon abdominal palpitation will be misleading and can result in hazardous exploratory surgery and a potentially lethal delay in specific antimicrobial therapy.

Patients develop a significant clinically apparent bacteremia with secondary septicemic plague reported in about 23% of those with bubonic plague. Blood cultures obtained prior to antimicrobial therapy will almost always be positive, but most do not have clinical evidence of septicemia. Those with blood colony counts higher than 100/mL have higher fatality rates, although a patient with 10^7/mL count did survive [51]. Untreated, the case fatality rate is 40–60%, but where therapy is used, this can be reduced to about 14% [52].

When *Y. pestis* infection with bacteremia occurs without the development of lymphadenopathy, primary septicemic plague is diagnosed, which is found in about 10–15% of presentations [53, 54]. Symptoms of septicemic plague resemble those of most Gram-negative bacteremias: fever, chills, headache, and malaise. Due to difficulties in diagnosis and thus delays in appropriate antimicrobial therapy, mortality rates are higher than for bubonic plague. Untreated, septicemic plague is almost always fatal. In the course of septicemic plague (primary or secondary), endovascular injury causes disseminated intravascular coagulopathy leading to arterial thrombosis, tissue necrosis, and bleeding into the skin. These manifest to produce the classical "Black Death" of plague.

Plague meningitis is characterized by fever, headache, stiff neck, delerium, and confusion progressing to coma. Gram-negative bacteria and polymorphonuclear leukocytes are visible in cerebrospinal fluid. Meningitis arises as a complication of bubonic and septicemic plague, usually in patients with axillary buboes with delayed antimicrobial therapy [55, 56].

Another uncommon presentation of plague is pharyngeal/enteric plague, which can arise as a result of exposure to infectious aerosols or by ingestion of infected meat [57]. Enteric infection does not lead to enteric pathology or result in fecal excretion of plague bacilli [58]. Pharyngeal plague may be asymptomatic or may present clinically similarly to viral pharyngitis, although with more severe cervical lymphadenopathy. Diagnosis usually requires laboratory identification, unless historical information indicates plague infection.

Overall, death from plague occurs as a result of shock, probably due to endotoxin, resulting in disseminated intravascular coagulation, multiple organ failure, and respiratory distress syndrome.

3.4.2 Clinical Presentation of Biowarfare Plague

Primary pneumonic plague (1% of natural plague presentations) arises as a result of inhalation of plague bacilli in infectious aerosols, such as would be produced when there are secondary pneumonic complications in bubonic plague. It is also a form of disease contracted from infected cats [59, 60]. Primary pneumonic plague is the form of the disease that would be most likely if *Y. pestis* were to be used in an aerosol as a biological weapon. Such an aerosol would be likely to be used in an indoor setting to avoid the outdoor UV radiation inactivation of the organism. Bubonic plague can also be a manifestation of biowarfare. During World War II [61], the infamous Japanese Unit 731 facilitated the dropping of a mixture of materials with infected fleas over China, resulting in cases of plague.

Primary plague pneumonia has a short incubation period of 1–3 days, after which there is sudden onset of flu-like symptoms including fever, chills, headache, generalized body pains, weakness, and chest discomfort. A cough develops with sputum production, which may be bloody, and increasing chest pain and difficulty in breathing. As the disease progresses, hypoxia and hemoptysis are prominent. The disease is invariably fatal unless antibiotic therapy commences within 24 h of exposure.

3.4.3 Radiographic Diagnosis

The presence of chest x-ray infiltrates in a patient with bubonic or septicemic plague does not necessarily confirm the diagnosis of plague pneumonia. Indeed, minimal and transient infiltrates have been found with bubonic plague [62] that may represent atelectasis. As many as a quarter of all individuals with bubonic plague manifest a cough without overt chest x-ray changes [63]. Diffuse alveolar pulmonary infiltrates are also well described [62], also as were seen in the

New York scenario case above, representing the pulmonary manifestations of systemic inflammatory response syndrome often found in severe septicemia.

3.4.4 Laboratory Diagnosis

Definitive laboratory diagnosis of *Y. pestis* infection is based on isolation of the pathogen from clinical specimens or on the demonstration of a diagnostic change in antibody titer in paired serum samples. Blood cultures obtained before treatment will usually result in isolation of the organism. Gram, Giemsa, Wright, or Wayson staining can provide supportive, but not presumptive or confirmatory, evidence of the plague bacillus by the presence of the typical bipolar, safety-pin uptake of stain. However, this staining characteristic other Gram-negative bacilli may display it. Routine specimens for smear and culture include blood, bubo aspirates, pharyngeal swabs, and sputum samples from suspected pneumonic plague patients and cerebrospinal fluid in cases of suspected plague meningitis.

Y. pestis can grow on most routine laboratory media, such as brain-heart infusion, sheep blood, or MacConkey agars. For the field, selective media have been developed to recover *Y. pestis* from the mixed bacterial flora in decaying carcasses of infected rodents [63A]. Incubation for 2 days at 37°C will produce visible opaque colonies with irregular edges. Automated bacteriological test systems have misidentified *Y. pestis* as organisms such as *Y. pseudotuberculosis, Shigella boydii*, and *Enterobacter agglomerans* [64]. Cultures, however, can be definitively identified as *Y. pestis* by specific phage lysis.

Direct detection of F1 antigen itself has also been used for diagnosis. Rapid tests based on a monoclonal antibody against F1 antigen, including an antigen capture ELISA and a dipstick format, have been developed and used successfully in the field [65, 66]. Both F1 antigen and antibodies against it should be assayed simultaneously, as patients will be positive for one while negative for the other [67]. Real-time PCR tests may contribute to rapid diagnosis of plague in the future. With a turnaround time of less than 5 h, as few as 10^2 colony-forming units can be detected [67A].

Even if *Y. pestis* is not being isolated, plague can be confirmed by serological responses to F1 antigen. A fourfold or greater increase shown by passive hemagglutination testing of paired serum specimens, bolstered by the F1 antigen hemagglutination-inhibition test, is confirmatory. ELISAs for IgG and IgM antibodies are used in laboratory diagnosis in early phases of infection [65, 67, 68]. Paired serum samples, either from acute and convalescent phases or from convalescent and post-convalescent phases, are optimal for these tests, but a singe serum sample can also provide presumptive evidence of plague. Most patients seroconvert between 7 and 14 days after the onset of disease. Occasionally a patient will seroconvert as early as 5 days, and up to 5% of patients fail to seroconvert at all [69].

CDC guidelines (www.cdc.gov/ncidod/dvbid/plague/lab-test-criteria.htm) suggest that naturally spread plague should be considered if clinical symptoms are observed that are compatible with plague in a person who resides in or has recently traveled to a plague endemic area, and small Gram-negative coccobacilli are seen on a smear taken from affected tissues.

Concern about a biological warfare event, however, may void any geographical considerations.

Presumptive diagnosis of plague can be made if immunofluorescence staining of smears or material is positive for the presence of F1 antigen and/or a single serum specimen is tested and the anti-F1 antigen titer by agglutination is >1:10. Agglutination testing must be shown to be specific to *Y. pestis* F1 antigen by hemagglutination inhibition.

Confirmed plague is only diagnosed if

1) the culture isolated is lysed by specific bacteriophage,
2) two serum specimens demonstrate a fourfold anti-F1 antigen titer difference by agglutination testing confirmed by hemagglutination inhibition, or
3) a single serum specimen tested by agglutination has a titer of over 1:128 without a known previous plague infection or vaccination history.

3.5 Therapeutic Interventions

If plague is suspected, antimicrobial treatment should be started immediately without waiting for laboratory confirmation. Patients must be placed in isolation initially to reduce the risk of spread in the event that pneumonic plague develops. Parenteral antimicrobial therapy is preferred initially for overt human infection with *Y. pestis*, and the aminoglycoside streptomycin has been the drug of choice (Table 3.1). Gentamicin, another aminoglycoside, is comparable with streptomycin in the treatment of plague [69A]. Due to the toxicity of the aminoglycosides, patients may be switched to another agent, often a tetracycline, 3 days after their temperature has returned to normal. A further advantage of tetracyclines is that they can be effective when given orally. In cases of plague meningitis, chloramphenicol is the drug of choice due to its tissue penetration. Fluoroquinolones such as ciprofloxacin have been shown to be effective in laboratory animals [70], The newer fluoroquinolones, gatifloxacin and moxifloxacin, appear effective for both prophylactic and therapeutic use in a murine model [71]. There is little published data showing its efficacy in human plague [72].

Other classes of antibiotics, such as penicillins, cephalosporins, and macrolides, are ineffective in treatment of plague. Antibiotic-resistant strains are rare, but a multiply antibiotic-resistant strain was reported in 1997 from Madagascar [73]. The plasmid-based resistance included streptomycin, tetracycline, sulfonamides, and chloramphenicol, but not trimethoprim. A streptomycin-resistant strain was isolated in 2001 again in Madagascar [74]. Fluoroquinolone

Table 3.1 Antimicrobial treatment of plague (adapted from ref. 6 and 45)

Important points
Begin as soon as diagnosis is suspected especially in primary pneumonic disease where delay of $\geq$18 h portends a quite high mortality rate
Treatment is generally to be continued for 10 days
Oral therapy with a tetracycline or other agent may be used initially only in very mild bubonic plague or in a mass casualty setting
If clinically appropriate, oral tetracycline can be substituted for parenteral therapy for the last 5 days of the course
Biowarfare strains may be selected for antimicrobial resistance
Preferred choices
Streptomycin
Adults: 1 g intramuscularly (IM) twice per day
Children: 15 mg/kg IM twice per day (up to adult dose)
(or) Gentamicin
Adults: 5 mg/kg IM or intravenously (IV) once per day or 2 mg/kg and then 1.7 mg/kg IM or IV three times per day
Children: 2.5 mg/kg IM or IV three times per day
Alternative choices
Doxycycline (other tetracyclines may be used at appropriate dosing)
Adults: 100 mg IV twice daily or 200 mg IV once per day
Children: (>45 kg or 100 lbs) adult dosing (<45 kg) 2.2 mg/kg IV twice per day (up to adult dose)
(or) Ciprofloxacin (other fluoroquinolones may be used at appropriate dosing)
Adults: 400 mg IV two times per day
Children: 15 mg/kg IV two times per day
(or) Chloramphenicol
All ages: 25 mg/kg IV four times per day (not for use in <2 years old) (observe for bone marrow suppression)
Doses may need adjustment in the presence of hepatic or renal disease or in infants. Blood levels of gentamicin and streptomycin should be obtained

resistance was not reported in either strain, but ciprofloxacin resistance can be selected for in the laboratory [75]. Efficient transfer of resistance genes to *Y. pestis* in the midgut of the flea has been demonstrated [76]. It is important to note that if *Y. pestis* is used as a biowarfare agent, the organism could have been engineered to be resistant to a variety of usually effective antimicrobial agents.

3.6 Preventive Measures

3.6.1 Infection Control

Persons who have been in contact with pneumonic plague patients or have been handling potentially infectious body fluids or tissues without appropriate protection should receive preventive antimicrobial therapy. The preferred

Table 3.2 Postexposure antimicrobial prophylaxis for prevention of plague pneumonia (adapted from ref. 6)

Important points
For close (≤6 m or 20 ft) contacts of a case of pneumonic plague or in a circumstance of a clandestine attack of aerosolized *Yersinia Pestis*
Chemoprophylaxis is to be continued for 7 days
Those who manifest fever ≥38.5°C or a new cough after exposure should receive parenteral, not oral, antimicrobial agents except in a setting of mass causalities
Biowarfare strains may be selected for antimicrobial resistance
Doxycycline (other tetracyclines may be used at appropriate dosing)
Adults: 100 mg orally two times per day
Children: >45 kg (100 lbs) use adult dosing (<45 kg) 2.2 mg/kg orally two times per day
(or) Ciprofloxacin (other fluoroquinolones may be used at appropriate dosing)
Adults: 500 mg orally twice per day
Children: 20 mg/kg orally twice per day (up to adult dose)
(or) Chloramphenicol
All ages: 25 mg/kg orally four times daily (not for use in <2 years old) (observe for bone marrow suppression)

Doses may need adjustment in the presence of hepatic or renal disease

antimicrobial agents for prophylaxis are tetracyclines, quinolones, or chloramphenicol (Table 3.2). If available, vaccination should be offered to these individuals. The lack of clear protection against pneumonic plague, and the number of months required to develop an immune response, suggest that vaccination is of little use in the early stages of a plague outbreak or following a deliberate release where pneumonic plague would predominate. Vaccination could, however, be useful in containing an ongoing plague outbreak.

Patients with primary pneumonic plague generate large quantities of infectious aerosols that pose a significant risk to close contacts. CDC guidelines identify contacts within 2 m as being at greatest risk and do not consider the organism likely to be carried through air ducts or vents [44]. Isolation precautions, such as hand washing, wearing latex gloves and gowns, and protection of mucous membranes, should be undertaken for all bubonic plague patients for 48 h. If no pneumonia is found or there are no draining lesions, isolation can be discontinued.

Pneumonic plague patients should also be managed under respiratory droplet precautions, including

1) accommodation in an individual room,
2) restriction of patient movement outside the room and access to the room, and
3) masking of both patient and health-care deliverers.

It is thought that the risk of transmission is ended after the completion of at least 4 days of therapy [45]. The Working Group on Civilian Biodefense recommends isolation during the first 48 h and until clinical improvement occurs [6].

Laboratory-acquired plague has been reported and can result in primary pneumonic plague. Probably initially reported in Wu's 1926 classic monograph on plague [77], the laboratory transmission of *Y. pestis* appears to be rare. A case report with a review of four other cases was published in the USA in 1962 [78]. *Y. pestis* has been found to maintain some viability for some periods of time (at least 5 days) on environmental surfaces under controlled conditions [79]. Such an environmental risk for humans is likely to be minimal, and environmental decontamination is not recommended [6].

3.6.2 Immunization

Historically, various live attenuated strains of *Y. pestis* have been used in humans in an attempt to prevent plague. It was known from early studies that an effective vaccine strain had to express F1 and V antigen to induce a protective immune response. For example, immunization with strain Tjiwidej, which does not produce V antigen, did not reduce the incidence of pneumonic plague, whereas strain EV, which does produce V antigen, was able to induce a protective immune response [15]. Sera from vaccinated individuals were able to protect passively immunized mice against plague. The degree of protection was dependent on titers of antibody directed against F1 antigen [15].

The EV series of strains has been most widely used for human vaccination, primarily in the former Soviet Union. These strains are descended from an attenuated strain isolated early in the twentieth century. Although laboratory passage led to heterogeneity in the strains [80], the primary basis for attenuation was loss of the pigmentation locus and the associated loss of an adjacent pathogenicity island. There were several problems associated with using such live vaccines. The immune response varied between individuals, and some vaccinees failed to respond, even to multiple inoculations. In addition, the side effects associated with the use of such strains may be severe, even to the point of a significant proportion of recipients requiring hospitalization [80]. For these reasons, vaccination with live attenuated strains of *Y. pestis* declined in the 1960s.

Killed whole-cell plague vaccines have been used in humans since 1946. The preparations used have been based on *Y. pestis* cells inactivated by either heat or formaldehyde. The history of the vaccine has been reviewed by Meyer [81]. The initial Haffkine vaccine caused a significant amount of local and systemic reaction, as it was thought, erroneously, that the degree of reactogenicity correlated with protection. An available vaccine, produced by the Commonwealth Serum Laboratories in Australia, consists of a suspension of agar-grown, heat-killed bacteria (approximately 3,000 cells/mL) in saline containing 0.5% phenol as a preservative. The vaccine is given subcutaneously as an initial course of two doses of 0.5 mL followed by six booster doses at monthly intervals. Side effects such as malaise, headache, fever, and lymphadenopathy occur in approximately 10% of recipients receiving the killed whole-cell plague vaccines, and are more frequent with increasing numbers of booster injections [82]. In this review of 1,219 vaccinees over 21 years, 29% had local reactions, 2% had systemic reactions, and only 0.1% of the total reactions were severe.

Although uncontrolled, the incidence of bubonic plague was ~1 case per 10^6 person-years of exposure in US troops during the Vietnam conflict as compared with ~333 cases per 10^6 person-years of exposure in Vietnamese civilians [83]. The inactivated vaccine appears to reduce the incidence of bubonic plague, but cases of pneumonic plague have been reported in immunized individuals [80, 84], a result that has been reproduced in a mouse model [85].

Because of variable degree of protection afforded by this vaccine and the high level of adverse side effects, it had been restricted to individuals such as veterinarians in endemic areas or laboratory workers who are at greatest risk of exposure to the organism. In the USA, the FDA-licensed inactivated whole-cell vaccine was available until 1999 when distribution was discontinued.

Research is underway to develop a more effective vaccine, capable of protecting against pneumonic plague, which would be suitable for more general use. Work has focused on formulations containing F1 and V antigens. The antigens have been produced as recombinant proteins, allowing a safe source for large-scale production. The monomeric unit of the F1 antigen has a molecular weight of 15.5 kDa, but aggregation of the monomers occurs, which produces large complexes in excess of 3 MDa [86]. This aggregation occurs spontaneously in solution. The V antigen has a molecular mass of 37 kDa and also spontaneously aggregates [87]. Folding of V antigen is important to immunogenicity, as studies have shown that B-cell epitopes in the protein are conformational. V antigen is more difficult to produce than F1 antigen due to inherent instability of the protein. It is produced as a fusion protein, which is purified and subsequently cleaved to give pure V antigen.

The F1 and V antigens have been shown to be able to induce a protective immune response individually, and a combination of the proteins had an additive effect. The optimum ratio for immunization was 2:1 (F1:V) [88]. At present, the antigens are being studied in clinical trials using alhydrogel as an adjuvant and are given intramuscularly. A combination of F1 and V vaccine has been found in a murine model to be fully protective for pneumonic plague as compared with 16% protection for the killed whole-cell vaccine [89]. A recombinant fusion protein vaccine with F1 and V antigens was also found to be protective in a flea transmission model [49].

Although this vaccine induces protection in mice against aerosol challenge, work is now underway to develop a vaccine that is mucosally delivered. In addition to inducing local immune responses in the respiratory tract, mucosal delivery has the advantage of being needle free. Much work has been undertaken to deliver antigens using biodegradable polymeric microencapsulation. A preparation suitable for nasal administration has been produced, which is fully protective against aerosol challenge in the mouse model after just two doses [90]. Using a live, recombinant *Salmonella typhimurium* strain (aroA), an F1 and V fusion protein produced a degree of protection in the mouse model as well [91].

Passive immunization may play a role in protection against epidemic plague. As an example, monoclonal antibodies directed against V and F1 antigens were protective alone or in combination synergistically in murine models of bubonic and pneumonic plague. The effect occurred even when given 48 h postexposure [92].

3.6.3 Rodent Control

Over 200 species of mammals have been reported to be susceptible to infection with *Y. pestis*. Of these, rodents are the most important hosts for plague, while other species, such as domestic cats, are important in being a potential source of infection for human contacts. Death of large numbers of rodents is one indication that plague is erupting in the local animal population. For example, rat deaths in large numbers were seen prior to the outbreak of human plague in India in 1994. Serological surveillance of animals is another method of monitoring plague activity in a given area. Texas, California, Colorado, and New Mexico all have ongoing surveillance programs for plague infection of rodents and carnivores. Insecticides must be used to kill fleas if rodent hosts are to be killed, and this must be done before rodenticides are employed. Such approaches are labor intensive, generally used only after a epizootic has begun and not particularly effective on a large scale in enzootic areas.

More effective are measures to eliminate habitat for rodents and reduce the appeal of residential areas to rodents, combined with treatment of domestic pets for fleas [93]. During an outbreak of plague in humans, however, it is important to control populations of both fleas and rodents. Again, flea populations must be reduced, therefore, before control of rodent reservoirs can be undertaken. Safe disposal of rodent corpses is a further priority in rodent control. Rural areas pose a specific problem in rodent control as removal of rodents from surrounding habitation can result in subsequent invasion by field rodents. Therefore, rodent proofing to prevent re-entry is important.

Vaccines may be utilized in animals such as rodents and cats to facilitate immunity to plague similar to the live, attenuated vaccine used to immunize feral animals against rabies. One such potential immunogen is a recombinant raccoon pox vaccine expressing F1 antigen that when given parenterally was protective in mice [94]. Voluntary oral administration of this vaccine in a palatable bait to black-tailed prairie dogs is immunogenic [95]. Inclusion of V antigen in this biologic may be an even more effective immunogen for feral reservoirs of the plague.

References

1. Thomas, K. S. Curbing a killer. *The Week*, Mar 3, 2002.
2. Anonymous. The plague epidemic of 1994. *Curr. Sci.*, 71, 781–806, 1994.
3. Ranga, S., Gulati, I., and Pandey, J. Plague – a review. *Indian J. Pathol. Microbiol.*, 38, 213–222, 1995.
4. World Health Organization. Plague. *Weekly Epidemiol. Rec.*, *70*, 35, 1995.
5. Fritz, C. L., Dennis, D. T., Tipple, M. A., et al. Surveillance for pneumonic plague in the United States during an international emergency: a model for control of imported emerging disease. *Emerg. Infect. Dis.*, 2, 30–36, 1996.
6. Inglesby, T. V., Dennis, D. T., Henderson, D. A., et al. Plague as a biological weapon – medical and public health management. *J. Am. Med. Assoc.*, 283, 2281–2290, 2000.
7. Davey, S. Removing Obstacles to Healthy Development, ed. Leotsakos, A.: World Health Organization, Geneva, 1999.
8. Centers for Disease Control and Prevention. Imported plague – New York City, 2002. *MMWR – Morbid. Mortal. Week. Rep.*, 52, 725–728, 2003.
9. Kellogg, W. H. An epidemic of pneumonic plague. *Am. J. Public. Health*, 10, 599–605, 1920.
10. Duplaix, N. Fleas – the lethal leapers. *Natl. Geogr.*, 173, 672–694, 1988.
11. Haddock, D. D., and Kiesling, L. The Black death and property rights. *J. Legal Stud.*, 31, S545–S587, 2002.
12. Moore, J. W. The crisis of feudalism – an environmental history. *Organ. Environ.* 15, 301–322, 2002.
13. Wheelis, M. Biological warfare at the 1346 Siege of Caffa. *Emerg. Infect. Dis.* 8, 971–975, 2002.
14. Brubaker, R. R. Factors promoting acute and chronic diseases caused by yersiniae. *Clin. Microbiol. Rev.*, 4, 309–324, 1991.
15. Burrows, T. W. Virulence of *Pasteurella pestis* and immunity to plague. In *Ergebnisse der Mikrobiologie Immunitatsforschung und Experimentellen Therapie* (Tomcsik, J. ed.), Springer-Verlag: Berlin, 1963, pp. 59–113.
16. Oyston, P. C. F., Russell, P., Williamson, E. D., and Titball, R. W. An *aroA* mutant of *Yersinia pestis* is attenuated in guinea-pigs, but virulent in mice. *Infect. Immun.*, 142, 1847–1853, 1966.
17. Achtman, M., Zurth, K., Morelli, C., et al. *Yersinia pestis*, the cause of plague, is a recently emerged clone of *Yersinia pseudotuberculosis*. *Proc. Natl. Acad. Sci. U.S.A.*, 96, 14043–14048, 1999.
18. Chain, P. S. G., Carniel, E., Larimer, F. W., et al. Insights into the evolution of *Yersinia pestis* through whole-genome comparison with *Yersinia pseudotuberculosis*. *Proc. Natl. Acad. Sci. U.S.A.*,101,13826–13831, 2004.
19. Devignat, R. Varietes de l'espece *Pasteurella pestis*. Nouvelle hyphothese. *Bull. World Health Org.*, 4, 247–263, 1951.
20. Parkhill, J., Wren, B. W., Thomson, N. R., et al. Genome sequence of *Yersinia pestis*, the causative agent of plague. *Nature*, 413, 523–527, 2001.
21. Deng, W., Burland, V., Plunkett, G., et al. Genome sequence of *Yersinia pestis* KIM. *J. Bacteriol.*, 184, 4601–4611, 2002.
22. Lindler, L. E., Plano, G. V., Burland, V., et al. Complete DNA sequence and detailed analysis of the *Yersinia pestis* KIM5 plasmid encoding murine toxin and capsular antigen. *Infect. Immun.*, 66, 5731–5742, 1998.
23. Hu, P., Elliott, J., McCready, P., et al. Structural organization of virulence-associated plasmids of *Yersinia pestis*. *J. Bacteriol.*, 180, 5192–5202, 1998.
24. Perry, R. D., Straley, S. C., Fetherston, J. D., et al. DNA sequencing and analysis of the low-Ca^{2+}-response plasmid pCD1 of *Yersinia pestis* KIM5. *Infect. Immun.*, 66, 4611–4623, 1998.

25. Cornelis, G. R. The *Yersinia* Yop virulon, a bacterial system to subvert cells of the primary host defense. *Folia Microbiol.*, 43, 253–261, 1998.
26. Titball, R. W., Hill, J., Lawton, D. G., and Brown, K. A. *Yersinia pestis* and plague. *Biochem. Soc. Trans.*, 31, 104–107, 2003.
27. Cornelis, G. R., Boland, A., Boyd, A. P., et al. The virulence plasmid of *Yersinia*, an antihost genome. *Microbiol. Mol. Biol. Rev.*, 62, 1315–1352, 1998.
28. Hueck, C. J. Type III protein secretion systems in bacterial pathogens of animals and plants. *Microbiol. Mol. Biol. Rev.*, 62, 379–433, 1998.
29. Tito, M. A., Miller, J., Griffin, K. F., et al. Macromolecular organization of the *Yersinia pestis* capsular F1 antigen: insights from time-of-flight mass spectrometry. *Protein Sci.*, 10, 2408–2413, 2001.
30. Du, Y. D., Rosqvist, R., and Forsberg, A. Role of fraction 1 antigen of *Yersinia pestis* in inhibition of phagocytosis. *Infect. Immun.*, 70, 1453–1460, 2002.
31. Davis, K. J., Fritz, D. L., Pitt, M. L., et al. Pathology of experimental pneumonic plague produced by fraction 1-positive and fraction 1-negative *Yersinia pestis* in African green monkeys (*Cercopithecus aethiops*). *Arch. Pathol. Lab. Med.*, 120, 156–163, 1996.
32. Karlyshev, A. V., Oyston, P. C. F., Williams, K., et al. Application of high-density array-based signature-tagged mutagenesis to discover novel *Yersinia* virulence-associated genes. *Infect. Immun.*, 69, 7810–7819, 2001.
33. Prior, J. L., Parkhill, J., Hitchen, P. G., et al. The failure of different strains of *Yersinia pestis* to produce lipopolysaccharide O-antigen under different growth conditions is due to mutations in the O-antigen gene cluster. *FEMS Microbiol. Lett.*, 197, 229–233, 2001.
34. Skurnik, M., Peippo, A., and Ervela, E. Characterization of the O-antigen gene clusters of *Yersinia pseudotuberculosis* and the cryptic O-antigen gene cluster of *Yersinia pestis* shows that the plague bacillus is most closely related to and has evolved from *Y. pseudotuberculosis* serotype O:1b. *Mol. Microbiol.*, 37, 316–330, 2000.
35. Sodeinde, O. A., Subrahmanyam, Y., Stark, K., et al. A surface protease and the invasive character of plague. *Science*, 258, 1004–1007, 1992.
36. Oyston, P. C. F., Prior, J. L., Kiljunen, S., et al. Expression of heterologous O-antigen in *Yersinia pestis* KIM does not affect virulence by the intravenous route. *J. Med. Microbiol.*, 52, 289–294, 2003.
37. Makoveichuk, E., Cherepanov, P., Lundberg, S., et al. pH6 antigen of *Yersinia pestis* interacts with plasma lipoproteins and cell membranes. *J. Lipid Res.*, 44, 320–330, 2003.
38. Huang, X. Z., and Lindler, L. E. The pH 6 antigen is an antiphagocytic factor produced by *Yersinia pestis* independent of *Yersinia* outer proteins and capsule antigen. *Infect. Immun.*, 72, 7212–7219, 2004.
39. Lindler, L. E., Klempner, M. S., and Straley, S. C. *Yersinia pestis* pH6 antigen – genetic, biochemical, and virulence characterization of a protein involved in the pathogenesis of bubonic plague. *Infect. Immun.*, 58, 2569–2577, 1990.
40. Groisman, E. A. The pleiotropic two-component regulatory system PhoP-PhoQ. *J. Bacteriol.*, 183, 1835–1842, 2001.
41. Oyston, P. C. F., Dorrell, N., Williams, K., et al. The response regulator PhoP is important for survival under conditions of macrophage-induced stress and virulence in *Yersinia pestis*. *Infect. Immun.*, 68, 3419–3425, 2000.
42. Hitchen, P. G., Prior, J. L., Oyston, P. C. F., et al. Structural characterization of lipo-oligosaccharide (LOS) from *Yersinia pestis*: regulation of LOS structure by the PhoPQ system. *Mol. Microbiol.*, 44, 1637–1650, 2002.
43. Gage, K. L., Dennis, D. T., Orloski, K. A., et al. Cases of cat-associated human plague in the western US, 1977–1998. *Clin. Infect. Dis.*, 30, 893–900, 2000.
44. Dennis, D. T., Gage, K. L., Grantz, N., et al. Plague Manual: Epidemiology, Distribution, Surveillance and Control. World Health Organization, Geneva, 1999.
45. McGovern, T. W., and Friedlander, A. M. Plague. In *Textbook of Military Medicine: Medical Aspects of Chemical and Biological Warfare* (Zajtchuk, R., and Bellamy, R. F.

eds.), Office of the Surgeon General, Borden Institute, Washington, D. C., 1997, pp. 479–502.

46. Burroughs, A. L. Sylvatic plague studies. The vector efficiency of nine species of plague compared with *Xenopsylla cheopis*. *J. Hyg.*, 45, 371–396, 1947.
47. Cavanaugh, D. C. Specific effect of temperature upon transmission of the plague bacillus by the oriental rat flea *Xenopsylla cheopis*. *Am. J. Trop. Med. Hyg.*, 20, 264–272, 1971.
48. Perry, R. D., Bobrov, A. G., Kirillina, O., et al. Temperature regulation of the hemin storage (hms+) phenotype of *Yersinia pestis* is postranscriptional. *J. Bacteriol.*, 186, 1638–1647, 2004.
49. Jarrett, C. O., Sebbane, F., Adamovicz, J. J., et al. Flea-borne transmission model to evaluate vaccine efficacy against naturally acquired bubonic plague. *Infect. Immun.*, 72, 2052–2056, 2004.
50. Wheeler, C. M., and Douglas, J. R. Sylvatic plague studies. V. The determination of vector efficiency. *J. Infect. Dis.*, 77, 4–12, 1945.
51. Perry, R. D., and Fetherston, J. D. *Yersinia pestis* – etiologic agent of plague. *Clin. Microbiol. Rev.*, 10, 35–66, 1997.
52. Craven, R. B., Maupin, G. O., Beard, M. L., et al. Reported cases of human plague infections in the United-States, 1970–1991. *J. Med. Entomol.*, 30, 758–761, 1993.
53. Hull, H. F., Montes, J. M., and Mann, J. M. Septicemic plague in New Mexico. *J. Infect. Dis.*, 155, 113–118, 1987.
54. Poland, J. D., and Barnes, A. M. Plague. In *CRC Handbook Series in Zoonoses. Section A. Bacterial, Rickettsial, and Mycotic Diseases* (Steele, J. H. ed.), CRC Press: Boca Raton, Florida, 1979, pp. 515–559.
55. Becker, T. M., Poland, J. D., Quan, T. J., et al. Plague meningitis – a retrospective analysis of cases reported in the United States, 1970–1979. *West. J. Med.*, 147, 554–557, 1987.
56. Christie, A. B., Chen, T. H., and Elberg, S. S. Plague in camels and goats: their role in human epidemics. *J. Infect. Dis.*, 141, 724–726, 1980.
57. Butler, T., Levin, J., Nguyen, N. L., et al. *Yersinia pestis* infection in Vietnam II. Quantitative blood cultures and detection of endotoxin in the cerebrospinal fluid of patients with meningitis. *J. Infect. Dis.*, 133, 493–499, 1976.
58. Butler, T., Fu, Y.-S., Furman, L., et al. Experimental *Yersinia pestis* infection in rodents after intragastric inoculation and ingestion of bacteria. *Infect. Immun.*, 36, 1160–1167, 1982.
59. Doll, J. M., Zeitz, P. S., Ettestad, P., et al. Cat-transmitted fatal pneumonic plague in a person who traveled from Colorado to Arizona. *Am. J. Trop. Med. Hyg.*, 51, 109–114, 1994.
60. Gasper, P. W., Barnes, A. M., Quan, T. J., et al. Plague (*Yersinia pestis*) in cats – description of experimentally induced disease. *J. Med. Entomol.*, 30, 20–26, 1993.
61. Williams, P., and Wallace, D. Unit 731: Japan's Secret Biological Warfare in World War II., The Free Press, New York, New York, 1989.
62. Alsofrom, D. J., Mettler, F. A., and Mann, J. M. Radiographic manifestations of plague in New Mexico, 1975–1980. *Radiology*, 139, 561–565, 1981.
63. Butler, T. A clinical study of bubonic plague. Observations of the 1970 Vietnam epidemic with emphasis on coagulation studies, skin histology and electrocardiograms. *Am. J. Med.*, 53, 268–276, 1972.

63A. Ber, R., Mamroud, E., Aftalion, M., et al. Development of an improved selective agar medium for isolation of *Yersinia pestis*. *Appl. Environ. Microbiol.*, 69, 5787–5792, 2003.

64. Wilmoth, B. A., Chu, M. C., and Quan, T. J. Identification of *Yersinia pestis* by BBL Crystal enteric/nonfementor identification system. *J. Clin. Microbiol.*, 34, 2829–2830, 1996.
65. Chanteau, S., Rahalison, L., Ratsitorahina, M., et al. Early diagnosis of bubonic plague using F1 antigen capture ELISA assay and rapid immunogold dipstick. *Int. J. Med. Microbiol.*, 290, 279–283, 2000.

66. Chanteau, S., Rahalison, L., Ralafiarisoa, L., et al. Development and testing of a rapid diagnostic test for bubonic and pneumonic plague. *Lancet*, 361, 211–216, 2003.
67. Williams, J. E., Gentry, M. K., Braden, C. A., et al. Use of an enzyme-linked immunosorbent-assay to measure antigenaemia during acute plague. *Bull. World Health Organ.*, 62, 463–466, 1984.
67A Loïez, C., Herwegh, S., Wallet, F., et al. Detection of *Yersinia pestis* in sputum by real-time PCR. *J. Clin. Microbiol.*, 41, 4873–4875, 2003.
68. Rasoamanana, B., Leroy, F., Boisier, P., et al. Field evaluation of an immunoglobulin G anti-F1 enzyme-linked immunosorbent assay for serodiagnosis of human plague in Madagascar. *Clin. Diagn. Lab. Immunol.*, 4, 587–591, 1997.
69. Butler, T., and Hudson, B. W. (1977) The serological response to *Yersinia pestis*. *Bull. World Health Organ.*, 55, 39–42, 1977.
69A Boulanger, L. L., Ettestad, P., Fogarty, J. D., Gentamicin and tetracyclines for the treatment of human plague: review of 75 cases in New Mexico, 1985–1999, *Clin. Infect. Dis.*, 38, 663–669, 2004.
70. Byrne, W. R., Welkos, S. L., Pitt, M. L., et al. Antibiotic treatment of experimental pneumonic plague in mice. *Antimicrob. Agents Chemother.*, 42, 675–681, 1998.
71. Steward, J., Lever, M. S., Russell, P., et al. Efficacy of the latest fluoroquinolones against experimental *Yersinia pestis*. *Int. J. Antimicrob. Agents.*, 24, 609–612, 2004.
72. Kuberski, T., Robinson, L., and Schurgin, A. A case of plague successfully treated with ciprofloxacin and sympathetic blockade for treatment of gangrene. *Clin. Infect. Dis.*, 36, 521–523, 2003.
73. Galimand, M., Guiyoule, A., Gerbund, G., et al. Multidrug resistance in *Yersinia pestis* mediated by a transferable plasmid. *N. Engl. J. Med.*, 337, 677–680, 1997.
74. Guiyoule, A., Gerbaud, G., Buchrieser, C., et al. Transferable plasmid-mediated resistance to streptomycin in a clinical isolate of *Yersinia pestis*. *Emerg. Infect. Dis.*, 7, 43–48, 2001.
75. Hartle, W., Lindler, L., Fan, W., et al. Detection and identification of ciprofloxacin-resistant *Yersinia pestis* by denaturing high-performance liquid chromatography. *J. Clin. Microbiol.*, 41, 3273–3283, 2003.
76. Hinnebusch, B. J., Rosso, M. L., Schwan, T. G., and Carniel, E. High-frequency conjugative transfer of antibiotic resistance genes to Yersinia pestis in the flea midgut. *Mol. Microbiol.*, 46, 349–354, 2002.
77. Wu, L-T. A Treatise on Pneumonic Plague. League of Nations, Geneva, 1926.
78. Burmeister, R. W., Tigertt, W. D., and Overholt, E. L. Laboratory-acquired pneumonic plague. Report of a case and review of previous cases. *Ann. Intern. Med.*, 56, 789–800, 1962.
79. Rose, L. J., Donlan, R., Banerjee, S. N., and Arduino, M. J. Survival of *Yersinia pestis* on environmental surfaces. *Appl. Environ. Microbiol.*, 69, 2166–2171, 2003.
80. Meyer, K. F. Effectiveness of live or killed plague vaccines in man. *Bull. World Health Organ.*, 42, 653–666, 1970.
81. Meyer, K. F., Cavanaugh, D. C., Bartelloni, P. J., and Marshall, J. D. Plague immunization. I. Past and present vaccines. *J. Infect. Dis.*, 129 (Suppl.), S13–S18, 1974.
82. Marshall, J. D., Bartelloni, P. J., Cavanaugh, D. C., et al. Plague immunization II. Relation of adverse clinical reactions to multiple immunizations with killed vaccine. *J. Infect. Dis.*, 129 (Suppl.), S19–S25, 1974.
83. Cavanaugh, D. C., Elisberg, B. L., Llewellyn, C. H., et al. Plague immunization. V. Indirect evidence of the efficacy of plague vaccine. J Infect. Dis. 129(Suppl.), S37–S40, 1974.
84. Cohen, R. J., and Stockard, J. L. Pneumonic plague in an untreated plague vaccinated individual. *J. Amer. Med. Assoc.*, 2, 365–366, 1967.
85. Russell, P., Eley, S. M., Hibbs, S. E., Manchee, R. J., Stagg, A. J., and Titball, R. W. (1995) A comparison of plague vaccine, USP and EV76 vaccine induced protection against *Yersinia pestis* in a murine model. *Vaccine*, 13, 1551–1556, 1995.

86. Miller, J., Williamson, E. D., Lakey, J. H., et al. Macromolecular organisation of recombinant *Yersinia pestis* F1 antigen and the effect of structure on immunogenicity. *FEMS Immunol. Med. Microbiol.*, 21, 213–221, 1998.
87. Titball, R. W., and Williamson, E. D. Vaccination against bubonic and pneumonic plague. *Vaccine*, 19, 4175–4184, 2001.
88. Williamson, E. D., Vesey, P. M., Gillhespy, K. J., et al. An IgG1 titre to the F1 and V antigens correlates with protection against plague in the mouse model. *Clin. Exp. Immunol.*, 116, 107–114, 1999.
89. Williamson, E. D., Eley, S. M., Stagg, A. J., et al. A single dose sub-unit vaccine protects against pneumonic plague. *Vaccine*, 19, 566–571, 2000.
90. Eyles, J. E., Sharp, G. J. E., Williamson, E. D., et al. Intranasal administration of poly-lactic acid microsphere co-encapsulated *Yersinia pestis* subunits confers protection from pneumonic plague in the mouse. *Vaccine*, 16, 698–707, 1998.
91. Leary, S. E., Griffin, K. F., Garmory, H. S., et al. Expression of an F1/V fusion protein in attenuated *Salmonella typhimurium* and protection of mice against plague. *Microb. Pathog.*, 23, 167–179, 1997.
92. Hill, J., Copse, C., Leary, S., et al. Synergistic protection of mice against plague with monoclonal antibodies specific for the F1 and V antigens of *Y. pestis*. *Infect. Immun.*, 71, 2234–2238, 2003.
93. Mann, J. M., Martone, W. J., Boyce, J. M., et al. Endemic human plague in New Mexico: risk factors associated with infection. *J. Infect. Dis.*, 140, 397–401, 1979.
94. Osorio, J. E., Powell, T. D., Frank, R. S., et al. Recombinant raccoon pox vaccine protects mice against lethal plague. *Vaccine*, 21, 1232–1238.
95. Mencher, J. S., Smith, S. R., Powell, T., D., et al. Protection of black-tailed prairie dogs (*Cynomys ludovicianus*) against plague after voluntary consumption of baits containing recombinant reccoon poxvirus vaccine. *Infect. Immun.*, 72, 5502–5505, 2004.

Chapter 4
Tularemia

Daniel S. Shapiro

4.1 Outbreak Scenario

A 50-year-old African-American male was admitted to an inner city hospital in Brooklyn, New York, with fever, chills, and cough of 2 days' duration. He was unemployed and spent most of his time in the neighborhood, which included a number of vacant lots. The man had a relatively rapid downhill course despite broad-spectrum antimicrobials and respiratory support, dying on the fourth hospital day. Postmortem, a blood culture revealed a Gram-negative coccobacillus that was subsequently identified as *Francisella tularensis*, the causative agent of tularemia. Despite aggressive investigations by several tiers of law enforcement personnel, no evidence was found to suggest that the case was anything other than an isolated case of pneumonic tularemia acquired from the local fauna of the vacant lots.

The most likely type of tularemia outbreak due to bioterrorism is caused as a result of the purposeful use of an aerosol of *F. tularensis* [1]. One large outbreak not due to bioterrorism, affecting 676 people in Sweden, was caused by either inhalation or skin contamination of hay dust related to farm work that had been contaminated by vole feces [2]. This was caused by the less virulent *F. tularensis* biovar palearctica (type B). Of note, the majority of the serologically proven cases thought to have been acquired via inhalation did not have documented pneumonia.

Although there have been waterborne outbreaks of tularemia [3–5], some of which have been relatively large in scope, water as a vehicle is not thought to be as likely a scenario for a bioterrorist attack with this agent as is aerosol delivery.

D.S. Shapiro
Clinical Microbiology Laboratory and Department of Infectious Diseases, Lahey Clinic, 41 Mall Rd., Burlington, MA, 01805 USA
e-mail: daniel.s.shapiro@lahey.org

L.I. Lutwick, S.M. Lutwick (eds.), *Beyond Anthrax*,
DOI: 10.1007/978-1-59745-326-4_4, © Springer Science+Business Media, LLC 2008

4.2 The Organism

Francisella tularensis, a Category A bioterrorism agent, is a fastidious, small, non-motile, Gram-negative, facultative coccobacillus. It may require cysteine supplementation for good growth on general laboratory media; of the commonly available laboratory media, it is worth noting that it can be isolated on buffered charcoal yeast extract agar (BCYE), which is generally used for the isolation of the bacterium causing legionellosis. In attempting to isolate the organism from sites that may have a normal flora, the use of a selective medium typically used for the isolation of the gonococcus, such as modified Thayer–Martin agar, may be helpful. Minimum, maximum, and optimal temperatures for the growth of *F. tularensis* are 24°C, 37°C, and 39°C, respectively [6].

As previously noted, *F. tularensis* has different subspecies, also called biovars. *F. tularensis* subsp. *holarctica* (biovar holarctica; also known as type B and as biovar palearctica and as subspecies *palearctica*) tends to produce milder disease and is representative of Eurasian strains and is also found in North America. *F. tularensis* subspecies *tularensis* (biovar nearctica; also known as type A and as subspecies *nearctica*) is a more virulent organism and is found primarily in North America. This organism has recently been found in Europe. An additional subspecies, *F. tularensis* subsp. *mediasiatica*, has been found in the central Asian republics of the former Soviet Union.

Misidentification of *F. tularensis* has been reported in a number of published papers, and there is no commercial "kit" system that is available for its identification in clinical laboratories. The organism has been misidentified as a *Haemophilus* species [7–9], *Actinobacillus actinomycetemcomitans* [10], and *Neisseria meningitidis* [10]. *F. tularensis* is characteristically isolated as small, poorly staining Gram-negative rods that on microscopy are seen most often as single cells. On growth, it often grows as pinpoint colonies on chocolate agar (and sometimes on sheep agar) at 48 h, does not grow on either MacConkey or eosin methylene blue agars, is oxidase-negative, and has a weakly positive or a negative catalase test. Perhaps most notably, the satellite test is negative with *F. tularensis*, a test that is now included in a flow chart in the current protocol for this organism for Sentinel (Level A) Laboratories in the United States [11]. Potential *F. tularensis* isolates should only be manipulated within biological safety cabinets by individuals wearing appropriate personal protective equipment, such as gloves and a gown. This includes those isolates that grow only on BCYE and chocolate agar. If the identification of *F. tularensis* cannot be excluded in a clinical laboratory that performs the protocol for this organism, the isolate should be sent without delay to a Level B laboratory, such as a State Public Health Laboratory, that is able to identify the organism.

There have been rare reports of *F. tularensis* strains that do not require cysteine [7], and strains that grow well on sheep blood agar and trypticase soy agar [10], though these are uncommon.

Concerns exist about engineered antibiotic resistance in *F. tularensis*. In the Soviet Union, efforts were reportedly made to engineer fully virulent strains with resistance to multiple antibiotics [12].

Given the very real concern about laboratory infection with *F. tularensis* and the difficulty in growing, isolating, and identifying this organism, there are a number of non-culture methods that are available for diagnostic purposes. Serologic diagnosis is commonly used, but may be suboptimal in the acute setting of an epidemic due to a bioterrorism event, as the time required for patients to produce diagnostic antibody levels is likely to result in delay. DFA, which is available through many Level B laboratories, can be performed rapidly on direct specimens such as sputum, conjunctival scrapings, lymph node aspirates, throat swabs, and bronchial washings. The polymerase chain reaction to establish the diagnosis of tularemia from clinical specimens and autopsy material is also available from specific laboratories within the Laboratory Response Network. It appears to be, if anything, more sensitive than is culture in the diagnosis of ulceroglandular tularemia in the published literature [13], though the sensitivity and specificity of the method used within the Laboratory Response Network has not been submitted to the peer review process and published.

In the event that there is a bioterrorism event, strain typing of *F. tularensis* will be of importance during the investigation of the incident and, potentially, in any subsequent law enforcement efforts. Molecular methods for strain typing have included multiple-locus, variable-number tandem repeat analysis [14], repetitive extragenic palindromic element PCR, enterobacterial repetitive intergenic consensus sequence PCR, and random amplified polymorphic DNA assays [15].

4.3 Epidemiology and Modes of Transmission

Tularemia is found in numerous mammals and is especially common in rabbits and hares. Individuals who hunt or skin infected animal carcasses may acquire tularemia. Ticks, mosquitoes, and biting flies have been implicated as vectors of tularemia. Contaminated hay, infected carcasses, chronically infected animals and, as noted above, both contaminated water and infectious aerosols, including aerosols resulting from lawn mowing [16, 17] and brush cutting [17], have been implicated as sources of infection. Person-to-person transmission has only been documented in a single instance. This was in the setting of an accidental inoculation during an autopsy [18].

Tularemia is a relatively uncommon disease in the United States. A total of 1,368 cases from 44 states were reported to the CDC from 1990 to 2000 [19]. The disease was more common in the earlier portion of the twentieth century.

Despite the relative infrequency of tularemia, in Pike's study of 3,921 cases of laboratory-associated infections it ranked second in the United States as a cause of laboratory-associated infections [20]. Infection does not confer immunity to reinfection [21]. It is important to point out again, however, that although generally looked at as a zoonotic infection occurring in more suburban and rural parts of the US, well documented urban tularemia infections (including pneumonic disease) have occurred in inner city environments such as New York City and Washington DC.

4.4 Clinical Presentation

The symptoms of tularemia are not unique. The incubation period is typically 3–5 days but may range from 1 to 14 days [1]. There are several different clinical presentations, the most common of which is ulceroglandular disease (45%–80%). In this clinical setting, following the introduction of bacteria percutaneously, such as via entry following the skinning of an infected animal or by the bite of an infected tick, bacterial replication causes the formation of a local ulcer. The bacteria are subsequently transported to regional nodes from which they may disseminate via the hematogenous route to distant sites. The onset of clinical symptoms is sudden. An infected individual will commonly have a fever of 38°C–40°C with nonspecific symptoms of chills, headache, body aches, pharyngitis, cough, and chest pain or tightness. Without treatment, these nonspecific symptoms will persist for weeks or even months, and result in progressive weakness and weight loss. Similar symptomatology may occur in cases of glandular tularemia, in which there is no cutaneous ulcer at the site of inoculation. Another form of tularemia, historically the first to be bacteriologically identified [22], is oculoglandular tularemia, in which direct inoculation of the organism via contaminated hands or via aerosol results in conjunctival involvement and localized lymphadenopathy of the draining lymph nodes [23]. Tularemic pneumonia is the form that is of most importance in the setting of a possible bioterrorism event and is associated with a significant mortality rate. It may have a variety of different radiologic appearances and pleural fluid is often present. Typhoidal tularemia, in which the source of the infection is not clinically apparent, may be complicated by bacteremic spread to lung or by septic shock. Pharyngeal involvement is common when the source of the organism is contaminated water [3–5]. Meningitis, though rare, has been reported [24–26].

A poor outcome in tularemia has been associated with serious underlying disease, the presence of bacteremia, an elevated CK level, and undiagnosed pneumonia [27]. Rhabdomyolysis is seen in some cases of tularemia [28] as is sterile pyuria [27]. The adult respiratory distress syndrome has been described in patients with tularemic pneumonia [29].

4.5 Bioterrorism Presentations and How They may Differ from Natural Disease

The anticipated presentation of tularemia in the setting of a bioterrorism incident is one in which there has been simultaneous exposure of a group of people to an infectious aerosol of *F. tularensis*. As a result, one would anticipate that epidemiologically there is likely to be a common geographical point of exposure, a defined window of time during which the exposure occurred, and that there is the potential for large numbers of people to be infected within one incubation period of the time of exposure (assuming that terrorists use the organism in aerosol form only a single time and not on multiple occasions). On the basis of the experience in the large aerosol outbreak in Sweden [2], it is likely that in addition to pulmonary involvement due to inhalation of the aerosol, there could be significant numbers of cases of oculoglandular and ulceroglandular tularemia. The number of people who will have serologic evidence of infection without clinical disease is uncertain, as one would anticipate that a virulent isolate would be used if it is available to terrorists.

Given the relative ease with which laboratory infections due to *F. tularensis* occur, an individual who presents with tularemia, especially in the absence of a known geographic focus of the disease, should raise a red flag not only as a possible index case for a bioterrorism incident, but also as a possible bioterrorist who was infected during the preparation of *F. tularensis* as a weapon.

4.6 Therapy

Although streptomycin is the drug of choice and has the highest reported cure rate for tularemia of any of the antibiotics with which there is significant experience [30], the possibility of engineered antibiotic-resistance must be considered in the setting of a bioterrorist event. Other antibiotics that have been tried with varying degrees of success have included gentamicin, tetracycline, chloramphenicol, tobramycin, tetracycline, imipenem, and ciprofloxacin [30]. In vitro studies have shown that fluoroquinolones other than ciprofloxacin appear to be active against *F. tularensis*, but clinical experience is even more limited than is the case with ciprofloxacin in the treatment of tularemia.

4.6.1 Preventative Measures (Infection Control, Antimicrobials, Vaccines)

There are limited data on the efficacy of prophylaxis against tularemia with tetracyclines. In a study involving human challenge to *F. tularensis*, 2 g of tetracycline given for 15 days was shown to be effective prophylaxis [31]. Oral doxycycline, which is dosed less frequently than is tetracycline, has been used as prophylaxis in the setting of laboratory exposure [32].

There is no currently available vaccine for the prevention of tularemia in the United States. The live vaccine strain (LVS) is no longer available in the United States. It was descended from strain 15, which was developed by the Soviet Union's Institute of Epidemiology and Microbiology Gamalcia Institute and sold to the US military in 1956 [33]. In the early 1960 s, the LVS strain had been further purified and studied for tularemia prevention in at-risk US military personnel [34, 35]. Efficacy studies in civilian laboratory employees at the military's Fort Detrick facility revealed that the vaccine was safe and significantly reduced the incidence of typhoidal tularemia from 5.70 to 0.27 cases per 1,000 at-risk employee-years [36]. Although the incidence of ulceroglandular tularemia was unchanged by the vaccines, the disease was found to be milder in the vaccine cohort. Worldwide, LVS has since been used as seed stock for tularemia vaccines [35].

Several limitations of the LVS tularemia vaccine have indicated a need to move forward on developing an improved vaccine. One limitation is the current mode of administration, which requires scarification that is both cumbersome and difficult to standardize. Further limitations deal with gaps in understanding the factors responsible for the virulence and genetic stability of *F. tularensis*, as well as which antigens are needed to produce an effective cell-mediated immunity. Apparently, only one of the two phenotypes of LVS, the blue colony type, appears to be immunogenic [34, 35]. Another issue relates to which arm of the immune system should be targeted. Although it has been thought that the humoral immune response is not important in protection against tularemia, a relatively recent report from the Fort Detrick group has suggested that this may not be the case [37]. Pooled sera from humans immunized with LVS were found to fully protect mice against a large lethal challenge of LVS organisms. LVS produced in the United States clearly show immunogenicity in human volunteers, producing both brisk cell-mediated and humoral immune responses [38]. In the future, techniques to optimize the appropriate humoral response may be used.

Strategies for development of a new generation of vaccines include identification of individual components of *F. tularensis*, such as the lipopolysaccharide (LPS) or various outer surface proteins as potential vaccine components (either native or recombinant). After identification, these components would then be used as immunogens, instead of using the entire organism. In laboratory studies, some of these cell components have been tested and found to have variable protection in mice. For instance, one of the membrane proteins of the *F. tularensis* that has been studied as a potential immunogen is a 17-kDa lipoprotein, TUL4. The gene for this antigen has been cloned into a *Salmonella typhimurium* mutant [39]. In mice immunized with this recombinant vector, both humoral and cell-mediated immune response to the antigen developed, and mice were protected from an LVS challenge.

References

1. Dennis DT, Inglesby TV, Henderson DA, et al. Tularemia as a biological weapon: medical and public health management. *JAMA* 2001;285:2763–73.
2. Dahlstrand S, Ringertz O, Zetterberg B. Airborne tularemia in Sweden. *Scand J Infect Dis* 1971;3:7–16.
3. Karpoff SA, Antonoff NI. The spread of tularemia through water, as a new factor in its epidemiology. *J Bacteriol* 1936;32:243–58.
4. Jellison WL, Epler DC, Kuhns E, Kohls GM. Tularemia in man from a domestic rural water supply. *Public Health Rep* 1950;65:1219–26.
5. Mignani E, Palmieri F, Fontana M, Marigo S. Italian epidemic of waterborne tulaeremia. *Lancet* 1988;2:1423.
6. McDowell JW, Scott HG, Stojanovich CJ, Weinburgh HB. *Tularemia.* Atlanta: U.S. Department of Health, Education, and Welfare, Public Health Service, Communicable Disease Center, Training Branch; 1964.
7. Bernard K, Tessier S, Winstanley J, Chang D, Borczyk A. Early recognition of atypical *Francisella tularensis* strains lacking a cysteine requirement. *J Clin Microbiol* 1994;32:551–3.
8. Fredricks DN, Remington JS. Tularemia presenting as community-acquired pneumonia. Implications in the era of managed care. *Arch Intern Med* 1996;156:2137–40.
9. Shapiro DS, Mark EJ. Case records of the Massachusetts General Hospital. Weekly clinicopathological exercises. Case 14-2000. A 60-year-old farm worker with bilateral pneumonia. *N Engl J Med* 2000;342:1430–8.
10. Clarridge JE, 3rd, Raich TJ, Sjosted A, et al. Characterization of two unusual clinically significant *Francisella* strains. *J Clin Microbiol* 1996;34:1995–2000.
11. Centers for Disease Control and Prevention. *Basic protocols for level A laboratories for the presumptive identification of Francisella tularensis.* Centers for Disease Control and Prevention, American Society for Microbiology, Association of Public Health Laboratories; 2001. Location is: http://www.asm.org/ASM/files/LEFTMARGINHEADERLIST/DOWNLOADFILENAME/0000000525/tularemiaprotocol[1].pdf.
12. Alibek K, Handelman S. *Biohazard: the chilling true story of the largest covert biological weapons program in the world, told from the inside by the man who ran it.* 1st edn. New York: Random House; 1999.
13. Johansson A, Berglund L, Eriksson U, et al. Comparative analysis of PCR versus culture for diagnosis of ulceroglandular tularemia. *J Clin Microbiol* 2000;38:22–6.
14. Farlow J, Smith KL, Wong J, Abrams M, Lytle M, Keim P. *Francisella tularensis* strain typing using multiple-locus, variable-number tandem repeat analysis. *J Clin Microbiol* 2001;39:3186–92.
15. de la Puente-Redondo VA, del Blanco NG, Gutierrez-Martin CB, Garcia-Pena FJ, Rodriguez Ferri EF. Comparison of different PCR approaches for typing of *Francisella tularensis* strains. *J Clin Microbiol* 2000;38:1016–22.
16. McCarthy VP, Murphy MD. Lawnmower tularemia. *Pediatr Infect Dis J* 1990;9:298–300.
17. Feldman KA, Enscore RE, Lathrop SL, et al. An outbreak of primary pneumonic tularemia on Martha's Vineyard. *N Engl J Med* 2001;345:1601–6.
18. Weilbacher JO, Moss ES. Tularemia following injury while performing post-mortem examination of a human case. *J Lab Clin Med* 1938;24:34–8.
19. Centers for Disease Control and Prevention. Tularemia – United States, 1990-2000. *Morb Mortal Wkly Rep* 2002;51:181–4.
20. Pike RM. Laboratory-associated infections: summary and analysis of 3921 cases. *Health Lab Sci* 1976;13:105–14.
21. Green TW, Eigelsbach HT. Immunity in tularemia: report of 2 cases of proved reinfection. *Arch Intern Med* 1950;85:777.

22. Wherry WB, Lamb BH. Infection of man with *Bacterium tularense*. *J Infect Dis*. 1914;15:331–40.
23. Hughes WT. Oculoglandular tularemia: transmission from rabbit, through dog and tick to man. *Pediatrics* 1965;36:270–2.
24. Bryant AR, Hirsch EF. Tularemic leptomeningitis. Report of a case. *Arch Pathol*. 1931;12:917–23.
25. Stuart BM, Pullen RL. Tularemic meningitis. Review of the literature and report of a case with postmortem analysis. *Arch Intern Med*. 1945;76:163–6.
26. Rodgers BL, Duffield RP, Taylor T, Jacobs RF, Schutze GE. Tularemic meningitis. *Pediatr Infect Dis J* 1998;17:439–41.
27. Penn RL, Kinasewitz GT. Factors associated with a poor outcome in tularemia. *Arch Intern Med* 1987;147:265–8.
28. Kaiser AB, Rieves D, Price AH, et al. Tularemia and rhabdomyolysis. *JAMA* 1985;253:241–3.
29. Sunderrajan EV, Hutton J, Marienfeld RD. Adult respiratory distress syndrome secondary to tularemia pneumonia. *Arch Intern Med*. 1985;145:1435–7.
30. Enderlin G, Morales L, Jacobs RF, Cross JT. Streptomycin and alternative agents for the treatment of tularemia: review of the literature. *Clin Infect Dis* 1994;19:42–7.
31. Sawyer WD, Dangerfield HG, Hogge AL, Crozier D. Antibiotic prophylaxis and therapy of airborne tularemia. *Bacteriol Rev* 1966;30:542–50.
32. Shapiro DS, Schwartz DR. Exposure of laboratory workers to *Francisella tularensis* despite a bioterrorism procedure. *J Clin Microbiol* 2002;40:2278–81.
33. Tigertt WD. Soviet viable *Pasteurella tularensis* vaccines. *Bacteriol Rev* 1962;26:354–73.
34. Sandstrom G. The tularemia vaccine. *J Chem Tech Biotechnol* 1994;59:315–20.
35. Cieslak T, Christopher GW, Kortepeter MG, et al. Immunization against potential biological warfare agents. *Clin Infect Dis* 2000;30:843–50.
36. Burke DS. Immunization against tularemia: analysis of the effectiveness of live *Francisella tularensis* vaccine in prevention of laboratory-acquired tularemia. *J Infect Dis* 1977;135:55–60.
37. Drabick JJ, Narayanan RB, Williams JC, Leduc JW, Nacy CA. Passive protection of mice against lethal *Francisella tularensis* (live tularemia vaccine strain) infection by the sera of human recipients of the live tularemia vaccine. *Am J Med Sci* 1994;308:83–7.
38. Waag DM, Galloway A, Sandstrom G, et al. Cell-mediated and humoral immune responses induced by scarification vaccination of human volunteers with a new lot of the live vaccine strain of *Francisella tularensis*. *J Clin Microbiol* 1992;30:2256–64.
39. Sjostedt A, Sandstrom G, Tarnvik A. Humoral and cell-mediated immunity in mice to a 17-kilodalton lipoprotein of *Francisella tularensis* expressed by *Salmonella typhimurium*. *Infect Immun* 1992;60:2855–62.

Chapter 5
Botulism

Jeremy Sobel

5.1 Documented Aerosol Exposure Through Laboratory Accident

In the early 1960s, as part of the German biowarfare program [1], laboratory workers exposed rabbits and guinea pigs to aerosolized botulinum toxin type A. The animals were enclosed in hermetically sealed containers during the exposures, and the workers wore "completely protective clothing. [2]" Following the exposures, the animals were transferred to other enclosures, and later, examinations were made by the workers with only protective gloves.

By the third day after the exposures, the workers developed pooling of secretions in the mouth, an influenza-like feeling, and some dysphagia to solids. The next day, increased weakness, difficulties with gait and speech, and oculomotor pareses were noted. All three were treated with botulinum antitoxin. Subsequently, they had slow recoveries and their serum was shown to contain type A toxin in a mouse assay.

5.2 *Clostridium botulinum*

5.2.1 Vegetative Forms

Clostridium botulinum in spore form is ubiquitously found in soil. The species comprises several clostridial organisms that produce seven immunologically distinct toxins, designated by the letters A through G but are not otherwise related [3]. Strains of *C. botulinum* vary according to proteolytic tendency, fermentative abilities, lipase production, and other characteristics. Culturally identical but nontoxigenic organisms exist and are designated as different species, for example, *C. sporogenes* and *C. novyi* [4].

J. Sobel
Foodborne and Diarrheal Diseases Branch, CDC, MS-A38, 1600 Clifton Rd., NE, Atlanta, GA 30333, USA
e-mail: jsobel@cdc.gov

L.I. Lutwick, S.M. Lutwick (eds.), *Beyond Anthrax*,
DOI: 10.1007/978-1-59745-326-4_5, © Springer Science+Business Media, LLC 2008

The species *C. botulinum* is divided into four groups based on culture and serological characteristics. The proteolytic or nonproteolytic character of a strain correlates with the severity of the paralytic syndrome produced by the strain's toxin in humans. Group I consists of all strains of type A (all are proteolytic) and proteolytic strains of types B and F. Group II consists of the nonproteolytic strains of types B and F and all type E strains. Group III includes all strains of types C alpha, C beta, and D. Group IV consists of all type G strains [5].

Rare non-botulinum clostridia produce botulinum toxins and are considered a fifth group. This group consists of *C. baratii* and *C. butyricum* that produce toxins of type F and E, respectively [6–8]. The genes encoding toxin types A, B, E, and F are located on the bacterial chromosome; genes of toxin types C and D are encoded by bacteriophages; and genes of type G are located on a plasmid [5]. All strains of *C. botulinum* are mesophilic, although considerable variation in growth temperatures is observed across groups. The organisms are strongly staining Gram-positive rods, with straight to slightly curved appearance, from 2 to 10 μm in length and 0.5–2 μm in width, with an oval, subterminal spore [4].

5.2.2 The Spore

Under stress, *C. botulinum* forms a spore that is the hardiest and most efficient biological entity in nature, capable of withstanding extreme environmental conditions. The spores can survive for 30 years in liquid medium and are likely capable of withstanding many months in conditions of outer space [4]. Consequently, *C. botulinum* spores can survive standard cooking and food processing measures and remain viable in preserved foods, where, under appropriate conditions, the spores could germinate and toxin production can occur. The technique of modern industrial canning (retort canning) was developed expressly for killing *C. botulinum* spores and is defined as the ability to achieve a 12 log kill of *C. botulinum* spores. This is accomplished by heating to 121°C at 15–20 lb/in.^{2} for at least 20 min [9, 10].

The types of *C. botulinum* are differentially distributed in the environment. Type A is found more commonly in the western United States and type B in the east [11]; in Europe and the Caucus, type B is the most common. These distributions are reflected in the toxin types that cause human disease [12]. Type E is found in aquatic environments (salt, fresh, and estuarine) as reflected in the strong association between human cases caused by toxin type E and foods of marine origin [13]. Toxin types C, D, F, and G are less commonly found in soil, and this may account in part for the rarity of human cases of type F and nearly utter absence of cases caused by types C, D, and G [14].

Conditions in the normal human intestine are not conducive to germination and vegetation of *C. botulinum*. Ubiquitous in soil, *C. botulinum* spores are routinely ingested and excreted by humans without germination, toxin production, or any harm to the person through whom they pass. The exceptions are the small number of infants who develop infant botulism and the handful of adults who develop adult toxemic infectious botulism.

5.2.3 The Toxins

Botulinum toxins are the most potent toxins known to man. The exact lethal dose (LD) is not known, but extrapolations can be made from primate studies. Commonly cited estimated LDs for purified crystalline botulinum toxin type A for a 70 kg man are as follows: 0.09–0.15 μg intravenously, 0.80–0.90 μg by inhalation, and 70 μg orally [15]. Considerably lower figures, however, have been generated by other studies [16, 17] and estimates from human cases [18]. Because a mouse bioassay is the standard for detection and quantification, the toxin is usually expressed in terms of biological activity in terms of mouse intraperitoneal LD_{50} ($MIPLD_{50}$).

The seven toxin types produced by *C. botulinum* are immunologically distinct but produce a clinically similar and highly recognizable syndrome by similar pharmacological mechanisms. The molecular site of action and some clinical features, however, differ. All the toxins are translated as single polypeptide chains of similar structure that are nicked by proteases. The protease nick yields a light chain of approximately 50 kD containing a catalytic subunit (a zinc-dependent metallo-endopeptidase) responsible for the toxic effects and a heavy chain of about 100 kD that binds to the target. Both clostridial proteolytic enzymes and human digestive enzymes such as trypsin can activate the toxin.

The toxins are released from *C. botulinum* in association with two other proteins, a hemagglutinin and a nontoxin, nonhemagglutinin [19]. The complex of the toxin and its covalently bound associated proteins is referred to as the progenitor toxin. These associated proteins, however, neither play a role in the symptoms of botulism nor are needed for binding or penetration.

All toxin types exert their action on the cholinergic system at the presynaptic motor-neuron terminal by blocking acetylcholine transmission across the neuromuscular junction [5, 14, 20, 21]. Toxins types A and E enzymatically cleave a specific presynaptic membrane-associated protein; toxin types B, D, F, and G cleave a synaptic vesicle-associated protein. Type C toxin cleaves both the membrane-associated protein targeted by types A and E and an additional protein associated with exocytosis. The effect in all cases is neuromuscular blockade resulting in flaccid paralysis. The toxins also affect the adrenergic system but apparently with insignificant consequences.

Toxin type A causes most cases of foodborne and wound botulism in the United States. The syndrome produced by toxin type A is most severe, with more rapid progression of paralysis and a higher proportion of patients requiring mechanical ventilation [22]. This may be the toxin type weaponized by Iraq, and before the 1972 treaty, the United States [23]. Type B is the predominant cause of illness in Europe. Both proteolytic and nonproteolytic forms of *C. botulinum* type B appear to cause milder disease than type A. Only two cases of human illness from toxin type C [24, 25] and one outbreak caused by toxin type D [26] have been reported. The reasons for the rarity of cases of these types are not understood. Small-scale animal experiments have established that primates are susceptible to ingested toxin type C and D [27]. Massive outbreaks of type C botulism in birds occur periodically [28], particularly in the Salton Sea area of southwest America, which is rich in *C. botulinum* type C [29].

Type E toxin, associated exclusively with foodborne botulism from aquatic-origin foods in man, produces a syndrome of variable severity [13]. This may reflect the differing effects of proteolytic and nonproteolytic strain toxins and how well trypsin activation of the toxin from some strains in the human gastrointestinal tract occurs [14]. Massive outbreaks of fish botulism from type E toxin in the Great Lakes region of the United States are well described, and in recent years they have been associated with large avian outbreaks as well [30, 31]. To date, however, no human cases have been associated with these animal die-offs. Although no human type G case has been reported, there is no pharmacological reason that would prevent it from causing botulism in man.

Botulinum toxins are variably sensitive to temperature, depending on toxin type and the matrix in which the toxin is located (e.g., the food), but all will be inactivated by heating to 85°C for 5 min [10]. Irradiation can destroy toxin, but this method is impractical for food treatment, as the required level would so alter the organoleptic characteristics of most foods to the point of unpalatability [4]. Little published information exists on the decay of botulinum toxin in the environment; thus it is difficult to predict exactly what risk might be posed by environmental exposure following aerosolized toxin release. It has been estimated that, under most atmospheric conditions, weaponized botulinum toxin would be inactivated at the rate of about 1–4% per hour, and would be inactivated completely within 48 h [32], although these estimates must be regarded as speculative. Similarly, it has been postulated that once settled onto surfaces, weaponized botulinum toxin is unlikely to re-aerosolize, but given the absence of published data, this too must be regarded as a guess. It is worth remembering that in the early stages of the investigation of the terroristic anthrax mailings in 2001, the possibility of re-aerosolization of the finely milled anthrax spores in contaminated buildings was dismissed, a supposition subsequently disproved. In laboratory settings, denaturation of toxin by treatment of surfaces with alkali solutions such as 0.1 M potassium hydroxide for 20 min is effective [10].

5.3 Modes of Transmission

Based on the setting for the introduction of *C. botulinum* or its toxin, four naturally occurring syndromes of botulism exist: foodborne, wound, infant, and adult intestinal toxemia. A fifth syndrome, inhalational botulism, does not occur naturally but could be produced by aerosolization of botulinum toxin by terrorists or in a battlefield setting. The viability of aerosolized toxin transmission has been documented in one laboratory accident involving three humans [1, 2] and in primate studies [33]. All clinical syndromes result from toxin uptake into circulation and subsequent binding at the neuromuscular junction, and therefore the clinical illness in each syndrome is essentially identical.

5.4 Diagnosis

5.4.1 Clinical Presentation

The clinical syndrome of botulism is highly distinctive, consisting of symmetrical cranial nerve palsies followed by symmetrical descending flaccid paralysis that may progress to respiratory arrest [11, 22]. For a sporadic (isolated) case, the differential diagnosis is short and the combination of neurological findings and common laboratory tests provide highly sensitive clinical diagnosis pending laboratory confirmation [15]. A cluster of two or more cases with compatible symptoms is essentially pathognomonic since the illnesses that resemble botulism do not produce outbreaks. The diagnosis in sporadic cases and even in small outbreaks is frequently missed, however, because botulism is a rare disease with which most clinicians are unfamiliar [34].

Every case of botulism is a public health emergency, and immediately upon suspecting the diagnosis, the clinician should report the suspected case to the 24-h emergency telephone number of the state health department [35]. The state health department will initiate an epidemiological investigation, and at the same time, will put the physician in contact with the 24-h botulism consultancy service of the Center for Disease Control and Prevention (CDC). The on-call CDC consultant will review the case with the clinician telephonically, and if indicated, will help arrange for laboratory confirmation by testing appropriate specimens either at the state public health laboratory or at CDC and for shipment of antitoxin, which in the United States is available exclusively from the CDC [10]. The state health departments of California and Alaska maintain their own botulism clinical consultation services.

The incubation period from exposure to onset of symptoms is best established for foodborne botulism. The median time from ingestion of toxin to first symptoms is 18–36 h, but has occurred as early as 6 h and as late as 8 days following ingestion. Primate experiments suggest that the incubation period following inhalation of aerosolized toxin would be similar [33].

Cranial nerve palsies are invariably the presenting symptoms of botulism. Their absence, or onset after other true neurological symptoms have made their appearance, almost entirely rules out the disease. Extraocular muscle paralysis is due to paralysis of cranial nerves III, IV, and VI and manifests as blurry vision or frank diplopia and the inability to accommodate near vision. Paralysis of cranial nerve VII produces expressionless facies, and dysphagia is caused by cranial nerve IX paralysis that may present as regurgitation, at times nasal, of masticated food or beverages. Dysarthria is prominent. In some cases, pharyngeal collapse secondary to cranial nerve paralysis may compromise the airway and require intubation in the absence of the failure of respiratory muscles.

Prominent autonomic symptoms include ptosis, dilated and fixed pupils, anhydrosis, which often manifests with pronounced mucosal erythema and pain and has been mistaken for pharyngitis, and postural hypotension. Rare cases of autonomic dysfunction as the most prominent symptom of botulism have been described [36].

In foodborne botulism, particularly of types B and E, gastrointestinal symptoms of nausea and vomiting may precede neurological symptoms. It is unknown if these are caused by direct action of botulinum toxin, other products of *C. botulinum*, or some other contaminant of spoiled food. These symptoms have never been reported in wound botulism [37] nor have corresponding signs been observed in primate experiments in which pure toxin was administered intragastrically or intravenously [16, 27, 33, 38–40]. Therefore, these symptoms may be absent in illness resulting from consumption of food deliberately contaminated with pure toxin.

Following manifestation of cranial nerve palsies, flaccid, descending, completely symmetric paralysis of voluntary muscles may occur, affecting in order the muscles of the neck, shoulders, and proximal and then distal upper extremities, followed by proximal-to-distal paresis of the lower extremities. Paralysis of the diaphragm and accessory breathing muscles results in respiratory compromise or arrest. Constipation is nearly universal.

Vital signs are usually normal, with preservation of normal-range blood pressure possibly manifesting in consequence of an equilibrium between vagal blockade and extensive peripheral vasodilatation, both caused by the toxin, but in some cases hypotension occurs. Deep tendon reflexes progressively disappear.

The ultimate extent of paralysis in untreated patients, and the rapidity of progression, are variable. Symptoms may be limited to a few cranial nerves or may progress to complete paralysis of all voluntary muscle paralysis. Symptoms may progress over hours to days, with the rate apparently proportional to dose. Toxin binding is noncompetitive and irreversible. Nerve terminals do regenerate slowly, allowing for eventual full recovery in 95% of cases in the United States. Paralysis resolves in weeks to months and often requires extended outpatient rehabilitation therapy.

The sensory system is unaffected. In some cases, sensory symptoms, principally parasthesias, have been reported (CDC, unpublished data); these may represent skin irritation from secondary immobility to paralysis. Intellectual function is preserved throughout. Patients are able to respond appropriately to all questions. Once intubated, they can continue communicating by signal using fingers or toes, so long as paralysis has not affected the digits. Tragically, in some instances the patient's ptosis, expressionless facies, and altered voice have been interpreted as signs of mental status changes from alcohol intoxication, recreational drug overdose, encephalitis, or meningitis; critical components of the history including potential sources of toxin were not sought by questioning. Because of skeletal muscle paralysis, patients experiencing respiratory distress do not present signs of agitation such as restlessness, tossing, gasping, thrashing, or flailing, and may appear placid and detached even as they near respiratory arrest. Death in untreated botulism patients is due to airway obstruction from pharyngeal muscle paralysis and inadequate tidal volume resulting from paralysis of diaphragmatic and accessory respiratory muscles.

Standard blood work and radiological studies are not useful in diagnosing botulism. On lumbar puncture, cerebrospinal fluid (CSF) values are normal, in particular the protein level, in contrast to Guillain-Barre Syndrome (see below). Brain imaging may help rule out rare stroke syndromes that produce non-lateralizing symptoms. The Tensilon test helps diagnose myasthenia gravis. In experienced hands, electromyography can be an exceedingly helpful adjunct to diagnosis. In affected muscles, findings consistent with neuromuscular junction blockage, normal axonal conduction, and potentiation with rapid repetitive stimulation are indicative of botulism [41].

In the setting of an outbreak, where several or many persons present with the signs and symptoms of botulism, the diagnosis readily suggests itself. The situation for the lone, or sporadic, botulism patient (who may, in fact, be but the first case in a larger outbreak) is more precarious because of general unfamiliarity with the syndrome. However, if the diagnosis is considered, the clinician should immediately call the state health department emergency number, and free expert consultation will be provided within minutes over the phone [35]. The differential diagnosis includes the diseases listed in Table 5.1.

Table 5.1 Partial differential diagnosis of botulism

Disease	Comment
Guillain-Barre syndrome (GBS)	Often occurs after acute infection; 95% of cases ascending, not descending [42], only occurs as sporadic (lone) cases, not clusters
Miller Fischer variant of GBS	5% of GBS is descending [43, 44]; only occurs as sporadic (lone) cases, not clusters
Myaesthenia gravis	Positive tensilon test, only occurs as sporadic (lone) cases, not clusters
Cerebrovascular accident	Asymmetry of paralysis; upper motor neuron signs; positive brain imaging studies; only occurs as sporadic (lone) cases, not clusters
Eaton Lambert syndrome	Proximal limb weakness; patient usually known to have cancer, only occurs as sporadic (lone) cases, not clusters
Tick paralysis	Feeding gravid female tick found on body; removal usually results in rapid resolution [45]; only occurs as sporadic (lone) cases, not clusters

Clusters of cases are overwhelmingly likely to be botulism

5.4.2 Epidemiology

5.4.2.1 Foodborne Botulism

Foodborne disease is caused by consumption of foods contaminated with botulinum toxin. Although spores of *C. botulinum* are ubiquitous in the environment [14], growth and elaboration of toxin occur rarely, only when the food presents conditions that include an anaerobic milieu, pH $<$ 4.5, low salt and sugar content, and temperatures above 4°C and below 121°C [46]. Heating contaminated food to 85°C for at least 5 min destroys the toxin, and spores are inactivated by heating to 121°C at 15–20 lb/in.^{2} for at least 20 min [10].

Canning and fermentation of foods are particularly conducive to the creation of anaerobic conditions that may allow the germination of *C. botulinum* spores. Commercially canned foods caused outbreaks in the nineteenth and the early twentieth centuries before standard methods for inactivating *C. botulinum* spores in cans were perfected [9]. Early in the twentieth century, the proportion of botulism outbreaks caused by commercially produced contaminated foods declined, and improperly made home-canned foods have long constituted a major source of intoxication in the continental United States [11, 47]. Since the 1970s, restaurant-associated botulism outbreaks may account for a large proportion of U.S. cases [48]. Traditional Alaskan native dishes, especially fermented foods like fish and fish eggs, seal, beaver, and whale, also pose a significant risk and account for the high incidence of botulism in Alaska [49]. These foods are prepared by allowing the products to putrefy at ambient temperatures and are often consumed without cooking.

In the United States during 1990–2000, the median number of cases per year was 23 (range 17–43) yielding an annual incidence of 0.1 per million. Most botulism cases are sporadic (not part of outbreaks); outbreaks are typically small, involving two or three persons. The largest outbreak in U.S. history included 55 cases. The highest incidence rates were in Alaska, Idaho, and Washington. During 1990–2000, 50% of cases were caused by toxin type A, 10% by toxin type B, 37% by toxin type E, and <1% by type F. The average age of patients was 44–50, and gender distribution was approximately even.

Outside Alaska, a food was implicated by laboratory detection of toxin or epidemiological investigation without laboratory confirmation in 77 (76%) events, of which 68 (67%) were caused by homemade foods, and of these, 47 (69%) were home canned. Of the nine events caused by non-homemade foods, five, affecting 10 people, were caused by commercial foods, and two, affecting 25 people, were caused by restaurant-prepared foods. In Alaska, all cases during this period were caused by Alaskan native foods such as fermented whale, beaver, or seal [50].

Obtaining a 3- to 5-day food history from the patient, with focused questions about home-canned foods or exotic or unusual foods prepared by fermentation, smoking, or other atypical methods, can specifically further the suspicion of foodborne botulism. A history of home-canned food consumption within the incubation period in a patient with compatible history and findings substantially enhances its probability. Close contacts who may have shared foods should also be noted. It is important that the clinician solicit this information early because if, despite supportive and specific therapy, the patient progresses to respiratory failure and mechanical ventilation, eliciting further information will be compromised.

Control of foodborne botulism outbreaks rests on early diagnosis of cases by clinicians, immediate reporting to public health authorities, rapid epidemiological investigation to identify the contaminated food(s) and their removal from circulation, and warning the public.

5.4.2.2 Wound Botulism

This form of the disease is caused by contamination of a wound with *C. botulinum* spores from the environment and their subsequent germination with production of toxin in the anaerobic milieu of a focal infection. The condition was first reported in 1943 and for several decades was usually associated with traumatic wounds. The condition was exceedingly rare until the early 1990s; since that time, the western United States has experienced a dramatic and continuing increase in incidence, virtually exclusively in injection drug users [36]. Almost all injection-drug-associated cases are users of so-called black tar heroin, a specific preparation of heroin, and they "skin-pop," that is, inject the black tar heroin into tissues, as opposed to veins [51]. The typical patient is an adult in the fourth or fifth decade of life with a long history of black tar heroin injection and residing in the western United States.

The incubation period is hard to establish as most patients inject several times daily. The clinical syndrome is indistinguishable from that of foodborne botulism. Quite often, the site of toxin production is a minor lesion, at times no more than a small furuncle or resembling mild cellulitis. Whenever possible, necrotic areas or abscesses should be cleaned and debrided, tissue material collected in anaerobic culture tubes for testing at public health laboratories, and appropriate antimicrobial therapy provided.

For the clinician, ascertaining a history of injection drug use, particularly of black tar heroin, is crucial; in combination with compatible presentation, it is highly predictive. As always, the case should be immediately reported to the state public health department.

5.4.2.3 Infant Botulism

Infant botulism results from absorption of toxin produced in situ by *C. botulinum* colonization of the intestine of certain infants less than 1 year of age [52]. This is the most common form of botulism, with about 80–100 cases reported annually in the United States [11]. Colonization is believed to occur because normal bowel flora that could compete with *C. botulinum* has not been fully established, a theory supported by animal studies. Studies have implicated honey consumption as a risk factor for illness, but honey consumption only accounts for up to 20% of cases [53]. For reasons unknown, the highest incidence is found in the vicinity of Philadelphia [54]. The clinical presentation resembles that of adult forms of the disease, with common symptoms including inability to suck and swallow, weakened voice, ptosis, and floppy neck, which may progress to generalized flaccidity and respiratory compromise [55]. Specific therapy for infant botulism is a newly licensed human-source antitoxin that halves the median hospitalization period from 6 to 3 weeks; with appropriate intensive care, survival is nearly 100% with or without antitoxin therapy [52].

5.4.2.4 Adult Intestinal Toxemia Botulism

Adult intestinal toxemia botulism is the consequence of absorption of toxin produced in situ by the rarely occurring intestinal colonization in a few adults by toxigenic clostridia. Typically, patients have some anatomical or functional bowel abnormality, which is postulated to permit normally fastidious clostridia protection from competition with normal bowel flora [7, 56–59]. Protracted symptoms and relapse in the face of antitoxin treatment due to ongoing intralumenal production of toxin may be observed. Diagnosis in a patient with sporadic botulism and no known food or wound source rests on demonstrating protracted excretion of organisms and toxin in the stool.

5.4.3 Laboratory Diagnosis and Confirmation

Confirmation of botulism rests on demonstration of the toxin in patient serum, gastric secretions, or stool or in a food sample [10]. Demonstration of *C. botulinum* in a patient's stool or in cultures of wound material is generally satisfactory for diagnosis of adult botulism syndromes and is considered definitive in infant botulism. Demonstration of toxin is by means of a bioassay involving intraperitoneal injection of toxin into mice and observing the development of botulism-specific symptoms. This remains the most sensitive test for the toxin and can detect concentrations on the order of 1 $MIPLD_{50}$/mL.

Toxin type is determined by injecting a panel of mice with mixtures of test sample and a monoclonal type-specific antitoxin (e.g., anti-A, anti-B, etc.) and observing which antitoxin confers protection on the mice. The mouse bioassay is carried out in a limited number of public health laboratories. From the time mice are injected, final results may not be available for 24 h or even 48 h. Accordingly, all clinical management decisions and initial public health interventions are determined solely on the basis of clinical diagnosis. Various enzyme-linked immunoabsorbent assays (ELISAs) for botulinum toxin are currently in advanced stages of validation. A micromechanosensor for botulism toxin type B has been described [60]. Although not as sensitive as the standard mouse assay, this assay allows toxin identification within minutes.

Clinical samples for suspected cases of foodborne botulism include serum; vomitus, or gastric secretions; stool; and suspect foods in original containers. For suspect wound botulism cases, samples include 10 mL of serum and anaerobic wound material; for infant botulism, stool is the preferred material [10]. The overall sensitivity of laboratory testing of clinical specimens has been reported as low as 33–44% [61, 62] but varies inversely with the time elapsed between symptom onset and sample collection. Accordingly, when syndromes other than infant botulism are suspected, serum (at least one 10 mL red top serum tube, spun and separated) should be drawn immediately and always before antitoxin administration. The antitoxin will neutralize all circulating toxin and render the test meaningless. If possible, the earliest available serum such as that from admission blood work should be salvaged and preserved for testing. Vomitus should be collected, and if a nasogastric tube is placed, gastric secretions should be collected immediately. Since constipation is the rule, stool should be collected by means of a sterile water enema. These samples should be kept refrigerated, but not frozen, pending shipping directions from public health officials. In general, ingested toxin is not demonstrable in serum more than a week after exposure, although exceptions have been reported. Toxin can be isolated from stool further in the course of illness, and the toxin is stable in many food matrices for considerably longer time. In the setting of a large outbreak, laboratory confirmation of every case would be unnecessary.

No standard protocols exist for diagnosis of botulism post mortem, but hepatic sections and stool should be collected and refrigerated. No standard protocols exist for environmental testing in case of suspected aerosolized release; nasal and surface swabs may be collected for experimental purposes if recommended by public health officials.

5.4.4 Botulism as a Biowarfare Event

5.4.4.1 The Threat

Governmental military programs, including those of the former Soviet Union, Nazi Germany, imperial Japan, and the United States [32], have extensively weaponized botulinum toxin. In violation of the 1972 Biological and Toxin Weapons Convention, the Soviet Union and Iraq continued large-scale production of botulinum toxin for offensive warfare purposes [15]. Reportedly, Soviet scientists attempted splicing the *C. botulinum* toxin gene into other bacterial species [63]. Before the Persian Gulf War of 1991, thousands of liters of concentrated botulinum toxin, according to the United Nations inspection team reports, were loaded by Iraq into munitions, including long-range missiles and bombs. Several thousand liters of concentrated botulinum toxin from the Iraqi program have never been accounted for [64]. Iran, Syria, and North Korea are believed to be developing or to have developed botulinum toxin as a weapon [65, 66].

What information that has been published regarding inhalation of anthrax in humans is summarized in the first scenario. In a small report in primates, within 12–18 h after exposure, mild motor weakness and extraocular muscle dysfunction were observed followed by more weakness and difficulty in breathing. Death occurred in some of the nine exposed primates between 2 and 4 days after exposure [33]. In an in vitro model for toxin inhalation [67], the nontoxic heavy chain of the toxin was shown to be specifically bound and transported, in an energy-dependent way, across rat primary alveolar epithelial cells.

Aum Shinrikyo, the Japanese cult whose members released sarin nerve gas in Tokyo subways in 1995, unsuccessfully attempted aerosolized release of botulinum toxin in downtown Tokyo and against U.S. military installations in Japan in 1990 and 1995 [68, 69]. The episode underscores the relative ease of producing toxin and potential technical difficulties to aerosolized dissemination. These difficulties have led some military analysts to downgrade the risk from botulinum toxin. These represent military concerns related to battlefield deployment of aerosolized toxin over many square kilometers by spraying from an airplane or dispersion by bombs [23]. However, what would constitute a militarily "ineffective" casualty rate, either by aerosolization or by contamination of food or water, could be attractive to terrorists. For example, while a military analyst may consider a 10% casualty rate at a range of 0.5 km from weaponized botulinum toxin militarily ineffective, this figure in a crowded urban population would be catastrophic [15].

While contamination of foods or beverages with botulinum toxin is not an important concern on the military battlefield, this mode of dissemination may serve a terrorist's aims of terrorizing a civilian population, decreasing confidence in the government's ability to protect the food supply, and perpetrating economic losses. Depending on a perpetrator's resources and intentions, deliberate food contamination could take any form, from small-scale tampering (which could still create considerable public anxiety and challenge the public health system) to a sophisticated contamination of a mass-produced, widely distributed food item resulting in mass casualties. Furthermore, as the anthrax mailings of 2001 demonstrated, a technically sophisticated terrorist may deploy a biological or chemical agent in novel ways, and modes of dispersion other than aerosolization and food or beverage contamination could be attempted [70].

There have been no known cases of botulism occurring related to a water supply contamination with botulinum toxin, naturally or criminally. This is unlikely to occur because the toxin is inactivated by standard water treatment methodology and, since the turnover of water in a reservoir is quite slow, very large quantities of toxin would be needed.

5.4.4.2 The Potential Role of Commercial Botulinum Toxin

Commercially available purified botulinum toxin A has been used at low dosage for the treatment of strabismus, dystonia, and other disorders of muscle spasticity, focal hyperhidrosis, and as an antiwrinkle therapy. Using single-fiber electromyography, local injections of recommended dosages of toxin have been found to have measurable effects in muscles distant from the treatment [71]. Although these measurable effects do not generally have clinical manifestations, generalized muscular weakness and even respiratory arrest have been reported with usual dosing [72–74]. A cluster of botulism with respiratory failure was reported in late 2004 involving four individuals [75]. The source of the toxin administered was thought to be an illicit one of much higher potency.

5.4.4.3 Recognizing the Intentional Nature of an Outbreak of Botulism

An outbreak of botulism due to deliberate dissemination of toxin can initially resemble an unintentional outbreak of foodborne botulism and may be detected by the public, astute clinicians, or local public health officials. Current surveillance practices typically result in rapid reporting of diagnosed cases to the public health system [70]. While epidemiological features alone cannot prove a terrorist event, deviation from established patterns of disease manifest in unusual relationships between patient, exposure vehicle, and toxin can provide clues of an unnatural event [76].

Given the rarity of botulism and the small size of unintentional outbreaks (median in the previous decade, one case; largest recorded, 55), even a small outbreak would be considered unusual. Any outbreak in which no common food exposure is apparent would raise the possibility of dissemination by aerosol or some other means. Epidemiological features consistent with aerosol dissemination may include victims' being in a common location such as a building or public area, attending an event, and especially exposure to a common ventilation system [15]. Unusual epidemiological features of a foodborne botulism outbreak might include implication of a commercial food, which is rare compared with home-canned or Alaskan native foods. Illness with toxin type E has been associated exclusively with aquatic foods [9]; illness from a non-aquatic source would be highly unusual. Individual cases or outbreaks caused by more than one toxin type are extraordinarily rare [77]; human cases caused by toxin types D, or G are unknown, and those of type F or C are very rare [10]. This said, new food vehicles and even toxin types are reported over time, and an unintentional foodborne botulism outbreak may have very unusual features, while a terroristic one may have natural ones; only a detailed investigation by epidemiologists, food safety regulators, and law enforcement can prove intentional contamination.

5.4.4.4 Responding to an Outbreak of Botulism of Intentional Origin

The public health response to a botulism event consists of two components. One is the epidemiological investigation to identify the agent and contaminated food and implement control measures. Public health agencies and their counterparts in food safety regulatory agencies address these tasks routinely in response to naturally arising foodborne disease outbreaks of assorted pathogens [70, 78, 79]. The second component is the medical response to casualties. Depending on the number of casualties, medical supplies and personnel might need to be transported rapidly to the outbreak site(s); alternatively, large numbers of patients might need to be evacuated. The complexity of the logistics involved requires integrated action by local, state, and federal agencies [70]. The objective of the epidemiological investigation of an outbreak would be confirmation of the toxin type(s), mode and vehicle of transmission, and manner of contamination, followed by timely implementation of control measures including, in the case of contaminated food, removal from circulation, and proper treatment of exposed people.

Resources and protocols for the medical response component, including rapid transport of medical supplies and personnel or patient evacuation, have been described [80]. Stocks of antitoxin, ventilators, and other supplies are maintained in stockpiles, and reserves of medical personnel must be available for immediate deployment to casualty locations. A contamination event that targets a food or foods distributed over a wide geographical area could challenge the assurance of adequate medical supplies and personnel in far-flung locations.

The central challenges to the medical response in a botulism event involving many casualties will be the requirement for immediate provision of intensive care–level treatment and mechanical ventilation [15]. Excess capacity beyond that available in hospitals might be required, including physical facilities, ventilators, and ancillary equipment. Appropriately trained nursing and medical staff would need to be available immediately and would need to remain dedicated to the care of victims for many weeks.

Respiratory compromise in botulism is due to muscular paralysis; alveolar gas exchange is unaffected. Therefore, the ventilatory requirement of the botulism patient in respiratory compromise can be met with small, portable, inexpensive ventilators using compressed air (not oxygen). Emergency response planners at all levels, and hospital emergency directors, should consider integrating such devices into their plans.

The government's ability to transport large amounts of antitoxin to the location(s) of victims and the capacity of the emergency medical infrastructure on site to evaluate and triage patients and administer the antitoxin will critically affect the need for ventilators, because early treatment may avert respiratory compromise in many cases.

5.5 Therapeutic Interventions

5.5.1 Supportive Intensive Care

During the first decades of the twentieth century in the United States, mortality among botulism patients was 60–70% even when equine antitoxin was administered in heroic doses. During the late 1940s and 1950s, mortality dropped precipitously, until it reached its current rate of 3–5% [47]. The difference is due largely to the development of modern intensive care techniques, principally mechanical ventilation. Persons with suspected botulism should be placed immediately in an intensive care setting, with frequent monitoring of vital capacity and institution of mechanical ventilation if required. Paralysis from botulism is protracted, lasting weeks to months, and meticulous intensive care is required during this period of debilitation.

5.5.2 *Antitoxin Therapy*

The only specific treatment for botulism is administration of botulinum antitoxin. Antitoxin can arrest the progression of paralysis or decrease the duration of paralysis and dependence on mechanical ventilation. Antitoxin should be given early in the course of illness, ideally within less than 24 h of symptom onset [81], because antitoxin neutralizes only toxin molecules yet unbound to nerve endings. Animal experiments confirm this relationship [16, 17, 33, 40]. Use of this equine-derived antitoxin is associated with side effects, including anaphylaxis, other hypersensitivity reactions, and serum sickness. Approximately 9% of persons treated in previous decades experienced hypersensitivity reactions [82], at a time that the recommended antitoxin dose was two- to fourfold higher than at present.

Of patients who were treated with one vial of antitoxin in the past few years, <1% experienced serious reactions. Before administration of antitoxin, skin testing should be performed to test for sensitivity to serum or antitoxin, a procedure that may be difficult in a massive outbreak with many casualties. With a positive skin test, desensitization protocols can be used for a nonmass casualty setting. Administration of one vial of botulism antitoxin produces serum levels of toxin-type-specific antibodies capable of neutralizing serum toxin concentrations many fold in excess of those reported for botulism patients [83].

Botulinum antitoxin is toxin-type specific, that is, antitoxin to toxin type A will only be effective for patients intoxicated by toxin type A, and so on. It is therefore critical to establish the toxin type(s) (A–G) involved in a bioterrorism event and to treat with the appropriate antitoxin(s). Both licensed (trivalent – A, B, and E) and IND-status preparations of equine-source and human-source botulinum antitoxin are in the possession of the U.S. Government. Antitoxin preparations currently not licensed can be used for patient treatment in a bioterrorist event under an emergency-use IND protocol [15]. An equine heptavalent antitoxin has been evaluated in which the Fc fragments have been removed ("despeciated"), leaving only F(ab)2 fragments [84].

Given the high predictive value of objectively noted symmetric cranial nerve palsies in previously healthy patients in the setting of a mass outbreak, all such patients should be diagnosed with probable botulism. Exposed persons should be observed closely, and if they develop symptoms compatible with botulism, they should be treated with antitoxin immediately.

Monoclonal antibodies have been produced against botulism toxin. A combination of three recombinant monoclonals (oligocolonal antibodies) had a 90 times greater potency than a hyperimmune globulin [85]. The effect was due to a large increase in functional antibody binding affinity.

5.6 Preventative Measures

5.6.1 Isolation and Infection Control

Standard precautions should be exercised when evaluating and treating patients. Botulinum toxin cannot be absorbed through intact skin but can be absorbed through mucosal surfaces, the eye, or non-intact skin. No case of person-to-person transmission of botulinum has ever been described, including in patient-care settings. Nevertheless, persons exposed to bodily fluids or stool of botulinum patients should be advised of the early signs of botulism and should report for evaluation if these are noted. Objects contaminated with toxin should be treated with 0.1 M sodium hydroxide [10].

5.6.2 Prophylactic Treatment

Persons who were exposed to botulinum toxin should be evaluated by a physician and carefully observed for the development of symptoms of botulism. If symptoms appear, the patient should be treated immediately with botulinum antitoxin.

5.6.3 Immunization

No licensed vaccine is currently available for botulism. An experimental toxoid (deactivated toxin vaccine) providing some immunity against toxin types A, B, C, D, and E is available from CDC for laboratorians working with botulinum toxin. The toxoid is administered by primary series of deep subcutaneous injections at 0, 2, and 12 weeks, a booster is given at 6 months, and repeated titer testing and frequent booster shots are required to maintain immunity. The vaccine has mild reactogenicity with some local reactions in 2–4% of primary injections and as much as 20% of booster injections. Because of the duration of the primary series and the need for titer determinations and boosters, this vaccine is not deemed a useful public health tool either in an acute event or for preparedness purposes.

Current potential, next-generation botulism vaccines utilize a number of modern technological advances. These methods include cloning the toxin's nontoxic heavy chain into an attenuated *Salmonella enterica* var. Typhimurium strain [86], a Venezuelan equine encephalitis replicon particle [87], or the methyltropic yeast *Pichia pastoris* [88]. Either the supernatant of the yeast culture or the vector in the first two methods produced protection against type-specific botulism toxin in the murine model. Botulinum toxin heavy chain administered intranasally also demonstrated protection against botulism in the mouse model [66].

5.7 Preparedness and Research Agenda

The rarity of botulism, thanks to food safety standards, has provided little impetus to advance standard diagnosis and treatment modalities beyond those of the early twentieth century – equine antitoxin and the mouse bioassay. Accordingly, preparedness entails optimizing the effectiveness of available technology for emergency response while vigorously developing improved therapeutics and diagnostics.

Preparedness and research priorities are shown in Table 5.2

Table 5.2 Preparedness and research botulism priorities

Preparedness priorities
Educate all emergency care and primary care healthcare providers about the signs and symptoms of botulism, and the need to contact public health authorities immediately if a case is suspected
Assure that emergency contacts for public health authorities are available at all emergency and primary care medical facilities
Enhance the capacity of local and state health departments to conduct outbreak investigations, most effectively by hiring and training appropriate staff
Address at the local level the options for substantially increased ventilator capacity. Identify facilities, trained personnel, ventilators and other equipment, and outside resources
Formalize and thoroughly drill the integration of federal, state, and local bioterrorism and emergency medical plans. Include hospitals and local care givers in planning and exercises to identify and close gaps when responsibility and material are transferred from one organization to another
Research priorities
Investigate the effectiveness of currently available adjunct therapies, including guanidine, activated charcoal, enemas, emetics, cathartics, and intralumenal intestinal toxin binding agents
Establish the effectiveness of alternatives to equine antitoxin therapy, including monoclonal and transgenic antitoxins (ongoing)
Develop and test the efficacy of new vaccines
Develop, validate, and license highly sensitive and specific rapid assays for detection of toxin in clinical specimens and foods
Develop, validate, and license highly sensitive and specific environmental monitors for botulinum toxins

References

1. Holzer, V. E. Botulismus durch inhalation. *Med. Klin.* 41, 1735–1738, 1962.
2. Middlebrook, J.L. and Franz, D.R. Botulinum toxins, in *Medical Aspects of Chemical and Biological Warfare*, Sidell, F.R., Takafuji, E.T., Franz, D.R., (eds.), 1997, Borden Institute, Walter Reed Army Medical Center: Washington, DC. p. 643–654.
3. Hatheway, C.L. Toxigenic clostridia. *Clin. Microbiol. Rev.* 3, 66–98, 1990.
4. Smith, L.D. *Botulism: The Organism, its Toxins, the Disease*. The Bannerstone Division of American Lectures in Clinical Microbiology, ed. Balows. A. 1977, Charles C Thomas: Springfiled.
5. Hatheway, C.L. *Clostridium botulinum* and other clostridia that produce botulinum neurotoxin, in *Clostridium botulinum. Ecology and Control in Foods*, Hauschild, A.H.S., Dodds, K.L., (eds.), 1992. Marcel Dekker, Inc.: New York, Basel, Hong Kong. p. 3–20.
6. Aureli, P., Di Cunto, M., Maffei, A., et al. An outbreak in Italy of botulism associated with a dessert made with mascarpone cream cheese. *Eur. J. Epidemiol.* 16, 913–918, 2000.
7. McCroskey, L., Hatheway, C.L., Woodruff, B.A., et al. Type F botulism due to neurotoxigenic *Clostridium baratii* from an unknown source in an adult. *J. Clin. Microbiol.* 29, 2618–2620, 1991.
8. Gupta, A., Sumner, C., Castor, M., et al. Adult botulism type F in the United States, 1981–2002. Interagency Botulism Research Coordinating Committee Conference (IBRCC): Atlanta, GA 2003.
9. Meyer, K. The protective measures of the state of California against botulism. *J. Prev. Med.* 5, 261–293, 1931.
10. Centers for Disease Control and Prevention. Botulism in the United States, 1899–1996, handbook for epidemiologists, clinicians and laboratory workers. Centers for Disease Control and Prevention: Atlanta, GA, 1998.
11. Shapiro, R., Hatheway, C., and Swerdlow, D.L. Botulism in the United States: a clinical and epidemiologic review. *Ann. Intern. Med.* 129, 221–228, 1998.
12. Meyer, K. The status of botulism as a world health problem. *Bull. World Health Org.* 15, 281–298, 1956.
13. Dolman, C.E. and Iida, H. Type E botulism: its epidemiology, prevention and specific treatment. *Can. J. Public Health* 54, 293–308, 1963.
14. Hauschild, A.H. *Clostridium botulinum*, in *Foodborne bacterial pathogens*, Doyle, M., Editor. 1989, Marcel Dekker: New York. p. 112–189.
15. Arnon, S.S., Schechter, R., Inglesby, T.V., et al. Botulism toxin as a biological weapon: medical and public health management. 285, 1059–1070, 2001.
16. Dack, G.M. and Wood, W.L. Serum therapy of botulism in monkeys. *J. Infect. Dis.* 42, 209–212, 1928.
17. Ono, T., Karashimada, T., and Iida, H. Studies on the serum therapy of type E botulism (Part III). *Japan J. Med. Sci. Biol.* 28, 177–191, 1970.
18. Morton H.E. The toxicity of *Clostridium botulinum* Type A toxin for various species of animals, including man. The Institute for Cooperative Research, University of Pennsylvania: Philadelphia, 1961.
19. Oguma, K., Fujinaga, Y., and Inoue, K. Structure and function of *Clostridium botulinum* toxins. *Microbiol. Immunol.* 39, 161–168, 1995.
20. Hatheway, C.L. *Clostridium botulinum*, in *Infectious Diseases*, Bartlett, J.G., Blacklow, N.R., (eds.), 1991, W. B. Saunders Company: Orlando, FL. p. 1583–1586.
21. Sugiyama, H. *Clostridium botulinum* neurotoxin. *Microbiol. Rev.* 44, 419–448, 1980.
22. Hughes, J.M., Blumenthal, J.R., Merson, M.H., et al. Clinical features of types A and B food-borne botulism. *Ann. Intern. Med.* 95, 442–445, 1981.
23. Patrick, W.C. Analysis of botulinum toxin, type A, as a biological warfare threat (unpublished report), 1998.

24. Prevot, A.R., Terrasse, J., Daumail, J., et al. Existence en France du botulisme humaine de type C. *Bull. Acad. Natl. Med.* 139, 355–358, 1955.
25. Matveev, J.I., Nefejeva, N., Bulatova, T.I., and Skolov, I.S. Epidemiology of botulism in the USSR, in Botulism 1966; Proceedings of the Fifth International Symposium on Food Microbiology. Ingrom, M., Roberts, T.A., (eds.), 1966, Chapman and Hall Ltd.: Moscow
26. Demarchi, J., Mourgues, E., Orio, J., and Prevot, A.R. Existence du botulisme humain de type D. *Bull. Acad. Natl. Med.* 142, 580–582, 1958.
27. Gunnison, J.B. and Mayer, K.F. Susceptibility of monkeys, goats and small animals to oral administration of botulinum toxin types B, C, and D. *J. Infect. Dis.* 46, 335–340, 1930.
28. Wobeser, G. Avian botulism – another perspective. *J. Wildlife Dis.* 33, 181–186, 1997.
29. Nol, P., Williamson, J.L., and Rocke, T.E. The epizootiology of type C botulism at the Salton sea. Interagency Botulism Research Coordinating Committee Meeting (IBRCC): Madison, WI 2002.
30. Rocke, T.E. and McLaughlin, G.S. Recent outbreaks of type E botulism in waterbirds in the Great Lakes. Interagency Botulism Research Coordinating Committee: Madison, WI 2002.
31. Brand, C.J., Schmitt, S.M., Duncan, R.M., and Cooley, T.M. An outbreak of type E botulism among common loons (*Gavia immer*) in Michigan's upper peninsula. *J. Wildlife Dis.* 24, 471–476, 1988.
32. Dorsey, E.L., Beebe, J.M., and Johns, E.E. Responses of airborne *Clostridium botulinum* toxin to certain atmospheric stresses. US Army Biological Laboratories: Frederick, MD, 1964.
33. Franz, D.R., Pitt, L.M., Clayton, M.A., et al. Efficacy of prophylactic and therapeutic administration of antitoxin for inhalation botulism, in *Botulinum and Tetanus Neurotoxins: Neurotransmission and Biomedicine Aspects*, Das Gupta, B.R., (ed.), 1993, Plenum Text: New York, p. 473–476.
34. St. Louis, M.E., Peck, S.H., Bowering, D., et al. Botulism from chopped garlic: delayed recognition of a major outbreak. *Ann. Intern. Med.* 108, 363–368, 1988.
35. Shapiro, L., Hatheway, C., Becher, J., and Swerdlow, D.L. Botulism surveillance and emergency response: a public health strategy for a global challenge. *J. Am. Med. Assoc.* 278, 433–435, 1997.
36. Merz, B., Bigalke, H., Stoll, G., and Naumann, M. Botulism type B presenting as pure autonomic dysfunction. *Clin. Auton. Res.* 13, 337–338, 2003.
37. Werner, S.B., Passaro, D.J., McGee, J., et al. Wound botulism in California, 1951–1998: recent epidemic in heroin injectors. *Clin. Infect. Dis.* 31, 1018–1024, 2000.
38. Herrero, B.A., Ecklund, A.E., Streett, C.S., et al. Experimental botulism in monkeys – a clinical pathological study. *Exp. Mol. Pathol.* 6, 84–95, 1967.
39. Stookey, J.L., Streett, C., and Ford, D.F. Preliminary studies on the disappearance of botulinum toxin from the circulating blood of rhesus monkeys. US Army Edgewood Arsenal Chemical Research and Development Laboratories: Edgewood Arsenal, 1965.
40. Oberst, F.W., Crook, J.W., Cresthull, P., and House, M.J. Evaluation of botulism antitoxin, supportive therapy, and artificial respiration in monkeys with experimental botulism. *Clin. Pharmacol. Ther.* 9, 209–214, 1968.
41. Cherington, M. Electrophysiologic methods as an aid in diagnosis of botulism: a review. *Muscle Nerve* 5, S28–S29, 1982.
42. Pascuzzi, R.M., and Fleck, J.D. Acute peripheral neuropathy in adults. Guillian-Barre syndrome and related disorders. *Neurol. Clin. North Am.* 15, 529–547, 1997.
43. Asbury, A. New concepts of Guillian-Barre syndrome. *J. Child. Neurol.* 15, 183–191, 2000.
44. Willison, H.J. and O'Hanlon, G.M. The immunopathogenesis of Miller Fisher Syndrome. *J. Neuroimmunol.* 100, 3–12, 1999.

45. Felz, M.W., Smith, C.D., and Swift, T.R. A six-year-old girl with tick paralysis. *N. Engl. J. Med.* 342, 90–94, 2000.
46. ICMSF. *Clostridium botulinum*, in *Micro-Organisms in Foods 5: Characteristics of Microbial Pathogens*. 1996, Blackie Academic & Professional: New York. p. 68–111.
47. Gangarosa, E.A. Botulism in the U.S., 1899–1969. *Am. J. Epidemiol.* 93, 93–101, 1971.
48. MacDonald, K.L., Cohen, M.L., and Blake, P.A. The changing epidemiology of adult botulism in the United States. *Am. J. Epidemiol.* 124, 794–799, 1986.
49. Wainright, R.B., Heyward, W.L., Middaugh, J.P., et al. Food-borne botulism in Alaska, 1947–1985: epidemiology and clinical findings. *J. Infect. Dis.* 157, 1158–1162, 1987.
50. Sobel, J., Tucker, N., McLaughlin, J., and Maslanka, S. Foodborne botulism in the United States, 1990–2000. *Emerg. Infect. Dis.* 10, 1606–1611, 2004.
51. Passaro, D.J., Werner, S.B., McGee, J., et al. Wound botulism associated with black tar heroin among injecting drug users. *J. Am. Med. Assoc.* 279, 859–863, 1998.
52. Arnon, S. Infant botulism, in *Textbook of Pediatric Infectious Diseases*, Feigen R.D., Cherry, J.D., (eds.), 1998, WB Saunders: Philadelphia. p. 1570–1577.
53. Spika J.S., Shafer N., Hargrett-Bean N. Risk factors for infant botulism in the United States. *Am. J. Dis. Child.* 143, 828–832, 1989.
54. Long, S. Epidemiologic study of infant botulism in Pennsylvania: report of the infant botulism study group. *Pediatrics* 75, 928–934, 1985.
55. Arnon, S.S., Midura, T.F., Clay, S.A., et al. Infant botulism: epidemiological, clinical, and laboratory aspects. *J. Am. Med. Assoc.* 237, 1946–1951, 1977.
56. Chia, J.K., Clark, J.B., Ryan, C.A., and Pollack, M., Botulism in an adult associated with food-borne intestinal infection with *Clostridium botulinum*. *N. Engl. J. Med.* 315, 239–254, 1986.
57. Arnon, S. Botulism as an intestinal toxemia, in *Infections of the Gastrointestinal Tract*, Blaser M. J., Ravdin, J. I., Greenberg, H.B., Gusrrant, R.L., (eds.), 1995, Raven Press: New York. p. 257–271.
58. Fenicia, L., Franciosa, G., Pourshaban, M., and Aureli, P. Intestinal toxemia botulism in two young people, caused by *Clostridium butyricum* type E. *Clin. Infect. Dis.* 29, 1381–1387, 1999.
59. Griffin, P.M., Hatheway, C., Rosenbaum, R.B., and Sokolow, R. Endogenous antibody production to botulinum toxin in an adult with intestinal colonization botulism and underlying Crohn's disease. *J. Infect. Dis.* 175, 633–637, 1997.
60. Liu, W., Montana, V., Chapman, E.R., et al. Botulinum toxin type B micromechanosensor. *Proc. Natl. Acad. Sci. USA* 100, 13621–13625, 2003.
61. Woodruff, B.A., Griffin, P.M., McCroskey, L.M., et al. Clinical and laboratory comparison of botulism from toxin types A, B, and E in the United States, 1975–1988. *J. Infect. Dis.* 166, 1281–1286, 1992.
62. Dowell, V.R., Jr., McCroskey, L.M., Hatheway, C.L., et al. Coproexamination for botulinal toxin and *Clostridium botulinum*. A new procedure for laboratory diagnosis of botulism. *J. Am. Med. Assoc.* 238, 1829–1832, 1977.
63. Alibek K., Handleman S. Biohazard. Random House: New York, 1999.
64. Ekeus, R. Report of the Secretary General on the status of the Implementation of the Special Commision's plan for the ongoing monitoring and verification of Iraq's compliance with relevant parts of Sector C of Security Council Resolution 687. 1991, United Nations Special Commision: New York.
65. Cordesman, A. Weapons of Mass Destruction in the Gulf and Greater Middle East: Force Trends, Strategy, Tactics and Damage Effects. Center for Strategic and International Studies: Washington DC. 1998, p. 18–52.
66. Bermudez, J. The Armed Forces of North Korea. IB Tauris: London, 2001.
67. Park, J.B. and Simpson, L.L. Inhalational poisoning by botulinum toxin and inhalation vaccination with its heavy chain component. *Infect. Immun.* 71, 1147–1154, 2003.
68. Tucker, J. Toxic Terror: Assessing the Terrorist Use of Chemical and Biological Weapons. MIT Press: Cambridge, 2000.

69. WuDunn, S., Miller, J., and Broad, W.J. How Japan germ terror alerted world, in *New York Times*. 1998: New York. p. A1, A10.
70. Sobel, J., Khan, A.S., and Swerdlow, D.L. Threat of a biological terrorist attack on the US food supply: the CDC perspective. *Lancet* 359, 874–880, 2002.
71. Sanders, D.B., Massey, E.W., and Buckley, E.G. Botulinum toxin for blepharospasm: single-fiber EMG studies. *Neurology*. 36, 545–547, 1986.
72. Bhatia, K.P., Münchau, A., Thompson, P.D., et al. Generalised muscular weakness after botulinum toxin injections for dystonia: a report of three cases. *J. Neurol. Neurosurg. Psych*. 67, 90–93, 1999.
73. Cobb, D.B., Watson, W.A., and Fernandez, M.C. Botulism-like syndrome after injections of botulinum toxin. *Vet. Hum. Toxicol*. 42, 163, 2000.
74. Tugnoli, V., Eleopra, R., Quatrale, R., et al. Botulism-like syndrome after botulinum toxin type A injections for focal hyerhidrosis. *Br. J. Dermatol*. 147, 808–809, 2002.
75. ProMED-mail. Botulism, human, botox related – USA (Florida): suspected. ProMED-mail 2004; 29 Nov: 20041129.3185. <http://www.promedmail.org.> Accessed 6 December 2004.
76. Treadwell, T.A., Koo, D., Kuker, K., and Khan, A.S. Epidemiologic clues to bioterrorism. *Public Health Rep*. 118, 92–98, 2003.
77. Barash, J.R. and Arnon, S.S. Dual toxin-producing strain of Clostridium botulinum type Bf isolated from a California patient with infantile botulism. *J. Clin. Microbiol*. 42, 1713–1715, 2004.
78. Khan, A.S., Swerdlow, D., and Juranek, D.D. Precautions against biological and chemical terrorism directed at food and water supplies. *Public Health Rep*. 116, 3–14, 2001.
79. Sobel, J., Griffin, P.M., Slutsker, L., et al. Investigation of mulstistate foodborne disease outbreaks. *Public Health Rep*. 117, 8–19, 2002.
80. Khan, A.S., Morse, S., and Lillibridge, S. Public-health preparedness for biological terrorism in the USA. *Lancet* 356, 1179–1182, 2000.
81. Tacket, C.O., Shandera, W.X., Mann, J.M., et al. Equine antitoxin use and other factors that predict outcome in type A foodborne botulism. *Am. J. Med*. 76, 794–798, 1984.
82. Black, R.E. and Gunn, R.A. Hypersensitivity reactions associated with botulinal antitoxin. *Am. J. Med*. 69, 567–570, 1980.
83. Hatheway, C.H., Snyder, J.D., Seals, J.E., et al. Antitoxin levels in botulism patients treated with trivalent equine botulism antitoxin to toxin types A, B, and E. *J. Infect. Dis*. 150, 407–412, 1984.
84. Hibbs, R.G., Weber, J.T., Corwin, A., et al. Experience with the use of an investigational F(ab')2 heptavalent botulism immune globulin of equine origin during an outbreak of type E botulism in Egypt. *Clin. Infect. Dis*. 23, 337–340, 1996.
85. Nowakowski, A., Wang, C., Powers, D.B., et al. Potent neutralization of botulinum neurotoxin by recombinant oligoclonal antibody. *Proc. Natl. Acad. Sci. USA* 99, 11346–11350, 2002.
86. Foynes, S., Holley, J.L., Garmory, H.S., et al. Vaccination against type F botulinum toxin using attenuated Salmonella enterica var Typhimurium strains expressing the BoNT/F H(C) fragment. *Vaccine* 7, 1052–1059, 2003.
87. Lee, J.S., Pushko, P., Parker, M.D., et al. Candidate vaccine against botulinum neurotoxin serotype A derived from a Venezuelan equine encephalitis virus vaccine system. *Infect. Immun*. 69, 5709, 2001.
88. Smith, L.A. Development of recombinant vaccines for botulinum neurotoxin. *Toxicon* 36, 1539–1548, 1998.

Chapter 6
The Viral Hemorrhagic Fevers

Daniel G. Bausch and C. J. Peters

6.1 Disease Outbreak Scenario

A 34-year-old male presents to the emergency room with a 4-day history of fever, headache, myalgia, nausea, and general malaise. Physical exam reveals hyperthermia, tachycardia, and diaphoresis. Laboratory tests show mild leucopenia and thrombocytopenia and elevated BUN and creatinine. A rapid test for influenza is negative. The patient is a clerk in the municipal county building. He has no significant past medical history, has not recently traveled outside of the United States, and reports no history of exposure to exotic pets or foods. Acetaminophen and oral rehydration solution are prescribed and the patient is discharged with a diagnosis of "viral syndrome."

The next morning, a 43-year-old woman presents with a similar clinical picture, but with a fine morbilliform rash over her face and chest. As the doctor working the shift is not the same from the day before, the coincidence that the woman also works at the municipal county building goes unnoticed. She is similarly discharged with a diagnosis of "viral syndrome." Later that afternoon, an ambulance arrives returning the 34-year-old man seen the previous day, whose condition has deteriorated to include severe abdominal pain and hematemesis. Physical exam now shows hypothermia, hypotension, tachycardia, and oozing of blood from the nose and gums. He is admitted to the critical care unit.

Two days later at a joint morning report held with physicians from all the hospitals in the area, one of the residents presents a case of a 28-year-old woman with fever and bleeding. When it is reported that the patient is a secretary at the municipal county building, the doctors begin to suspect a common source. They contact the city public health officials who, through further inquiry with emergency rooms throughout the city, identify five more workers from the municipal county building with recent febrile syndromes over the past week, one with a

D.G. Bausch
Department of Tropical Medicine, Tulane School of Public Health and Tropical Medicine, SL-17, 1430 Tulane Avenue, New Orleans, LA 70112-2699, USA
e-mail: dbausch@tulane.edu

L.I. Lutwick, S.M. Lutwick (eds.), *Beyond Anthrax*,
DOI: 10.1007/978-1-59745-326-4_6, © Springer Science+Business Media, LLC 2008

rash and another with bleeding. City public health officials are concerned about a bioterrorist attack with a hemorrhagic fever (HF) virus.

6.2 Introduction

The term "viral HF" refers to an acute systemic illness classically involving fever, a constellation of initially nonspecific signs and symptoms, and a propensity for bleeding and shock. Viral HFs may be caused by more than 25 different viruses from four families: *Filoviridae, Arenaviridae, Bunyaviridae*, and *Flaviviridae* (Table 6.1). Characteristics of the viral HFs with regard to their potential for use as biological weapons are presented in Table 6.2. Many of the HF viruses have been placed on the CDC's Select Agents list of pathogens that pose a potential bioterrorism threat [1]. The HF viruses of highest concern are Ebola and Marburg (filoviruses), Lassa, Junin, Machupo (arenaviruses), Rift Valley Fever (RVF), and Crimean-Congo HF (CCHF) (bunyaviruses). The reasons that some HF viruses are of lesser concern with regard to the potential for bioterrorism include availability of an effective vaccine, low potential for person-to-person transmission, low associated mortality, or difficulty in production in the laboratory. This chapter will focus specifically on the potential of HF viruses as potential biological weapons. The reader is referred to various published reviews for a more comprehensive background of all viral HFs [2, 3].

6.3 History of the Weaponization of HF Viruses

Although there is no record of deployment of a HF virus as a weapon, research and development to weaponize various HF viruses, including Ebola, Marburg, Lassa, Machupo, and Junin viruses is reported to have taken place in the ex-Soviet Union during the cold war and, to a lesser degree, in the United States prior to the abolishment of its biological warfare program in 1969 [4]. No country is presently recognized as actively developing HF viruses as weapons, but concerns persist over clandestine activity, such as the reported attempt by the Japanese cult group Aum Shinrikyo to acquire Ebola virus, and the whereabouts of virus stocks produced during the Soviet era.

6.3.1 The Viruses

All viral HFs are caused by small, lipid-enveloped, single-stranded RNA viruses. Most of the HF viruses can be cultured in a variety of vertebrate or mosquito cell lines, depending on the specific virus (Table 6.2) [5, 6]. Laboratory animal systems for isolating and propagating HF viruses in mice, hamsters, or guinea pigs also exist, again depending upon the specific virus. Pathogenicity

Table 6.1 Principal viruses causing hemorrhagic fevers

Virus	Disease	Biosafety level	Principal reservoir/vector	Geographic distribution of reservoir/vector	Geographic distribution of human disease	Annual cases	Disease-to-infection ratio
Filoviridae							
Ebola	Ebola HF	BSL-4	Unknown, bat suspected	Sub-Saharan Africa, Philippines?	Sub-Saharan Africa	–[a]	1:1
Marburg	Marburg HF	BSL-4	Unknown, bat suspected	Sub-Saharan Africa	Sub-Saharan Africa	–[a]	1:1
Arenaviridae[b]							
Lassa	Lassa fever	BSL-4	Rodent ("multimammate rat" or *Mastomys natalensis*)	Sub-Saharan Africa	West Africa	100,000– 300,000	1:5–10
Junin	Argentine HF	BSL-4	Rodent ("corn mouse" or *Calomys musculinus*)	South America	Argentine pampas	~100	1:1.5
Machupo	Bolivian HF	BSL-4	Rodent ("large vesper mouse" or *Calomys callosus*)	South America	Beni department, Bolivia	<50	1:1.5
Guanarito	Venezuelan HF	BSL-4	Rodent ("cane mouse" or *Zygodontomys brevicauda*)	South America	Portuguesa state, Venezuela	<50	1:1.5
Sabiá[c]	Proposed name: Brazilian HF	BSL-4	Unknown, rodent suspected	Unknown	Rural area near Sao Paulo, Brazil?	–[c]	1:1.5
Flexal[d]	None	BSL-3	Rodent (*Oryzomys* species)	South America	Brazilian Amazon	–[d]	Unknown
Bunyaviridae							
Hantaan, Seoul,	HF with renal syndrome	BSL-3	Rodent (Hantaan: "striped field	Striped field mouse:	Hantaan: northeast	50,000–150,000	Hantaan: 1:1.5; Others: 1:20

Table 6.1 (continued)

Virus	Disease	Biosafety level	Principal reservoir/vector	Geographic distribution of reservoir/vector	Geographic distribution of human disease	Annual cases	Disease-to-infection ratio
Puumala, Dobrava, others			mouse" or *Apodemus agrarius*; Seoul: "Norway rat" or *Rattus norvegicus*; Puumala: "bank vole" or *Clethrionomys glareolus*; Dobrava: "yellow-necked field mouse" or *Apodemus flavicollis*)	northeast Asia; Norway rat: worldwide; bank vole: northern Europe; yellow-necked field mouse: southern Europe	Asia; Seoul: urban areas worldwide; Puumala and Dobrava: Europe		
Rift Valley fever	Rift Valley fever	BSL-3	Domestic livestock/mosquitoes (*Aedes* and others)	Worldwide	Africa, Middle East	100–100,000[a]	1:100
Crimean-Congo HF	Crimean-Congo HF	BSL-4	Wild and domestic vertebrates/tick (*Hyalomma* species)	Worldwide?	Africa, Southern Europe and Russia, eastern Asia	~500	1:1–2
Flaviviridae							
Yellow fever	Yellow fever	BSL-3	Monkey/mosquito (*Aedes aegypti*, other *Aedes* and *Haemagogus* species)	Tropics and subtropics worldwide	Sub-Saharan Africa, South America	5,000–200,000[e]	1:2–20
Dengue	Dengue fever and dengue HF	BSL-2	Human/mosquito (*Aedes aegypti*)	Tropics and subtropics worldwide	Tropics and subtropics worldwide	Dengue fever: 100 million; Dengue HF: 100,000–200,000[e]	1:10–100 depending on age, previous infection, genetic background, and infecting serotype

Table 6.1 (continued)

Virus	Disease	Biosafety level	Principal reservoir/vector	Geographic distribution of reservoir/vector	Geographic distribution of human disease	Annual cases	Disease-to-infection ratio
Omsk HF	Omsk HF	BSL-4	Rodent/tick (*Ixodes*), maintenance cycle incompletely understood	Worldwide	Western Siberia	100–200	Unknown
Kyasanur Forest disease	Kyasanur Forest disease	BSL-4	Vertebrate (rodents, bats, birds, monkeys, others)/ tick (*Ixodes*)	Karnataka state, India	Karnataka state, India	400–500	Unknown
Alkhumra HF[f]	Proposed name: Alkhumra HF	BSL-4	Unknown, ticks suspected	Unknown	Saudi Arabia	<50	Unknown

BSL biosafety level, *HF* hemorrhagic fever

[a] Although some endemic transmission of the filoviruses (Ebola>Marburg) and Rift Valley fever virus occurs, these viruses have most often been associated with epidemics. Epidemics of Ebola hemorrhagic typically involve <500 people and Marburg <200. Filovirus epidemics have been recognized with increasing frequency during the period 1994–2008

[b] Although evidence of infection with the North American arenavirus Whitewater Arroyo has been noted in sick persons, its role as a pathogen has not been clearly established

[c] Only three cases (one fatal) of Sabiá virus infection have been noted since discovery of the virus in 1990. Two of them were related to laboratory infection. Disease from this virus is presumed to be similar to the other South American arenavirus HFs

[d] A single case of human infection (nonfatal) with Flexal virus has been reported from a presumed laboratory exposure in Belem, Brazil, in 1978

[e] Based on estimates from the World Health Organization. Significant underreporting occurs. Incidence may fluctuate widely depending on epidemic activity

[f] Alkhumra virus is considered by some to be a variant of Kyasanur Forest disease virus. Controversy exists over the proper spelling of the virus, written as "Alkhurma" in some publications

Table 6.2 Characteristics of the hemorrhagic fever viruses with regard to potential for use as bioweapons

Virus	Case fatality	Potential for person-to-person transmission	Infectious dose	Aerosol infectivity between humans in nature	Aerosol infectivity in laboratory experiments?	Vaccine available?	Potential to cause panic	Ease of acquiring virus	Feasibility of production	Reported or suspected history of development as a bioweapon?
Filoviridae										
Ebola	55%–85%, depending upon species	High	Low	Low or none	Yes	No	High	Difficult	Grows easily in primate cell lines. Dangerous to manipulate outside of a high containment facility.	Yes, ex-Soviet Union
Marburg	25%–85%	High	Low	Low or none	Yes	No	High	Difficult	Grows easily in primate cell lines. Dangerous to manipulate outside of a high containment facility.	Yes, ex-Soviet Union
Arenaviridae										
Lassa	2%–50%	Moderate	Moderate	Low or none	Yes	No	High	Relatively easy	Grows easily in primate cell lines.	Yes, ex-Soviet Union

Table 6.2 (continued)

Virus	Case fatality	Potential for person-to-person transmission	Infectious dose	Aerosol infectivity between humans in nature	Aerosol infectivity in laboratory experiments?	Vaccine available?	Potential to cause panic	Ease of acquiring virus	Feasibility of production	Reported or suspected history of development as a bioweapon?
									Dangerous to manipulate outside of a high containment facility.	
South America HF viruses	15%–30%	Low	Moderate	Low or none	Yes	Yes[a]	Moderate	Relatively easy	Grow easily in primate cell lines. Dangerous to manipulate outside of a high containment facility.	Yes (Machupo and Junin), ex-Soviet Union
Bunyaviridae										
HF with renal syndrome	<1%–50%, depending on specific virus	None	Low	None	No	Yes[b]	Moderate	Relatively easy	Difficult to culture	No
Rift Valley fever (HF syndrome)	50%	None	Moderate	Low or none	Yes	No[c]	Moderate	Moderate	Grows easily in primate cell lines.	No

Table 6.2 (continued)

Virus	Case fatality	Potential for person-to-person transmission	Infectious dose	Aerosol infectivity between humans in nature	Aerosol infectivity in laboratory experiments?	Vaccine available?	Potential to cause panic	Ease of acquiring virus	Feasibility of production	Reported or suspected history of development as a bioweapon?
									Dangerous to manipulate outside of a high containment facility.	
Crimean-Congo HF	15%–30%	High	Low	Low or none	Yes	No	Moderate	Moderate	Grows easily in various cell lines. Dangerous to manipulate outside of a high containment facility.	Yes, ex-Soviet Union
Flaviviridae										
Yellow fever	20%–50%	None	High	None	No	Yes	Moderate	Moderate	Grows easily in mosquito cell lines and in eggs.	No
Dengue HF	Untreated: 10%–15% Treated: <1%:	None	High	None	No	No	Low	Relatively easy	Grows easily in mosquito cell lines.	No

Table 6.2 (continued)

Virus	Case fatality	Potential for person-to-person transmission	Infectious dose	Aerosol infectivity between humans in nature	Aerosol infectivity in laboratory experiments?	Vaccine available?	Potential to cause panic	Ease of acquiring virus	Feasibility of production	Reported or suspected history of development as a bioweapon?
Omsk HF	1%–3%	Not reported	Unknown	Unknown	No data	No	Low	Moderate	Grows easily in various cell lines.	No
Kyasanur Forest disease	3%–5%	Not reported, but laboratory infections have occurred	Unknown	Unknown	No data	Yes[b]	Low	Moderate	Grows easily in various cell lines.	No
Alkhumra HF		Not reported	Unknown	Unknown	No data	No	Low	Moderate	Unknown (virus recently discovered)	No (virus recently discovered)

The data in this table are based on published research or consensus opinion of experts regarding the respective wild-type viruses. Genetic modification of the virus and/or the use of advanced physical dissemination mechanisms could alter the stated principles

HF hemorrhagic fever

[a] A live attenuated vaccine, Candid #1, licensed only in Argentina, has been shown to decrease morbidity and mortality associated with Argentine HF [163]. Laboratory studies suggest that Candid #1 may also be effective in Bolivian HF, although it does not appear to cross-protect against Guanarito or Sabiá viruses [Jahrling, P. B., Personal Communication]

[b] Vaccines for HF with renal syndrome (due to Hantaan virus) and Kyasanur forest disease are in use in other countries, but have not been licensed in the United States

[c] Vaccines for Rift Valley fever virus infection are licensed for use in animals, but not yet humans

varies among viruses and can also differ between species and strains of the same virus.

6.3.1.1 Natural Maintenance and Transmission

HF viruses are primarily maintained in nature in mammalian reservoirs (Table 6.1). The geographic distribution of any given HF virus is restricted by the distribution of its natural reservoir and/or arthropod vector. Human infection is generally rare. Humans are dead-end hosts, playing no role in the natural maintenance of any HF virus, with the exception of dengue.

Arenaviruses are maintained in nature via chronic asymptomatic infection in rodents, with a strict pairing between the specific arenavirus and the rodent species [7–11]. Virus is transmitted to humans primarily via exposure to rodent excreta [12]. The highest virus titers are in urine [12, 13]. Although the precise mechanism of human infection is unknown, the arenaviruses are relatively stable and infectious to nonhuman primates in aerosol form, suggesting that humans may be infected from primary aerosols produced when rodents urinate [14, 15]. Secondary aerosol generation is notoriously inefficient so disturbing shed urine is a less likely mechanism of infection. Direct inoculation into the conjunctivae or mucous membranes or, rarely, through a rodent bite, may also occur. In West Africa, Lassa virus is sometimes contracted through exposure to contaminated excreta and blood when rodents are trapped and prepared for consumption [16]. Oral infection may also occur, perhaps through a gastric portal, although there are few data on the subject [17].

Bats are suspected to be the reservoir for the filoviruses, although this remains to be definitively proven [18–20]. Humans can also contract these viruses from exposure to infected nonhuman primates which are, like humans, dead-end hosts [181, 182].

The bunya- and flaviviruses are arboviruses, spread to humans primarily by mosquitoes and ticks, depending on the specific virus.

Secondary human-to-human transmission occurs most commonly with the filoviruses, CCHF, and Lassa virus (Table 6.2). Contrary to popular belief, secondary attack rates are generally low, probably because transmission between humans usually requires direct contact with contaminated body fluids [21, 22]. Tertiary transmission is unusual and, for unclear reasons, often associated with milder disease [23–25].

Human infection probably usually occurs through oral or mucous membrane exposure, most often in the context of providing care to a sick family member (community) or patient (nosocomial transmission) [21, 26]. Funeral rituals which entail the touching of the corpse prior to burial have also played a significant role in transmission [27]. Infection through fomites cannot be ruled out, although virus culture and PCR were usually negative from environmental samples taken in a isolation ward for Ebola HF unless the samples were obviously contaminated with blood or body fluids [28, 29]. With the exception of the flavivirus and hantavirus infections, the viremia and infectivity of persons with viral HFs generally parallels their clinical state. Persons are especially infectious late in the course of severe disease, especially when bleeding. The risk of transmission during the incubation period or from asymptomatic persons is negligible.

6.3.1.2 Infectious Dose and Route of Infection

Based on limited data, the infectious dose for most HF viruses appears to be low on the order of a few virions or less [30]. Few data exist on the effect of the dose or route of infection on the clinical presentation of viral HF in humans. Furthermore, it is difficult to extrapolate results of studies performed using laboratory-adapted virus strains in mice and guinea pig models, in which the pathogenesis often differs significantly, to nonhuman primates and humans [30–32].

Epidemiologic and some limited laboratory-based data do not suggest aerosol transmission of the HF viruses between humans in natural settings [21, 33–37]. However, infectious and moderately stable aerosols have been artificially produced in the laboratory [14, 15, 38–44]. Aerosol transmission of Ebola–Reston virus appears to have occurred between caged monkeys, although infection through large-droplet deposition on mucous membranes cannot be excluded [41]. Aerosol spread of Lassa virus was speculated to occur in the first recognized outbreaks of Lassa fever, but extensive experience since then has not supported this hypothesis [45].

6.4 Possible Strategies for the Dissemination of HF Viruses as Bioweapons

Three dissemination strategies that bioterrorists might attempt, either singly or in combination, can be envisioned:

6.4.1 "Implantation" of Infected Humans in the Community or Hospitals to Initiate Person-to-Person Transmission

Although seemingly the easiest approach for those with access to HF viruses, experience from naturally occurring transmission suggests that this strategy would be unlikely to initiate a large outbreak in industrialized countries, at least if the initial number of implanted persons was small, perhaps less than the 10–20 people that could be accommodated by most hospital emergency rooms. Endemic transmission of CCHF, Lassa, and some of the South American HF viruses occurs in various resource-poor settings where community sanitation is substandard and laboratory confirmation is unavailable or delayed [12, 23, 24, 46–48]. Nevertheless, large community-based outbreaks are unusual. Despite being probably the most transmissible of all HF viruses, the secondary attack rate associated with an outbreak of Ebola virus in a community in sub-Saharan Africa was only 16%, despite the low level of sanitation (i.e., no running water) and little access to protective materials [21]. Similar attack rates have been noted during outbreaks of Marburg virus [183]. This number would likely be still lower in industrialized countries with heightened levels of sanitation and hygiene.

Large nosocomial outbreaks under the scenario of implanted cases are similarly unlikely. Hospital outbreaks of viral HFs have virtually always been associated with substandard infection control practices and have been rapidly curtailed with their improvement [25, 37, 49, 50]. When importation of a case of viral HF has occurred in modern hospitals with well-maintained barrier nursing precautions, little secondary transmission has resulted, even when the diagnosis of viral HF appears not to have been considered [21, 34, 37, 51]. Between 1975 and 2007 over 30 cases of laboratory-confirmed viral HF have been exported from Africa to various countries around the globe, resulting in just three secondary transmission events (one case each for Marburg, Ebola, and Lassa viruses – all in healthcare workers), despite thousands of contacts collectively occurring before the diagnosis was made and protective measures implemented [52] (A. Sanzone, manuscript in preparation). Similarly, although unwitting importations of persons infected with Ebola or Marburg viruses has occasionally resulted in fatalities, extensive secondary spread has not occurred [51, 53, 54].

The simultaneous implantation of a larger number of infected persons might exceed the surge capacity of a given facility, resulting in a breakdown of infection control measures and increased likelihood of significant secondary transmission. However, such an event would be unlikely to go undetected for very long. Contemporaneous measures to impair the response capacity of the public health system, such as simultaneous use of other biological or conventional weapons, attacks on hospitals and healthcare workers, or measures to disrupt communications or incite public panic, could significantly enhance secondary transmission regardless of the size of the initially implanted group. Attention required to the "worried well," those with "sociogenic illness," and to the safe burial of corpses would further stress the surge capacity [55].

Lastly, although terrorists often show little reluctance to die for their cause, the clinical course of most viral HFs can be incredibly painful, perhaps requiring a level of sacrifice even above that of those who are willing to die instantaneously through the detonation of explosives. Furthermore, even with the most lethal HF viruses, some of the terrorist implantees would survive and likely become prisoners who could be interrogated as a source of information for intelligence agencies.

6.4.2 Release of an Infected Reservoir or Vector

This strategy could be aimed directly at causing human infection or at infecting the domestic or wild animal population to disrupt the food supply and economy. Strategies aimed at direct human infection would have to overcome a host of natural impediments. The strict pairing of many HF viruses with specific reservoirs limits the potential for propagation in a new environment. HF virus infection of a non-host species usually results in transient asymptomatic infection and subsequent immunity. With the exception of dengue virus (for which the host is effectively humans) and some of the potential hosts for RVF virus, no reservoir for a HF virus is endemic in North America (Table 6.1). Widespread dissemination would thus require either the adaptation of the natural host species of a given HF virus to a new environment or a "species jump" in which the foreign virus would be introduced and chronically shed by a new reservoir. Even if these events were to occur, subsequent transmission of virus to humans would be far from certain, as transmission of the rodent-borne HF viruses to humans appears to be relatively inefficient, occurring infrequently even in areas where infected rodents are common [56, 57].

An alternative and perhaps more dangerous strategy might be to attempt to transiently infect a large number of animals with which humans would subsequently have close contact, such as domestic livestock destined for slaughter, pets, or research animals. Although not terrorist acts, various past and recent events illustrate the danger. The unwitting importation of monkeys infected with Marburg virus to Germany and the former Yugoslavia for harvesting of organs for use in vaccine production resulted in 26 primary and six secondary human infections with seven deaths [58, 59]. Although not a viral HF, cases of human monkeypox in the United States in 2004 have been traced to the importation of infected Gambian rats from Ghana with subsequent spread to North American prairie dogs sold as pets [60].

Introduction of a zoonotic virus could be especially devastating if the appropriate animal reservoir or arthropod vector is already endemic in the region, permitting autochthonous transmission and the potential establishment of a permanent endemic focus. The introduction of yellow fever or dengue viruses into endogenous populations of *Aedes aegypti* or *Ae. albopictus* in the southern United States would be of particular concern. Mosquito control measures and vaccination for yellow fever would eventually eliminate transmission, but perhaps not before significant human morbidity and mortality would occur. The sometimes limited availability of yellow fever vaccine could further compound the situation [61].

The introduction of a HF virus into the domestic livestock in industrialized countries could have grave consequences. Industrial scale farming practices predominant in North America and Western Europe render these regions particularly vulnerable. Even if no significant human morbidity or mortality results, the economic consequences of a declaration of a serious infectious agent in a country's livestock can be devastating, as illustrated by recent zoonotic outbreaks of avian influenza, Nipah virus, and foot and mouth disease. Although the HF viruses generally score low on the selection criteria for biological agents likely to be used against animals, a few of these viruses do pose a threat [62]. RVF virus is the agent of most concern because of its ability to infect a wide variety of wild and domestic animals, including ruminant livestock, and to be spread by many species of mosquitoes present in North America and Europe [63]. Mechanical transmission from several arthropods may also occur [64]. Although not an act of bioterrorism, the epidemic spread of RVF virus after its introduction into Egypt in 1977, resulting in over 100,000 human infections, 18,000 clinical cases, and 2,000 deaths, as well as 100,000s of thousands of deaths in livestock, is an example of the danger [65].

6.4.3 Direct Dissemination Through Artificially Produced Aerosols or Fomites

The most dangerous scenario is that of artificial aerosol dissemination of a HF virus resulting in the simultaneous infection of hundreds or even thousands of people. Decay, meteorological conditions, the effects of buildings, and other variables would impact virus dissemination [66]. Dissemination could theoretically be enhanced through genetic manipulation ("bioengineering") of the virus to alter transmission properties and/or the use of artificial devices, such as "crop duster" airplanes, backpack sprayers, or even small perfume atomizers. The aerosol stability of Marburg virus has been shown to be enhanced by the simple addition of glycerol [33]. The most dangerous, but also most technically difficult, approach would perhaps aim at engineering a chimeric agent possessing, for example, the aerosol transmissibility of smallpox and the virulence of Ebola virus, still further enhanced by a physical mass-dissemination device. The Soviet Union's bioweapon program may have encompassed such aims, but the data were either lost in the subsequent upheaval of the country or, for obvious reasons, are not available for public scrutiny [4].

6.5 Clinical Presentation

6.5.1 The Illness

The rare and sporadic nature of most viral HFs, along with their predominance in resource-poor settings, has impeded systematic clinical observations. Most descriptions are thus of an anecdotal nature. Although the pathophysiology of the viral HFs varies with the specific virus, certain common hallmarks can be identified, namely microvascular instability and impaired hemostasis. Contrary to popular thought, mortality usually results not directly from exsanguination, but rather from a process akin to septic shock, with insufficient effective circulating intravascular volume leading to cellular dysfunction and multi-organ system failure. In fact, external bleeding is seen in a minority of cases. Viral HF is seen in both genders and all age groups, with a spectrum from relatively mild or even asymptomatic infection to severe vascular permeability resulting in shock, multi-organ system failure, and death.

Although the clinical presentation may differ for each of viral HF as it progresses, in most cases the limited data do not permit clear distinctions, especially in the early phases of disease. At presentation most patients show nonspecific signs and symptoms difficult to distinguish from a host of other febrile illnesses (Table 6.3). Illness typically begins with fever and constitutional symptoms, including general malaise, anorexia, headache, chest or retrosternal pain, sore throat, myalgia, arthralgia, lumbosacral pain, and dizziness (Table 6.4). Relative bradycardia and orthostatic hypotension are often noted [56, 67–72]. The pharynx may be erythemic or, less frequently, exudative, especially in Lassa fever, incorrectly leading to a diagnosis of streptococcal pharyngitis. Gastrointestinal signs and symptoms readily ensue, including nausea and vomiting, epigastric and abdominal pain and tenderness (especially over the liver in Ebola HF, presumed to be due to stretching of the liver capsule), and diarrhea. Viral HF has sometimes been mistaken for acute appendicitis or other abdominal emergencies. Hepatosplenomegaly is frequently seen, but it is unknown whether this is specific to the viral HF or simply represents the high underlying prevalence of hepatosplenomegaly in populations in sub-Saharan Africa where most clinical observations have been made. A dry cough, sometimes accompanied by a few scattered rales on auscultation, is frequently noted, but prominent pulmonary symptoms or the presence of productive sputum early in the course of disease are uncommon. Conjunctival injection or hemorrhage is seen in about a third of the patients but is not typically accompanied by itching, discharge, or rhinitis. Various forms of skin rash, including morbilliform, maculopapular, petechial, and ecchymotic, may be seen, depending upon the specific viral HF. The presence of a maculopapular rash on the torso or face may be one early relatively specific, although insensitive, indicator of Ebola or Marburg HF [29]. For unclear reasons, a rash is almost always seen in whites with Lassa fever, but almost never in blacks.

In severe cases, patients progress to vascular instability and hemorrhage. Evidence of vascular instability may include conjunctival injection/hemorrhage, facial flushing, edema, bleeding, hypotension, shock, and proteinuria. The likelihood of clinically discernible hemorrhage varies with the infecting virus and may be manifested as hematemesis, melena, hematochezia, metrorrhagia, petechiae, purpura, epistaxis, and bleeding from the gums and venipuncture sites. Hemoptysis and hematuria are infrequently seen. Hemorrhage is almost never present in the first 48 h of illness. Central nervous system manifestations, including disorientation, tremor, gait anomalies, convulsions, and hiccups may be noted in end-stage disease, and are especially common in the South American HFs [73, 74]. Renal insufficiency or failure may occur, especially in HF with renal syndrome, as the name implies. Pregnant women often present with spontaneous abortion and vaginal bleeding [77–79]. With the exception of yellow fever, jaundice is not typical of the viral HFs.

The clinical course of viral HF usually unfolds quite rapidly, with death in fatal cases 7–10 days after symptom onset. Distinct phases of disease and recovery are classically described for HF with renal syndrome, yellow fever, and dengue HF, although not seen in all cases. Encephalitis and retinitis may

Table 6.3 Differential diagnosis of the viral hemorrhagic fevers

Disease	Distinguishing Characteristics and Comments
Parasites	
Malaria	Classically shows paroxysms of fever and chills. Hemorrhagic manifestations less common. Malaria smears or rapid test usually positive. Responds to anti-malarials.
Amebiasis	Hemorrhagic manifestations other than bloody diarrhea generally not seen. Amoebic trophozoites identified in the stool. Responds to antiparasitics.
Giardiasis	
African trypanosomiasis (acute phase)	Acute stages may mimic viral HF if neurologic syndrome not prominent.
Bacteria	
Typhoid fever	Hemorrhagic manifestations other than bloody diarrhea generally not seen. Responds to antibiotics.
Bacillary dysentery (including shigellosis, campylobacteriosis, salmonellosis, and enterohemorrhagic *Escherichia coli* and others)	Hemorrhagic manifestations other than bloody diarrhea generally not seen. Respond to antibiotics.
Meningococcemia	Bacterial-induced DIC may mimic the bleeding diathesis of viral HF. Large ecchymoses typical of meningococcemia are unusual in the viral HFs except for CCHF. May respond to antibiotics.
Staphylococcemia	Bacterial-induced DIC may mimic the bleeding diathesis of viral HF. May respond to antibiotics.
Septicemic plague	Bacterial-induced DIC may mimic the bleeding diathesis of viral HF. Large ecchymoses typical of plague are unusual in the viral HFs except for CCHF. May respond to antibiotics.
Streptococcal pharyngitis (may mimic the exudative pharyngitis sometimes seen in Lassa fever)	
Tularemia	
Acute abdominal emergencies (appendicitis and peritonitis)	
Pyelonephritis and post-streptococcal glomerulonephritis (may mimic HF with renal syndrome)	
Anthrax (inhalation or gastrointestinal)	
Psittacosis	Pulmonary symptoms often not present until late in the illness. Responds to antibiotics.

Table 6.3 (continued)

Disease	Distinguishing Characteristics and Comments
Viruses	
Influenza	Prominent respiratory component to clinical presentation. No hemorrhagic manifestations. Influenza rapid test may be positive. May respond to anti-influenza drugs.
Arbovirus infection (including dengue, yellow fever, and West Nile fever)	Encephalitis unusual, but when present may mimic the viral HFs with significant neurologic involvement (Kyasanur forest disease, Omsk HF). Usually less severe than viral HF. Hemorrhage not reported.
Viral hepatitis (including hepatitis A, B, and E, Epstein-Barr, and cytomegalovirus)	Jaundice atypical in HF except YF. Serologic tests for hepatitis positive.
Measles	Rash may mimic that seen in early stages of some viral HFs. Prominence of coryza and upper respiratory symptoms in measles should help differentiate. Vaccine preventable.
Rubella	Rash may mimic that seen in early stages of some viral HFs. Usually a mild disease. Vaccine preventable.
Hemorrhagic or flat smallpox	Diffuse hemorrhagic or macular lesions. In contrast to the viral HFs, the rash may involve the oral mucosa, palms, and soles. Smallpox in the wild has been eradicated.
Alphavirus infection (including chikungunya and o'nyong-nyong)	
Other viral HFs	Recent travel to tropics (YF, dengue HF). Jaundice common in YF but atypical in the other viral HFs. See Tables 6.1–6.3.
Spirochetes, Rickettsia, Ehrlichia, and Coxiella	
Relapsing fever	Recurrent fevers and flu-like symptoms, with direct neurologic involvement and splenomegaly. Spirochetes visible in blood while febrile. Responds to antibiotics.
Leptospirosis	Jaundice, renal failure, and myocarditis in severe cases. Responds to antibiotics.
Spotted fever group rickettsia (including Rocky Mountain spotted fever, Boutonneuse fever, African tick bite fever)	Necrotic lesion (eschar) at site of tick bite in some forms. Respond to antibiotics.
Typhus group rickettsia (including murine- and louse-borne typhus)	

Table 6.3 (continued)

Disease	Distinguishing Characteristics and Comments
Q fever	
Ehrlichiosis	
Non-infectious etiologies	
Idiopathic and thrombotic thrombocytopenic purpura (ITP/TTP)	Presentation usually less acute than viral HF. May have prominent neurologic symptoms in TTP. Coagulation factors normal and DIC absent. Often respond to corticosteroids (ITP) or plasma exchange (TTP).
Acute glaucoma (may mimic the acute ocular manifestations of Rift Valley fever)	
Leukemia (may resemble the leukemoid reaction occasionally seen in HF with renal syndrome)	

CCHF Crimean-Congo hemorrhagic fever, *DIC* disseminated intravascular coagulopathy, *HF* hemorrhagic fever, *YF* yellow fever

develop in RVF [76]. Deafness during convalescence is frequently noted after Lassa virus infection and has also been reported in Venezuelan HF [72, 75]. Common indicators of a poor prognosis include shock, bleeding, neurological manifestations, high viremia (or surrogate measurements of antigen or genome copies), and elevated levels of aspartate aminotransferase (>150 IU/L). Maternal and fetal mortality are elevated in pregnancy, especially during the third trimester [77–79]. However, mild and even asymptomatic cases have been reported even for what are considered the most virulent viral HFs. Reasons for the heterogeneity in severity are largely unknown, although differences in route and dose of infection, underlying comorbid illness, and genetic predisposition have been postulated. An association between certain major histocompatibility markers and severity of disease has been reported for hantavirus infections [184].

Common clinical laboratory findings are summarized in Table 6.5. Although data are limited, radiographic and EKG findings appear to be nonspecific and usually correlate with the physical exam [80, 81].

6.5.2 Bioterrorism Presentation

Bioterrorism strategies that rely on propagation through the usual contact with body fluids would be expected to result in a clinical presentation identical to that noted during naturally occurring outbreaks. If supra-normal infectious doses could be generated, the course of the disease would likely be accelerated.

Table 6.4 Clinical aspects of viral hemorrhagic fevers

Disease	Incubation period (days)	Onset	Bleeding	Rash	Jaundice	Heart	Lung	Kidney	CNS	Eye	Clinical Management
Filoviridae											
Ebola HF	3–21	Abrupt	+ +	+ + +	+	+ +?	+	+	+	+	Supportive
Marburg HF	3–21	Abrupt	+ +	+ + +	+	+ +?	+	+	+	+	Supportive
Arenaviridae											
Lassa fever	5–16	Gradual	+	+ +	0	+ +	+	0	+	0	Ribavirin
South American HFs[a]	7–14	Gradual	+ + +	0	0	+ +	+	0	+ + +	0	Convalescent plasma, ribavirin
Bunyaviridae											
HF with renal syndrome	9–35	Abrupt	+ + +	0	0	+ +	+	+ + +	+	0	Ribavirin
Rift Valley fever[b]	2–5	Abrupt	+ + +	+	+ +	+?	0	+	+ +	+ +	Ribavirin?
Crimean-Congo HF	3–12	Abrupt	+ + +	0	+ +	+?	+	0	+	0	Ribavirin
Flaviviridae											
Yellow fever	3–6	Abrupt	+ + +	0	+ + +	+ +	+	+ +	+ +	0	Supportive
Dengue HF	3–15	Abrupt	+ +	+ + +	+	+ +	+	0	+	0	Supportive
Omsk HF	3–8	Abrupt	+ +	0	0	+	+ +	0	+ + +	+	Supportive
Kyasanur forest disease	3–8	Abrupt	+ +	0	0	+	+ +	0	+ + +	+	Supportive
Alkhumra HF[c]	3–8	Abrupt	+ +	+	+	+	+	0	+ +	+	Supportive

HF hemorrhagic fever, *0* sign not typically noted/organ not typically affected, + sign occasionally noted/organ occasionally affected, + + sign commonly noted/organ commonly affected, + + + sign characteristic/organ involvement severe.

[a] Data are insufficient to distinguish between Argentine, Bolivian, Venezuelan, and Brazilian HF. They are thus frequently grouped as the "South American hemorrhagic fevers."

[b] HF, encephalitis, and retinitis may be seen in Rift Valley fever independently of each other

[c] Based on preliminary observations. Less than 100 cases have been reported

Table 6.5 Clinical laboratory findings in the viral hemorrhagic fevers. Laboratory derangements are estimated by arrows on a 1–3 scale, with 1 being occasional or mild and three indicating characteristic and often severe

Disease	Platelets	Leukocyte count	Clotting times (PT/PTT)	DIC	Transaminases	Azotemia
Filoviridae						
Ebola and Marburg HF	↓↓↓	↓/↑	↑↑	↑↑	↑↑	↑↑
Arenaviridae						
Lassa fever	↓ (with impaired aggregation)	↓	↑	↑	↑	↑
South American HFs	↓↓↓ (with impaired aggregation)	↓↓↓	↑↑	↑	↑	↑
Bunyaviridae						
HF with renal syndrome	↓↓↓ (with impaired aggregation)	↑↑	↑↑	↑↑	↑	↑↑↑
Rift Valley fever	↓↓↓	↓↓	↑↑	↑↑	↑↑	↑↑
Crimean-Congo HF	↓↓↓	↓↓	↑↑↑	↑↑↑	↑↑↑	↑↑
Flaviviridae						
Yellow fever	↓↓ (with impaired aggregation)	↓↓	↑↑	↑↑	↑↑↑ (also ↑↑↑ bilirubin)	↑↑
Dengue HF	↓↓↓ (with impaired aggregation)	↓↓ (neutropenia, atypical lymphocytes)	↑↑	↑↑	↑↑	↑
Omsk HF, Kyasanur Forest disease, Alkhumra HF	↓↓	↓↓	↑	↑?	↑↑	↑

PT prothrombin time, *PTT* partial thromboplastin time, *DIC* disseminated intravascular coagulopathy, *CSF* cerebrospinal fluid, *CNS* central nervous system

A bioengineered virus causing aerosol infection might be expected to result in more predominant pulmonary symptoms and infiltrates than typically seen, especially early in the course. Interestingly, in recent experiments of aerosol challenge of filoviruses in non-human primates, the disease course appeared to be slightly delayed realtive to that seen with intramuscular challenge (Thomas Geisbert, personal communication).

6.5.3 Differential Diagnosis

The nonspecific clinical presentation of most viral HFs makes them extremely difficult to diagnose clinically, especially early in the course of the disease when hemorrhage is usually absent. The differential diagnosis includes a broad array of febrile illnesses (Table 6.3). The situation becomes even more complex in the bioterrorism context when the most valuable clues – a history of recent travel to an endemic area, exposure to exotic animals, or possible laboratory exposure to the HF viruses – are eliminated, although this would also readily allow the exclusion from the differential diagnosis of many other tropical pathogens as long as they are not also considered potential agents of bioterrorism.

6.5.4 Laboratory Diagnosis

Consultation with an infectious disease specialist and local and federal public health officials should occur as soon as a diagnosis of viral HF is entertained. The difficulty in making a clinical diagnosis makes prompt laboratory testing imperative [82]. Enzyme-linked immunosorbent assays (ELISA) for viral antigen and specific IgM and the reverse transcriptase polymerase chain reaction (RT-PCR) form the mainstay of diagnosis [83–90]. Although generally associated with sensitivities and specificities of over 90%, the rarity of most viral HFs has precluded extensive standardization and validation [91]. Immunofluorescent antibody tests may also be employed, but are not as routinely sensitive or specific [83, 92]. Due to their sensitivity, careful attention should be paid to the potential for laboratory contamination resulting in false-positive results on RT-PCR, especially considering the significant ramifications of such false alarms in the bioterrorism context. Sequencing of PCR products to distinguish them from reference strains, targeting different portions of the genome, and/or the use of multiple supporting diagnostic methods can minimize the risk. Post mortem diagnosis for many viral HFs can be established by pathology examination with immunohistochemical staining of formalin fixed tissue [93, 94]. Research aimed at increasing the rapidity, sensitivity, and specificity of diagnostic assays for the viral HFs is ongoing. Assays under investigation include various forms of real-time and multiplex PCR, immunoblot tests, flow cytometry, and microarrays [87, 88, 95–98].

6.6 Therapeutic Interventions

Treatment of the viral HFs can be divided into four categories: general supportive measures, specific antiviral drugs, convalescent immune plasma, and immunomodulating drugs (Table 6.4). Detailed guidelines for clinical management can be found in recent publication [185, 186].

6.6.1 Supportive Measures

The treatment of most viral HFs is supportive. Management should take place in an intensive care unit if possible, since a patient's clinical status may abruptly and rapidly deteriorate. Electrolytes should be monitored closely, as third spacing, vomiting, diarrhea, and decreased fluid intake may result in significant imbalance. Judicious use of electrolyte and colloid containing solutions, supplemental oxygen, blood products, vasopressor agents, and hemodialysis may all be indicated. The anorexia, vomiting, and diarrhea of viral HF frequently result in hypokalemia, so regular potassium supplementation may be needed [Rollin, P.E., unpublised data]. Intramuscular and subcutaneous injections and the use of salicylates and non-steroidal anti-inflammatory drugs should be avoided if possible because of the risk of bleeding. Although invasive hemodynamic monitoring through the placement of arterial or a Swan-Ganz catheter would seem to be in order, with the exception of peripheral intravenous lines, indwelling vascular devices should probably be considered contraindicated due to the risk of bleeding at the site, although they have been occasionally placed without reported complications. The decision whether to place an indwelling catheter or reply on blood pressure cuff values should probably be made on a case-by-case basis.

Opiates or other analgesics for pain, and psychoactive or sedative medications such as diphenhydramine or benzodiazepines for agitation may be indicated. Careful attention must be present to these medications' potential to aggravate hypotension through their vasodilatory side effects. Anti-epileptic medications can be indicated in patients with advanced diseased who seize or show signs of hypertonicity, but should not be given empirically. It is reasonable to cover a patient suspected of having a viral HF with appropriate antibacterial and/or antiparasitic therapy until the diagnosis can be confirmed or when secondary infection is suspected. Uterine evacuation may be effective in decreasing maternal mortality in pregnant women with viral HFs [77–79].

The fluid management of patients with viral HFs poses a particular challenge. Vascular instability and permeability dictate a need for aggressive fluid replacement, which may also prevent disseminated intravascular coagulopathy. Over-aggressive and unmonitored rehydration, however, may lead to significant third spacing and pulmonary edema, especially given the decreased cardiac function in some viral HFs. Early use of vasopressors when blood pressure support is required may diminish the risk of fluid overload. Internal bleeding may be difficult to recognize. A 10% drop in hematocrit once fluid balance has been achieved should be taken as a sign of significant internal bleeding meriting transfusion. Careful diuresis may be needed to avoid pulmonary edema during the transfusion.

6.6.2 Antiviral Drugs

The arenavirus infections and CCHF are the only viral HFs for which an effective antiviral drug, the guanosine analogue ribavirin, is known. The most data are available for the arenaviruses, especially Lassa fever, for which intravenous ribavirin given within the first 6 days of illness reduced mortality from 55% to around 5% [99–103]. Ribavirin has in vitro activity against CCHF virus and appears to be efficacious in the treatment of clinical disease, although prospective evaluations of ribavirin in CCHF have yet to be undertaken [105–110]. Immune plasma and interferon have sometimes been used in CCHF but no data are available on their efficacy [108]. Ribavirin has in vitro activity against RVF virus and has been shown to be efficacious in some animal models, but use in human infections has met with mixed results [Khan, A.S. personal communication][110]. The drug has in vitro activity against Omsk HF virus as well [116].

The precise mechanism of action of ribavirin is uncertain, but may include both direct antiviral as well as immunomodulatory effects [115, 116]. Extensive investigation of the most efficacious dose has not been undertaken, but most sources recommend the 10-day intravenous regimen employed for Lassa fever, which consists of a single 30 mg/kg loading dose (maximum 2 g) followed by 16 mg/kg (maximum 1 g) every 6 h for 4 days and then 8 mg/kg (maximum 500 mg) every 8 h for 6 days [100]. The main side effect of ribavirin is a reversible, dose-dependent, mild-to-moderate hemolytic anemia that infrequently necessitates transfusion. Although conflicting results have been reported, findings of teratogenicity and fetal loss in rodent experiments have rendered ribavirin technically contraindicated in pregnancy [117–120]. Its use in pregnant women, however, must still be considered given the extremely high maternal and fetal mortality associated with most viral HFs.

Despite its potential benefits, treatment with intravenous ribavirin is fraught with significant logistical problems. The intravenous form of the drug is available for the viral HFs only on a compassionate use, investigational new drug format. The sole producer in the United States is ICN pharmaceuticals in Costa Mesa, California. Supplies of intravenous ribavirin are limited, making the drug unlikely to be available in sufficient speed or quantity in response to a bioterrorism event of any significant magnitude unless ribavirin is included in the strategic national stockpile. Commercially available oral ribavirin has been advocated as a substitute, but there are few data on the drug's efficacy in this format.

No specific antiviral therapy is available for the filoviruses or flaviviruses, although various chemical compounds are under study [121–127].

6.6.3 Convalescent Immune Plasma

Transfusion of appropriately titered immune plasma appears to be effective in the arenavirus infections, reducing the case-fatality rate of Argentine HF from

15% to 30% to less than 1% when administered within the first 8 days after symptom onset [130, 131]. However, the use of immune plasma in the treatment of Argentine HF has been associated with a convalescent phase neurologic syndrome characterized by fever, cerebellar signs, and cranial nerve palsies in 10% of those treated [130, 132]. The syndrome occurs after a period of 7–80 days (mean 20 days) after recovery and differs from the neurologic manifestations seen in the acute disease. Immune plasma may be of benefit in Lassa fever if the plasma has a high titer of neutralizing antibody and is appropriately matched to the infecting strain [133–137]. Although successful in some mouse and guinea pig models, the most well controlled investigations of immune plasma for treatment of the filoviruses in nonhuman primates have not shown the therapy to be efficacious [138–145]. Transfusion of whole blood from convalescent patients with Ebola HF appeared to reduce mortality, but conclusions on the treatment's efficacy are clouded by the fact that most transfusions occurred after the typical mean time to death for fatal Ebola HF and after many patients had already begun making antibody [146]. This strategy has not been shown protective in studies with nonhuman primates [147]. Few data are available on the use of immune plasma for CCHF or RVF, although it appears to be efficacious [109, 148].

The use of immune plasma for the viral HFs is complicated by significant logistical challenges. Sera must contain a high titer of neutralizing antibody to the specific viral HF in question, which is not always the case even in survivors, and sometimes must even be matched to the geographic source of the infecting strain [137]. No such bank of immune plasma is presently available nor could be collected from populations in North America or Europe where, with the exception of Seoul hantavirus and CCHF, none of the HF viruses are endemic. The risk of transmission of blood-borne pathogens such as HIV and the hepatitis viruses with immune therapy is also a concern. Given these challenges, it is unlikely that a strategy of large-scale treatment with immune plasma could be undertaken. Animal sources of targeted hyperimmune serum might be sought, but their efficacy has not yet been shown and the logistics of production and cold storage would be formidable.

6.6.4 Immunomodulating Drugs

Recent advances in the understanding of the pathogenesis of shock and hemorrhage have engendered new therapeutic strategies aimed at modulating the underlying immune processes inherent in most severe shock syndromes, including the viral HFs [149–151]. A key realization is that inflammation, derangements in the coagulation cascade, and shock are often linked [152]. One of the advantages of this syndromic approach is that it could allow effective treatment to be initiated prior to the identification of the specific offending pathogen. Administration of a recombinant inhibitor of factor VIIa/tissue factor to Ebola virus-infected rhesus monkeys diminished mortality by 33% and should be tested in the viral HFs in which DIC appears to play a major role (Table 6.5) [153]. Activated protein C has been shown to be effective in humans with septic shock and plans are underway to evaluate its efficacy in nonhuman primates experimentally infected with filoviruses [154]. Various other immunomodulatory compounds, including interferon and anti-tumor necrosis factor, have also undergone limited investigation in various viral HFs [144, 155–160]. Clinical trials have not been undertaken for the use of heparin or corticosteroids in most viral HFs. Until proven otherwise, steroids should best be considered contra-indicated, with the exception of their administration along with mannitol should signs of cerebral edema develop.

The difficulty in rapid clinical diagnosis and distinguishing one viral HF from another and the lack of availability of intravenous ribavirin and immune plasma make empiric therapy difficult. Until a regular supply of these products and algorithms for their use are established, treatment should be reserved for laboratory confirmed cases.

6.7 Preventative Measures and Infection Control

6.7.1 Prophylaxis

Ribavirin is the only drug potentially indicated for post-exposure prophylaxis for the HF viruses although there are no data on efficacy, dose, or duration of administration of the drug for this purpose. Given the necessity for direct contact with blood and body fluids for transmission of HF viruses, the generally low secondary attack rates, the risk of adverse effects (most often nausea and vomiting), and the lack of efficacy data, the administration of post-exposure ribavirin should be reserved for those with clear direct unprotected contact with blood or bodily fluids from a person with a confirmed symptomatic arenavirus, CCHF, or RVF virus infection. This applies most often to family members and healthcare workers in contact with an infected person prior to diagnosis. Doses of oral ribavirin for post-exposure prophylaxis have not been standardized and range from 1 to 4 g total per day divided into two or four doses, usually for a duration of 10 days. Various experimental vaccines show promise for use as prophylaxis for the filoviruses, but probably would need to be administered within hours after exposure to have effect [187].

6.7.2 Patient Isolation

Infection control of the HF viruses relies on classic public health principles of isolation of infected persons. Given the difficulty of clinical diagnosis, all patients with a syndrome clinically compatible with a viral HF should be presumed infectious and isolated until a specific diagnosis is made. Although specific viral

HF isolation precautions to prevent parenteral and droplet exposure to blood and body fluids are advised for added security, experience has shown that the observance of routine strict universal precautions is probably protective in most cases [22, 161, 162]. The effectiveness of such simple precautions tends to deteriorate, however, when the limits of the surge capacity are reached. Despite the lack of evidence for natural aerosol transmission between humans, it is prudent to place the patient in a negative airflow room when available. Small particle aerosol precautions, such as the use of HEPA filter masks, should be employed when performing procedures that may generate aerosols, such as endotracheal intubation. Disinfection of items coming into direct contact with the patient, including chemical or heat inactivation of human waste, is advised.

6.7.3 Contact Tracing

Persons with unprotected direct contact with someone during the symptomatic phase of a viral HF should be followed daily for evidence of disease for the duration of the longest possible incubation period. Those who develop fever or other signs and symptoms suggestive of viral HF should be immediately isolated until the diagnosis of viral HF can be ruled out.

6.7.4 Vaccines

Vaccines for the viral HFs are considered to be in the experimental stages. The Candid #1 live attenuated vaccine is effective in decreasing the morbidity and mortality of Argentine HF and may also protect against Bolivian and the other South American HFs [163]. The vaccine is not approved in the United States, however, and supplies are insufficient even in Argentina, the sole country in which the vaccine is produced. A trial of an adenovirus-vectored vaccine expressing the glyco- and nucleoproteins of Ebola virus has been shown to be protective in nonhuman primates [164]. Phase I human trials are planned. A vaccinia virus-vectored vaccine expressing Lassa virus glycoproteins has also proved protective in studies in nonhuman primates [165]. Although approved for human use, the formalin inactivated vaccine for RVF is not generally available [166, 167]. A live attenuated vaccine for RVF has been tested in both ruminants and nonhuman primates, with promising results [168–170]. A formalin inactivated Kyasanur forest disease appears to be effective [171].

6.7.5 Environmental Clean-up

There is virtually no published literature on the airflow dynamics or viability of the HF viruses once released into the environment, especially data that could be applied outside of the laboratory, as would be required for the sanitation of a contaminated environment after a bioterrorism attack. The lipid envelope of the HF viruses is generally easily disrupted. The survival of arenaviruses in rodent urine is probably affected by factors such as the animal's diet, and urinary pH and protein. The environmental stability of most HF viruses shed naturally in body fluids, which would then dry, appears to be on the order of hours to days [33, 188]. Viruses can be inactivated by exposure to temperatures above 60°C, disinfectants containing phenolic compounds, hypochlorite, quaternary amines, acidic or basic pH, ultraviolet light, gamma irradiation and surfactant nanoemulsions [28, 172–176]. However, HF viruses have been isolated from samples kept for weeks at ambient temperatures if stored hydrated in a biological buffer, such as blood or serum [115]. Freeze drying of pure virus cultures could potentially produce a stable concentrate which could be surreptitiously transported and reconstituted [39].

6.8 Surveillance

6.8.1 Human Disease

The early nonspecific presentation of the viral HFs poses a serious challenge to effective epidemiologic surveillance. Circulation of a HF virus as a bioterrorist act may be detected by rigorous syndromic surveillance for clusters of patients with compatible syndromes or by recognition of a single case by a clinician [177]. Critical components of such a surveillance system should include:

1. astute clinicians armed with an appropriate index of suspicion, and sound knowledge of the epidemiology and clinical presentation of the viral HFs;
2. ready access to consultants and other up-to-date information for guidance; and
3. a mechanism for real-time integration of data from diverse sources to readily detect trends.

It should be considered that many patients may initially seek care in ambulatory facilities and thus may not be registered by hospital based surveillance systems. The difficult task will be striking a balance between the high number of false alarms that would result from clusters of the early nonspecific HF syndrome, which may be easily confused with many other diseases, and delayed detection if one waits for the more specific manifestations. The size and dispersion of the population in question along with the season (such as influenza season or not) will be significant factors [177].

Surveillance aimed at the detection of disease in the early stages should focus on patients presenting with worsening febrile systemic syndromes accompanied by leucopenia, thrombocytopenia, and elevated hepatic transaminases, although it must be recognized that even these characteristics are not uniform to all viral HFs (Table 6.5). Inclusion of a rash in the case definition would add to the specificity of the diagnosis, but sacrifice sensitivity. Leucocytosis, bleeding, shock, and multi-organ failure would be more obvious clues as disease progresses. Bioterrorism should be suspected if the above clinical criteria are fulfilled in the absence a history of travel or work-related exposure to HF viruses.

6.8.2 Environmental Sampling

The absence of endemic transmission of most HF viruses in North America and Europe makes environmental sampling a theoretically useful tool for the detection of the release of such agents for malicious aims in these areas, perhaps using microarrays or real-time PCR. The specificity of these tests would have to be high to avoid the considerable alarm and expenditure of resources which a false-positive result would initiate.

6.9 How Likely is a Bioterrorist Attack with a HF Virus?

Perhaps even more than for the other potential agents of bioterrorism, the likelihood of use of a HF virus as a biological weapon is virtually impossible to predict. Setting public health priorities as well as providing guidance for the individual healthcare worker classically relies on a thorough analysis of the risk a given disease poses to the population. Precise quantification of risks from the deliberately clandestine activities of bioterrorists is obviously difficult, however, and opinions vary from the alarmist to the dismissive, even among experts [178–181].

On one hand, the relative rarity and instability of most HF viruses in nature (especially the more virulent ones), low secondary attack rates, lack of natural aerosol transmissibility between humans, high public profile, and relative virulence for those performing unprotected manipulation would seem to make the HF viruses a poor choice for would-be terrorists, at least in the absence of the most sophisticated and well funded network. The manipulation of HF viruses and delivery mechanisms to invoke large-scale dissemination and fatality would likely require a degree of knowledge and technology presently known to exist in only a handful of sites worldwide. Furthermore, most HF viruses have never been widely disseminated in research laboratories, making them relatively difficult to obtain and clandestinely develop, although the development of reverse genetic systems, through which a HF virus could potentially be created, is a concern.

On the other hand, the dangers of pathogens generally associated with high case-fatality ratios, a rapid progression of disease, and the absence of a readily available therapy or vaccine should not be underestimated. Furthermore, the absence of an endemic presence of most HF viruses in industrialized countries of North America and Europe presumably renders virtually 100% of their populations immunologically naïve and thus susceptible. Regardless of the actual biological risk presently attributable to use of the HF viruses for bioterrorism, the potential for widespread panic and diversion of resources due to the fear that the viral HFs invoke cannot be overlooked [182]. Fortunately, intensive research over the last decade shows promise for improved detection methods, treatment, and vaccine prevention for the viral HFs that may soon be of benefit to those concerned with their potential use in bioterrorism as well as in areas of endemic transmission.

References

1. Centers for Disease Control and Prevention. Emergency Preparedness and Response, Bioterrorism Agents/Diseases. Centers for Disease Control and Prevention, Atlanta, GA; 2004.
2. Bausch, D. G. and Ksiazek, T. G. Viral hemorrhagic fevers including hantavirus pulmonary syndrome in the Americas. Clin. Lab. Med. 22,981–1020, 2002.
3. Peters, C. J. and Zaki, S. R. Viral hemorrhagic fevers: an overview. In: Guerrant, R. L., Walker, D. H. and Weller, P. F., editors. Tropical Infectious Diseases: Principles, Pathogens, and Practice. W.B. Saunders Co., New York, NY; 1999, p. 1180–1188.
4. Alibek, K. and Handelman, S. Biohazard, 1st edn. Random House, New York; 1999.
5. Buchmeier, M. and Bowen, M. Arenaviridae: The viruses and their replication. In: Fields' Virology, 4th edn. Lippincott, Williams, and Wilkins, Philadelphia, PA; 2001, p. 1635–1668.
6. Ksiazek, T. G., Rollin, P. E., Williams, A. J., et al. Clinical virology of Ebola hemorrhagic fever (EHF): virus, virus antigen, and IgG and IgM antibody findings among EHF patients in Kikwit, Democratic Republic of the Congo, 1995. J. Infect. Dis. 179 Suppl 1,S177–S187, 1999.
7. Bowen, M. D., Peters, C. J. . Nichol, S. T. Phylogenetic analysis of the Arenaviridae: patterns of virus evolution and evidence for cospeciation between arenaviruses and their rodent hosts. Mol. Phylogenet. Evol. 8,301–16, 1997.
8. Johnson, K. M., Kuns, M. L., Mackenzie, R. B., et al. Isolation of Machupo virus from wild rodent *Calomys callosus*. Am. J. Trop. Med. Hyg. 15,103–106, 1966.
9. Fulhorst, C. F., Bowen, M. D., Salas, R. A., et al. Natural rodent host associations of Guanarito and Pirital viruses (family Arenaviridae) in central Venezuela. Am. J. Trop. Med. Hyg. 61,325–330, 1999.
10. Childs, J. E. and Peters, C. J. Ecology and epidemiology of arenaviruses and their hosts. In: Salvato, M. S., editor. The Arenaviridae. Plenum Press, New York; 1993, p. 331–384.
11. Mills, J. N., Bowen, M. D. and Nichol, S. T. African arenaviruses – coevolution between virus and murid host? Belg. J. Zool. 127,19–28, 1997.
12. McCormick, J. B. and Fisher-Hoch, S. P. Lassa fever. Curr. Top. Microbiol. Immunol. 262:75–109, 2002.
13. Fulhorst, C. F., Ksiazek, T. G., Peters, C. J. and Tesh, R. B. Experimental infection of the cane mouse *Zygodontomys brevicauda* (family Muridae) with Guanarito virus (Arenaviridae), the etiologic agent of Venezuelan hemorrhagic fever. J. Infect. Dis. 180,966–969, 1999.
14. Stephenson, E. H., Larson, E. W. and Dominik, J. W. Effect of environmental factors on aerosol-induced Lassa virus infection. J. Med. Virol. 14,295–303, 1984.
15. Kenyon, R. H., McKee, K. T., Jr., Zack, P. M., et al. Aerosol infection of rhesus macaques with Junin virus. Intervirology 33,23–31, 1992.

16. ter Meulen, J., Lukashevich, I., Sidibe, K., et al. Hunting of peridomestic rodents and consumption of their meat as possible risk factors for rodent-to-human transmission of Lassa virus in the Republic of Guinea. Am. J. Trop. Med. Hyg. 55,661–666, 1996.
17. Rai, S. K., Micales, B. K., Wu, M. S., et al. Timed appearance of Lymphocytic Choriomeningitis virus after gastric inoculation of mice. Am. J. Pathol. 151, 633–639, 1997.
18. Towner, J. S., Pourrut, X., Albarino, C. G. et al. Marburg virus infection detected in a common African bat. PLoS ONE 2:e764, 2007.
19. Swanepoel, R., Smit, S. B., Rollin, P. E., et al. Studies of reservoir hosts for Marburg virus. Emerg. Infect. Dis. 12,1847–1851, 2007.
20. Leroy, E. M., Kumulungui, B., Pourrut, X., et al. Fruit bats as reservoirs of Ebola virus. Nature 438,575–576, 2005.
21. Dowell, S. F., Mukunu, R., Ksiazek, T. G., et al. Transmission of Ebola hemorrhagic fever: a study of risk factors in family members, Kikwit, Democratic Republic of the Congo, 1995. Commission de Lutte contre les Epidemies a Kikwit. J. Infect. Dis. 179 (Suppl 1),S87–S91, 1999.
22. Fisher-Hoch, S. Stringent precautions are not advisable when caring for patients with viral haemorrhagic fevers. Med. Virol. 3,7–13, 1993.
23. Centers for Disease Control. Crimean-Congo hemorrhagic fever – Republic of South Africa. MMWR Morb. Mortal. Wkly. Rep. 34,94,99–101, 1985.
24. Burney, M. I., Ghafoor, A., Saleen, M., et al. Nosocomial outbreak of viral hemorrhagic fever caused by Crimean hemorrhagic fever-Congo virus in Pakistan, January 1976. Am. J. Trop. Med. Hyg. 29,941–947, 1980.
25. Khan, A. S., Tshioko, F. K., Heymann, D. L., et al. The reemergence of Ebola hemorrhagic fever, Democratic Republic of the Congo, 1995. Commission de Lutte contre les Epidemies a Kikwit. J. Infect. Dis. 179 (Suppl 1),S76–S86, 1999.
26. Jaax, N. K., Davis, K. J., Geisbert, T. J., et al. Lethal experimental infection of rhesus monkeys with Ebola-Zaire (Mayinga) virus by the oral and conjunctival route of exposure. Arch. Pathol. Lab. Med. 120,140–155, 1996.
27. Centers for Disease Control and Prevention. Outbreak of Ebola hemorrhagic fever Uganda, August 2000-January 2001. MMWR Morb. Mortal. Wkly. Rep. 50,73–77, 2001.
28. Chepurnov, A. A., Chuev Iu, P., P'Iankov, O. V. and Efimova, I. V. The effect of some physical and chemical factors on inactivation of the Ebola virus (Russian). Vopr. Virusol. 40,74–76, 1995.
29. Bausch, D. G., Towner, J. S., Dowell, S. F., Kaducu, F., et al. Assessment of the risk of Ebola virus transmission from bodily fluids and fomites. *J Infect Dis* 196 (Suppl 2),S142–S147, 2007.
30. Bray, M., Davis, K., Geisbert, T., et al. A mouse model for evaluation of prophylaxis and therapy of Ebola hemorrhagic fever. J. Infect. Dis. 179 (Suppl 1),S248–S258, 1999.
31. Mahanty, S., Gupta, M., Paragas, J., et al. Protection from lethal infection is determined by innate immune responses in a mouse model of Ebola virus infection. Virology 312,415–424, 2003.
32. Lukashevich, I. S., Djavani, M., Rodas, J. D., et al. Hemorrhagic fever occurs after intravenous, but not after intragastric, inoculation of rhesus macaques with lymphocytic choriomeningitis virus. J. Med. Virol. 67,171–186, 2002.
33. Belanov, E. F., Muntyanov, V. P., Kryuk, D., et al. Survival of Marburg virus on contaminated surfaces and in aerosol (Russian). Prog. Virol. 1:47–50, 1997.
34. World Health Organization. Ebola haemorrhagic fever in Sudan, 1976. Report of a WHO/International study team. Bull. World Health Organ. 56,247–270, 1978.
35. World Health Organization. Ebola haemorrhagic fever in Zaire, 1976. Bull. World Health Organ. 56,271–293, 1978.

36. Baron, R. C., McCormick, J. B. and Zubeir, O. A. Ebola virus disease in southern Sudan: hospital dissemination and intrafamilial spread. Bull. World Health Organ. 61,997–1003, 1983.
37. Ndambi, R., Akamituna, P., Bonnet, M. J., et al. Epidemiologic and clinical aspects of the Ebola virus epidemic in Mosango, Democratic Republic of the Congo, 1995. J. Infect. Dis. 179 (Suppl 1),S8–S10, 1999.
38. Pokhodiaev, V. A., Gonchar, N. I. and Pshenichnov, V. A. An experimental study of the contact transmission of the Marburg virus (Russian). Vopr. Virusol. 36,506–508, 1991.
39. Bazhutin, N. B., Belanov, E. F., Spiridonov, V. A., et al. The influence of the methods of experimental infection with Marburg virus on the course of illness in green monkeys (Russian). Vopr. Virusol. 37,153–156, 1992.
40. Johnson, E., Jaax, N., White, J. and Jahrling, P. Lethal experimental infections of rhesus monkeys by aerosolized Ebola virus. Int. J. Exp. Pathol. 76,227–236, 1995.
41. Jaax, N., Jahrling, P., Geisbert, T., et al. Transmission of Ebola virus (Zaire strain) to uninfected control monkeys in a biocontainment laboratory. Lancet 346, 1669–1671, 1995.
42. Miller, W. S., Demchak, P., Rosenberger, C. R., et al. Stability and infectivity of airborne yellow fever and Rift Valley fever viruses. Am. J. Hyg. 77,114–121, 1963.
43. Jahrling, P. B., Geisbert, T. W., Jaax, N. K., et al. Experimental infection of cynomolgus macaques with Ebola-Reston filoviruses from the 1989–1990 U.S. epizootic. Arch. Virol. 11 (Suppl),115–134, 1996.
44. McKinney, R. W., Barkley, W. E. and Wedum, A. G. The hazards of infectious agents in microbiological laboratories. In: Block, S. S., editor. Disinfections, Sterilization, and Preservation, 4th edn. Lea and Febiger, Philadelphia, PA; 1991, p. 748–756.
45. Carey, D. E., Kemp, G. E., White, H. A., et al. Lassa fever. Epidemiological aspects of the 1970 epidemic, Jos, Nigeria. Trans. R. Soc. Trop. Med. Hyg. 66,402–408, 1972.
46. Suleiman, M. N., Muscat-Baron, J. M., Harries, J. R., et al. Congo/Crimean haemorrhagic fever in Dubai. An outbreak at the Rashid Hospital. Lancet 2,939–941, 1980.
47. Mackenzie, R. B. Epidemiology of Machupo virus infection. I. Pattern of human infection, San Joaquin, Bolivia, 1962–1964. Am. J. Trop. Med. Hyg. 14,808–813, 1965.
48. Weissenbacher, M. C., Sabattini, M. S., Avila, M. M., et al. Junin virus activity in two rural populations of the Argentine hemorrhagic fever (AHF) endemic area. J. Med. Virol. 12,273–280, 1983.
49. Muyembe-Tamfum, J. J., Kipasa, M., Kiyungu, C. and Colebunders, R. Ebola outbreak in Kikwit, Democratic Republic of the Congo: discovery and control measures. J. Infect. Dis. 179 (Suppl 1),S259–262, 1999.
50. Fisher-Hoch, S. P., Tomori, O., Nasidi, A., et al. Review of cases of nosocomial Lassa fever in Nigeria: the high price of poor medical practice. Br. Med. J. 311,857–859, 1995.
51. Gear, J. S., Cassel, G. A., Gear, A. J., et al. Outbreak of Marburg virus disease in Johannesburg. Br. Med. J. 4,489–493, 1975.
52. Gunther, S., Emmerich, P., Laue, T., et al. Imported Lassa fever in Germany: molecular characterization of a new Lassa virus strain. Emerg. Infect. Dis. 6,466–476, 2000.
53. Formenty, P., Hatz, C., Le Guenno, B., et al. Human infection due to Ebola virus, subtype Cote d'Ivoire: clinical and biologic presentation. J. Infect. Dis. 179 (Suppl 1), S48–S53, 1999.
54. Richards, G. A., Murphy, S., Jobson, R., et al. Unexpected Ebola virus in a tertiary setting: clinical and epidemiologic aspects. Crit. Care Med. 28,240–244, 2000.
55. Alexander, D. A. Bioterrorism: preparing for the unthinkable. J. R. Army Med. Corps 149,125–130, 2003.
56. Bausch, D. G., Demby, A. H., Coulibaly, M., et al. Lassa fever in Guinea: I. Epidemiology of human disease and clinical observations. Vector Borne Zoonotic Dis. 1, 269–281, 2001.

57. Demby, A. H., Inapogui, A., Kargbo, K., et al. Lassa fever in Guinea: II. Distribution and prevalence of Lassa virus infection in small mammals. Vector Borne Zoonotic Dis. 1, 283–297, 2001.
58. Siegert, R., Shu, H. L. and Slenczka, W. Detection of the "Marburg Virus" in patients. Ger. Med. Mon. 13,521–524, 1968.
59. Martini, G. A., Knauff, H. G., Schmidt, H. A., et al. A hitherto unknown infectious disease contracted from monkeys. "Marburg-virus" disease. Ger. Med. Mon. 13, 457–470, 1968.
60. Reed, K. D., Melski, J. W., Graham, M. B., et al. The detection of monkeypox in humans in the Western Hemisphere. N. Engl. J. Med. 350, 342–350, 2004.
61. Nathan, N., Barry, M., Van Herp, M. and Zeller, H. Shortage of vaccines during a yellow fever outbreak in Guinea. Lancet 358,2129–2130, 2001.
62. Blancou, J. and Pearson, J. E. Bioterrorism and infectious animal diseases. Comp. Immunol. Microbiol. Infect. Dis. 26,431–443, 2003.
63. Meegan, J. M. and Bailey, C. L. Rift Valley fever. In: Monath, T. P., editor. The Arboviruses: Epidemiology and Ecology. CRC, Boca Raton, FL; 1988, p. 51–76.
64. Hoch, A. L., Gargan, T. P., 2nd and Bailey, C. L. Mechanical transmission of Rift Valley fever virus by hematophagous Diptera. Am. J. Trop. Med. Hyg. 34,188–193, 1985.
65. World Health Organisation. Rift Valley fever: an emerging human and animal problem. World Health Organisation, Geneva; 63, 1982, p. 1–69.
66. Cox, C. S. Inactivation kinetics of some microorganisms subjected to a variety of stresses. Appl. Environ. Microbiol. 31,836–846, 1976.
67. Bwaka, M. A., Bonnet, M. J., Calain, P., et al. Ebola hemorrhagic fever in Kikwit, Democratic Republic of the Congo: clinical observations in 103 patients. J. Infect. Dis. 179 (Suppl 1),S1–S7, 1999.
68. McCormick, J. B., King, I. J., Webb, P. A., et al. A case-control study of the clinical diagnosis and course of Lassa fever. J. Infect. Dis. 155,445–455, 1987.
69. Egbring, R., Slenczka, W. and Baltzer, G. Clinical manifestations and mechanism of the haemorrhagic diathesis in Marburg virus disease. In: Martini, G. A. and Siegert, R., editors. Marburg Virus Disease. Springer-Verlag, Berlin; 1971, p. 42–49.
70. Lisieux, T., Coimbra, M., Nassar, E. S., et al. New arenavirus isolated in Brazil. Lancet 343,391–392, 1994.
71. Stinebaugh, B. J., Schloeder, F. X., Johnson, K. M., et al. Bolivian hemorrhagic fever. A report of four cases. Am. J. Med. 40,217–230, 1966.
72. de Manzione, N., Salas, R. A., Paredes, H., et al. Venezuelan hemorrhagic fever: clinical and epidemiological studies of 165 cases. Clin. Infect. Dis. 26,308–313, 1998.
73. Biquard, C., Figini, H. A., Monteverde, D. A., et al. Neurological manifestations of Argentine hemorrhagic fever. Medicina (Buenos Aires) 37 (Suppl. 3),193–199, 1977.
74. Cummins, D., Bennett, D., Fisher-Hoch, S. P., et al. Lassa fever encephalopathy: clinical and laboratory findings. J. Trop. Med. Hyg. 95,197–201, 1992.
75. Cummins, D., McCormick, J. B., Bennett, D., et al. Acute sensorineural deafness in Lassa fever. JAMA 264,2093–2096, 1990.
76. Madani, T. A., Al-Mazrou, Y. Y., Al-Jeffri, M. H., et al. Rift Valley fever epidemic in Saudi Arabia: epidemiological, clinical, and laboratory characteristics. Clin. Infect. Dis. 37,1084–1092, 2003.
77. Briggiler, A. M., Levis, S., Enria, D. A., et al. Fiebre hemorragica Argentina (FHA) en la mujer embarazada (Spanish). Medicina (Buenos Aires) 50,443, 1990.
78. Mupapa, K., Mukundu, W., Bwaka, M. A., et al. Ebola hemorrhagic fever and pregnancy. J. Infect. Dis. 179 (Suppl 1),S11–S12, 1999.
79. Price, M. E., Fisher-Hoch, S. P., Craven, R. B. and McCormick, J. B. A prospective study of maternal and fetal outcome in acute Lassa fever infection during pregnancy. Br. Med. J. 297,584–587,1988.
80. Ketai, L., Alrahji, A. A., Hart, B., et al. Radiologic manifestations of potential bioterrorist agents of infection. Am. J. Roentgenol. 180,565–575, 2003.

81. Smyth, A. G. and Powell, G. M. The electrocardiogram in hemorrhagic fever. Am. Heart J. 47,218–240, 1954.
82. Rotz, L. D., Khan, A. S., Lillibridge, S. R., et al. Public health assessment of potential biological terrorism agents. Emerg. Infect. Dis. 8, 225–230, 2002.
83. Bausch, D. G., Rollin, P. E., Demby, A. H., et al. Diagnosis and clinical virology of Lassa fever as evaluated by enzyme-linked immunosorbent assay, indirect fluorescent-antibody test, and virus isolation. J. Clin. Microbiol. 38,2670–2677, 2000.
84. Ksiazek, T. G., West, C. P., Rollin, P. E., et al. ELISA for the detection of antibodies to Ebola viruses. J. Infect. Dis. 179 (Suppl 1),S192–S198, 1999.
85. Leroy, E. M., Baize, S., Lu, C. Y., et al. Diagnosis of Ebola haemorrhagic fever by RT-PCR in an epidemic setting. J. Med. Virol. 60,463–467, 2000.
86. Niklasson, B., Peters, C. J., Grandien, M. and Wood, O. Detection of human immunoglobulins G and M antibodies to Rift Valley fever virus by enzyme-linked immunosorbent assay. J. Clin. Microbiol. 19,225–229, 1984.
87. Drosten, C., Gottig, S., Schilling, S., et al. Rapid detection and quantification of RNA of Ebola and Marburg viruses, Lassa virus, Crimean-Congo hemorrhagic fever virus, Rift Valley fever virus, dengue virus, and yellow fever virus by real-time reverse transcription-PCR. J. Clin. Microbiol. 40,2323–2330, 2002.
88. Towner, J. S., Rollin, P. E., Bausch, D. G., et al. Rapid diagnosis of Ebola hemorrhagic fever by reverse transcription-PCR in an outbreak setting and assessment of patient viral load as a predictor of outcome. J. Virol. 78,4330–4341, 2004.
89. Palacios, G., Briese, T., Kapoor, V., et al. MassTag polyermase chain reaction for differential diagnosis of viral hemorrhagic fevers. Emerg. Infect. Dis. 12,692–695, 2006.
90. Riera, L. M., Feuillade, M. R., Saavedra, M. C. and Ambrosio, A. M. Evaluation of an enzyme immunosorbent assay for the diagnosis of Argentine haemorrhagic fever. Acta Virol. 41,305–310, 1997.
91. Niedrig, M., Schmitz, H., Becker, S., et al. First international quality assurance study on the rapid detection of viral agents of bioterrorism. J. Clin. Microbiol. 42,1753–1755, 2004.
92. Van der Waals, F. W., Pomeroy, K. L., Goudsmit, J., et al. Hemorrhagic fever virus infections in an isolated rainforest area of central Liberia. Limitations of the indirect immunofluorescence slide test for antibody screening in Africa. Trop. Geogr. Med. 38,209–214, 1986.
93. Zaki, S. R., Shieh, W. J., Greer, P. W., et al. A novel immunohistochemical assay for the detection of Ebola virus in skin: implications for diagnosis, spread, and surveillance of Ebola hemorrhagic fever. Commission de Lutte contre les Epidemies a Kikwit. J. Infect. Dis. 179 (Suppl 1),S36–S47, 1999.
94. Burt, F. J., Swanepoel, R., Shieh, W. J., et al. Immunohistochemical and in situ localization of Crimean-Congo hemorrhagic fever (CCHF) virus in human tissues and implications for CCHF pathogenesis. Arch. Pathol. Lab. Med. 121,839–846, 1997.
95. ter Meulen, J., Koulemou, K., Wittekindt, T., et al. Detection of Lassa virus antinucleoprotein immunoglobulin G (IgG) and IgM antibodies by a simple recombinant immunoblot assay for field use. J. Clin. Microbiol. 36,3143–3148, 1998.
96. Garcia, S., Crance, J. M., Billecocq, A., et al. Quantitative real-time PCR detection of Rift Valley fever virus and its application to evaluation of antiviral compounds. J. Clin. Microbiol. 39,4456–4461, 2001.
97. Gibb, T. R., Norwood, D. A., Jr., Woollen, N. and Henchal, E. A. Development and evaluation of a fluorogenic 5′ nuclease assay to detect and differentiate between Ebola virus subtypes Zaire and Sudan. J. Clin. Microbiol. 39,4125–4130, 2001.
98. Weidmann, M., Muhlberger, E. and Hufert, F. T. Rapid detection protocol for filoviruses. J. Clin. Virol. 30,94–99, 2004.
99. McCormick, J. B., King, I. J., Webb, P. A., et al. Lassa fever. Effective therapy with ribavirin. N. Engl. J. Med. 314,20–26, 1986.

100. Barry, M., Russi, M., Armstrong, L., et al. Brief report: treatment of a laboratory-acquired Sabia virus infection. N. Engl. J. Med. 333,294–296,1995.
101. Kilgore, P. E., Ksiazek, T. G., Rollin, P. E., et al. Treatment of Bolivian hemorrhagic fever with intravenous ribavirin. Clin. Infect. Dis. 24,718–722, 1997.
102. Enria, D. A. and Maiztegui, J. I. Antiviral treatment of Argentine hemorrhagic fever. Antiviral Res. 23,23–31, 1994.
103. McKee, K. T., Jr., Huggins, J. W., Trahan, C. J. and Mahlandt, B. G. Ribavirin prophylaxis and therapy for experimental Argentine hemorrhagic fever. Antimicrob. Agents Chemother. 32,1304–1309, 1988.
104. Watts, D. M., Ussery, M. A., Nash, D. and Peters, C. J. Inhibition of Crimean-Congo hemorrhagic fever viral infectivity yields in vitro by ribavirin. Am. J. Trop. Med. Hyg. 41,581–585, 1989.
105. Mardani, M., Jahromi, M. K., Naieni, K. H. and Zeinali, M. The efficacy of oral ribavirin in the treatment of Crimean-Congo hemorrhagic fever in Iran. Clin. Infect. Dis. 36,1613–1618, 2003.
106. Ergonul, O., Celikbas, A., Dokuzoguz, B., et al. Characteristics of patients with Crimean-Congo hemorrhagic fever in a recent outbreak in Turkey and impact of oral ribavirin therapy. Clin. Infect. Dis. 39,284–287, 2004.
107. Fisher-Hoch, S. P., Khan, J. A., Rehman, S., et al. Crimean Congo-haemorrhagic fever treated with oral ribavirin. Lancet 346,472–475, 1995.
108. van Eeden, P. J., van Eeden, S. F., Joubert, J. R., et al. A nosocomial outbreak of Crimean-Congo haemorrhagic fever at Tygerberg Hospital. Part II. Management of patients. S. Afr. Med. J. 68,718–721, 1985.
109. Athar, M. N., Baqai, H. Z., Ahmad, M., et al. Short report: Crimean-Congo hemorrhagic fever outbreak in Rawalpindi, Pakistan, February 2002. Am. J. Trop. Med. Hyg. 69,284–287, 2003.
110. Huggins, J. W. Prospects for treatment of viral hemorrhagic fevers with ribavirin, a broad-spectrum antiviral drug. Rev. Infect. Dis. 11 (Suppl 4),S750–S761, 1989.
111. Peters, C. J., Reynolds, J. A., Slone, T. W., et al. Prophylaxis of Rift Valley fever with antiviral drugs, immune serum, an interferon inducer, and a macrophage activator. Antiviral Res. 6,285–297, 1986.
112. Huggins, J. W., Jahrling, P. B., Kende, M. and Canonico, P. G. Efficacy of ribavirin against virulent RNA virus infections. In: Smith, J. A. D., editor. Clinical Applications of Ribavirin. Academic Press, New York; 1984, p. 49–63.
113. Stephen, E. L., Jones, D. E., Peters, C. J., et al. Ribavirin treatment of toga-, arena-, and bunyavirus infections in subhuman primates and other animal species. In: Kirkpatrick, W., editor. Ribavirin: A Broad Spectrum Antiviral Agent. Academic Press, New York; 1980, p. 169–183.
114. Loginova, S., Efanova, T. N., Koval'chuk, A. V., et al. [Effectiveness of virazol, realdiron and interferon inductors in experimental Omsk hemorrhagic fever]. Vopr. Virusol. 47,27–30, 2002.
115. Tam, R. C., Lau, J. Y. and Hong, Z. Mechanisms of action of ribavirin in antiviral therapies. Antivir. Chem. Chemother. 12,261–272, 2001.
116. Hong, Z. and Cameron, C. E. Pleiotropic mechanisms of ribavirin antiviral activities. Prog. Drug. Res. 59,41–69, 2002.
117. Kilham, L. and Ferm, V. H. Congenital anomalies induced in hamster embryos with ribavirin. Science 195,413–414, 1977.
118. Hoffmann, S. H., Wade, M. J., Staffa, J. A., et al. Dominant lethal study of ribavirin in male rats. Mutat. Res. 188,29–34, 1987.
119. Prows, C. A. Ribavirin's risks in reproduction – how great are they? MCN Am. J. Matern. Child. Nurs. 14,400–404, 1989.
120. Hegenbarth, K., Maurer, U., Kroisel, P. M., et al. No evidence for mutagenic effects of ribavirin: report of two normal pregnancies. Am. J. Gastroenterol. 96,2286–2287, 2001.

121. Huggins, J., Zhang, Z. X. and Bray, M. Antiviral drug therapy of filovirus infections: S-adenosylhomocysteine hydrolase inhibitors inhibit Ebola virus in vitro and in a lethal mouse model. J. Infect. Dis. 179 (Suppl 1),S240–S247, 1999.
122. Bray, M., Driscoll, J. and Huggins, J. W. Treatment of lethal Ebola virus infection in mice with a single dose of an S-adenosyl-L-homocysteine hydrolase inhibitor. Antiviral Res. 45,135–147, 2000.
123. Barrientos, L. G., O'Keefe, B. R., Bray, M., et al. Cyanovirin-N binds to the viral surface glycoprotein, GP1,2 and inhibits infectivity of Ebola virus. Antiviral Res. 58,47–56, 2003.
124. Tikunova, N. V., Kolokol'tsov, A. A., Chepurnov, A. A. Recombinant monoclonal human antibodies against Ebola virus. Dokl. Biochem. Biophys. 378,195–197, 2001.
125. Maruyama, T., Rodriguez, L. L., Jahrling, P. B., et al. Ebola virus can be effectively neutralized by antibody produced in natural human infection. J. Virol. 73,6024–6030, 1999.
126. Parren, P. W., Geisbert, T. W., Maruyama, T., et al. Pre- and postexposure prophylaxis of Ebola virus infection in an animal model by passive transfer of a neutralizing human antibody. J. Virol. 276,6408–6412, 2002.
127. Borisevich, G. V., Lebedev, V. N., Pashchenko Iu, I., et al. [The use of monoclonal antibodies in studying the causative agents of viral hemorrhagic fevers]. Vopr. Virusol. 48,4–8, 2003.
128. Maiztegui, J. I., Fernandez, N. J. and de Damilano, A. J. Efficacy of immune plasma in treatment of Argentine haemorrhagic fever and association between treatment and a late neurological syndrome. Lancet 2,1216–1217, 1979.
129. Enria, D. A., Briggiler, A. M., Fernandez, N. J., et al. Importance of dose of neutralising antibodies in treatment of Argentine haemorrhagic fever with immune plasma. Lancet 2,255–256, 1984.
130. Enria, D. A., de Damilano, A. J., Briggiler, A. M., et al. [Late neurologic syndrome in patients with Argentinian hemorrhagic fever treated with immune plasma]. Medicina (B Aires) 45,615–620, 1985.
131. Leifer, E., Gocke, D. J. and Bourne, H. Lassa fever, a new virus disease of man from West Africa. II. Report of a laboratory-acquired infection treated with plasma from a person recently recovered from the disease. Am. J. Trop. Med. Hyg. 19,677–679,1970.
132. Frame, J. D., Verbrugge, G. P., Gill, R. G., et al. The use of Lassa fever convalescent plasma in Nigeria. Trans. R. Soc. Trop. Med. Hyg. 78(3),319–324, 1984.
133. Jahrling, P. B., Peters, C. J. and Stephen, E. L. Enhanced treatment of Lassa fever by immune plasma combined with ribavirin in cynomolgus monkeys. J. Infect. Dis. 149,420–427, 1984.
134. Jahrling, P. B. and Peters, C. J. Passive antibody therapy of Lassa fever in cynomolgus monkeys: importance of neutralizing antibody and Lassa virus strain. Infect. Immun. 44,528–533, 1984.
135. Jahrling, P. B., Frame, J. D., Rhoderick, J. B. and Monson, M. H. Endemic Lassa fever in Liberia. IV. Selection of optimally effective plasma for treatment by passive immunization. Trans. R. Soc. Trop. Med. Hyg. 79,380–384, 1985.
136. Donchenko, V. V., Lebedev, V. N., Markin, V. A. and Firsova, I. V. [Effectiveness of virus-specific proteins in immunogenesis during experimental Marburg fever]. Vopr. Virusol. 41,216–218, 1996.
137. Gupta, M., Mahanty, S., Bray, M., et al. Passive transfer of antibodies protects immunocompetent and immunodeficient mice against lethal Ebola virus infection without complete inhibition of viral replication. J. Virol. 75,4649–4654, 2001.
138. Kudoyarova-Zubavichene, N. M., Sergeyev, N. N., Chepurnov, A. A. and Netesov, S. V. Preparation and use of hyperimmune serum for prophylaxis and therapy of Ebola virus infections. J. Infect. Dis. 179 (Suppl 1),S218–S223, 1999.
139. Knobloch, J., Dietrich, M., Peters, D., et al. [Maridi haemorrhgic fever: a new viral disease (author's transl)]. Dtsch. Med. Wochenschr. 102,1575–1581, 1977.

140. Borisevich, I. V., Mikhailov, V. V., Krasnianskii, V. P., et al. [Development and study of the properties of immunoglobulin against Ebola fever]. Vopr. Virusol. 40,270–273, 1995.
141. Mikhailov, V. V., Borisevich, I. V., Chernikova, N. K., et al. [The evaluation in hamadryas baboons of the possibility for the specific prevention of Ebola fever]. Vopr. Virusol. 39,82–84, 1994.
142. Jahrling, P. B., Geisbert, T. W., Geisbert, J. B., et al. Evaluation of immune globulin and recombinant interferon-alpha2b for treatment of experimental Ebola virus infections. J. Infect. Dis. 179 (Suppl 1),S224–S234, 1999.
143. Jahrling, P. B., Geisbert, J., Swearengen, J. R., et al. Passive immunization of Ebola virus-infected cynomolgus monkeys with immunoglobulin from hyperimmune horses. Arch. Virol. 11 (Suppl),135–140, 1996.
144. Mupapa, K., Massamba, M., Kibadi, K., et al. Treatment of Ebola hemorrhagic fever with blood transfusions from convalescent patients. International Scientific and Technical Committee. J. Infect. Dis. 179 (Suppl 1),S18–S23, 1999.
145. Jahrling et al., Ebola Hemorrhagic Fever: Evaluation of Passive Immunotherapy in Nonhuman Primates. JID 196 (Suppl 2), S400–S403, 2007.
146. Peters, C. J., Jones, D., Trotter, R., et al. Experimental Rift Valley fever in rhesus macaques. Arch. Virol. 99,31–44, 1988.
147. Bray, M. and Mahanty, S. Ebola hemorrhagic fever and septic shock. J. Infect. Dis. 188,1613–1617, 2003.
148. Mahanty, S., Bausch, D. G., Thomas, R. L., et al. Low levels of interleukin-8 and interferon-inducible protein-10 in serum are associated with fatal infections in acute Lassa fever. J. Infect. Dis. 183,1713–1721, 2001.
149. Sanchez, A., Lukwiya, M., Bausch, D., et al. Analysis of human peripheral blood samples from fatal and nonfatal cases of Ebola (Sudan) hemorrhagic fever: cellular responses, virus load, and nitric oxide levels. J. Virol. 78,10370–10377, 2004.
150. Esmon, C. T. Role of coagulation inhibitors in inflammation. Thromb. Haemost. 86,51–56, 2001.
151. Geisbert, T. W., Hensley, L. E., Jahrling, P. B., et al. Treatment of Ebola virus infection with a recombinant inhibitor of factor VIIa/tissue factor: a study in rhesus monkeys. Lancet 362,1953–1958, 2003.
152. Bernard, G. R., Vincent, J. L., Laterre, P. F., et al. Efficacy and safety of recombinant human activated protein C for severe sepsis. N. Engl. J. Med. 344,699–709, 2001.
153. Kolokol'tsov, A. A., Davidovich, I. A., Strel'tsova, M. A., et al. The use of interferon for emergency prophylaxis of Marburg hemorrhagic fever in monkeys. Bull. Exp. Biol. Med. 132,686–688, 2001.
154. Kaliberov, S. A., Ignat'ev, G. M., Pereboeva, L. A. and Kashentseva, E. A. [Experimental study of the possibility of emergency prophylaxis of Bolivian hemorrhagic fever]. Vopr. Virusol. 40,211–215,1995.
155. Sergeev, A. N., Lub, M., P'Iankova, O. G. and Kotliarov, L. A. [The efficacy of the emergency prophylactic and therapeutic actions of immunomodulators in experimental filovirus infections]. Antibiot. Khimioter. 40,24–27, 1995.
156. Ignatyev, G., Steinkasserer, A., Streltsova, M., et al. Experimental study on the possibility of treatment of some hemorrhagic fevers. J. Biotechnol. 83,67–76, 2000.
157. Morrill, J. C., Czarniecki, C. W. and Peters, C. J. Recombinant human interferon-gamma modulates Rift Valley fever virus infection in the rhesus monkey. J. Interferon. Res. 11,297–304, 1991.
158. Morrill, J. C., Jennings, G. B., Cosgriff, T. M., et al. Prevention of Rift Valley fever in rhesus monkeys with interferon-alpha. Rev. Infect. Dis. 11 (Suppl 4),S815–S825, 1989.
159. Centers for Disease Control and Prevention. Update: management of patients with suspected viral hemorrhagic fever – United States. MMWR Morb. Mortal. Wkly. Rep. 44,475–479, 1995.

160. Peters, C. J., Jahrling, P. B. and Khan, A. S. Patients infected with high-hazard viruses: scientific basis for infection control. Arch. Virol. 11 (Suppl),141–168, 1996.
161. Maiztegui, J. I., McKee, K. T., Jr., Barrera Oro, J. G., et al. Protective efficacy of a live attenuated vaccine against Argentine hemorrhagic fever. AHF Study Group. J. Infect. Dis. 177,277–283, 1998.
162. Sullivan, N. J., Geisbert, T. W., Geisbert, J. B., et al. Accelerated vaccination for Ebola virus haemorrhagic fever in non-human primates. Nature 424,681–684, 2003.
163. Fisher-Hoch, S. P., Hutwagner, L., Brown, B. and McCormick, J. B. Effective vaccine for Lassa fever. J. Virol. 74,6777–6783, 2000.
164. Frank-Peterside, N. Response of laboratory staff to vaccination with an inactivated Rift Valley fever vaccine – TSI-GSD 200. Afr. J. Med. Med. Sci. 29,89–92, 2000.
165. Pittman, P. R., Liu, C. T., Cannon, T. L., et al. Immunogenicity of an inactivated Rift Valley fever vaccine in humans: a 12-year experience. Vaccine 18,181–189, 1999.
166. Morrill, J. C. and Peters, C. J. Pathogenicity and neurovirulence of a mutagen-attenuated Rift Valley fever vaccine in rhesus monkeys. Vaccine 21,2994–3002, 2003.
167. Morrill, J. C., Mebus, C. A. and Peters, C. J. Safety and efficacy of a mutagen-attenuated Rift Valley fever virus vaccine in cattle. Am. J. Vet. Res. 58,1104–1109, 1997.
168. Baskerville, A., Hubbard, K. A. and Stephenson, J. R. Comparison of the pathogenicity for pregnant sheep of Rift Valley fever virus and a live attenuated vaccine. Res. Vet. Sci. 52,307–311, 1992.
169. Dandawate, C. N., Desai, G. B., Achar, T. R. and Banerjee, K. Field evaluation of formalin inactivated Kyasanur forest disease virus tissue culture vaccine in three districts of Karnataka state. Indian J. Med. Res. 99,152–158, 1994.
170. Mitchell, S. W. and McCormick, J. B. Physicochemical inactivation of Lassa, Ebola, and Marburg viruses and effect on clinical laboratory analyses. J. Clin. Microbiol. 20,486–489, 1984.
171. Elliott, L. H., McCormick, J. B. and Johnson, K. M. Inactivation of Lassa, Marburg, and Ebola viruses by gamma irradiation. J. Clin. Microbiol. 16,704–708, 1982.
172. Chepurnov, A. A., Bakulina, L. F., Dadaeva, A. A., et al. Inactivation of Ebola virus with a surfactant nanoemulsion. Acta Trop. 87,315–320, 2003.
173. Lupton, H. W. Inactivation of Ebola virus with 60Co irradiation. J. Infect. Dis. 143,291, 1981.
174. Logan, J. C., Fox, M. P., Morgan, J. H., et al. Arenavirus inactivation on contact with N-substituted isatin beta-thiosemicarbazones and certain cations. J. Gen. Virol. 28,271–283, 1975.
175. Buehler, J. W., Berkelman, R. L., Hartley, D. M. and Peters, C. J. Syndromic surveillance and bioterrorism-related epidemics. Emerg. Infect. Dis. 9.1197–1204, 2003.
176. Haas, C. N. The role of risk analysis in understanding bioterrorism. Risk Anal. 22,671–677, 2002.
177. Cohen, H., Sidel, V. and Gould, R. Preparedness for bioterrorism? N. Engl. J. Med. 345,1423, 2001.
178. Danzig, R. and Berkowsky, P. B. Why should we be concerned about biological warfare? JAMA 278,431–432, 1997.
179. Marklund, L. A. Patient care in a biological safety level-4 (BSL-4) environment. Crit. Care Nurs. Clin. North Am. 15,245–255, 2003.
180. Slovic, P. Perception of risk. Science 236,280–285, 1987.
181. Georges, A. J., Leroy, E. M., Renaut, A. A., et al. Ebola hemorrhagic fever outbreaks in Gabon, 1994–1997: Epidemiologic and health control issues. J. Infect. Dis. 179 (Suppl 1),S65–S75, 1999.
182. Formenty, P., Hatz, C., Le Guenno, B., et al. Human infection due to Ebola virus, subtype Cote d'Ivoire: clinical and biologic presentation. J. Infect. Dis. 179 (Suppl 1),S48–S53, 1999.

183. Borchert M, Mulangu S, Swanepoel R, et al. Serosurvey on household contacts of Marburg hemorrhagic fever patients. Emerg. Infect. Dis. 12,433–439, 2006.
184. Mustonen, J., Partanen, J., Kanerva, M., et al. Genetic susceptibility to severe course of nephropathia epidemica caused by Puumala hantavirus. Kidney Int. 49(1),217–221, 1996.
185. Bausch D.G. Viral Hemorrhagic Fevers. In Schlossberg D (ed): Clinical Infectious Disease. New York, NY, Cambridge University Press, 2008, pp 1319–1332.
186. Bausch D.G. (2007). Marburg and Ebola viruses. PIER: The Physicians' Information and Education Resource. American College of Physicians, electronic publication: pier. acponline.org/physicians/diseases/d891/d891.htmlhttp://pier.acponline.org/physicians/diseases/d891/d891.html.
187. Paragas J. and Geisbert T.W. Development of treatment strategies to combat Ebola and Marburg viruses. Expert. Rev. Anti. Infect. Ther. 4,67–76, 2006.
188. Pfau C.J. Biochemical and biophysical properties of the arenaviruses. Prog. Med. Virol. 18,64–80, 1974.

Chapter 7
Melioidosis

Pooja Tolaney and Larry I. Lutwick

7.1 Clinical Scenarios

These cases illustrate the potentially fulminant nature of this infection that may lie dormant for years and the propensity of the organism to cause metastatic abscesses.

7.1.1 Acute Fulminant Disease

A 21-year-old soldier deployed to Vietnam during the Vietnam conflict was admitted to a military hospital with the chief complaints of fever, chills, malaise and chest pain [1]. Historically, he had been well enough to play in a softball game the previous evening.

On initial examination, he was found to have a fever of 40°C. and clear lungs upon auscultation. By the end of the first day, however, the patient had developed a cough and a chest radiograph was reported to reveal bilateral pulmonary infiltrates. Scattered cutaneous pustules were observed on the trunk. Despite penicillin, chloramphenicol and streptomycin, progressive respiratory insufficiency and cyanosis ensued and he died 72 h after admission.

One day prior to death, a sputum culture revealed a Gram-negative bacillus that was subsequently identified as *Pseudomonas* (now *Burkholderia*) *pseudomallei*. On the day of death, the same organism was isolated from a pustule. Necrotizing bronchitis and pneumonia with Gram-negative bacilli were found at postmortem examination.

L.I. Lutwick
Infectious Diseases (IIIE), VA New York Harbor Health Care System, 800 Poly Place, Brooklyn, NY 11209, USA
e-mail: larry.lutwick@va.gov

L.I. Lutwick, S.M. Lutwick (eds.), *Beyond Anthrax*,
DOI: 10.1007/978-1-59745-326-4_7,

7.1.2 Reactivation Fatal Disease

A 64-year-old man was admitted to a hospital 16 years after a tour of duty in Vietnam [2]. With an underlying history of chronic lung disease and cigarette use, he had developed fever to 39.8°C. and chills 2 days prior to admission and was found to have a left upper lobe infiltrate/mass on chest x-ray. The x-ray had been normal 5 months before. His sputum culture revealed normal mouth flora and his temperature became normal during therapy with intravenous erythromycin. He was discharged on oral erythromycin to be readmitted in 2 weeks for further evaluation.

Several days prior to the scheduled readmission, a fever to 40°C. and a cough productive of rusty sputum precipitated hospital evaluation. His peripheral white blood cell count was elevated and there was pyuria, neither abnormality had been present during the recent stay and his infiltrate had expanded. The patient was begun on intravenous penicillin. Sputum culture again revealed normal flora and no evidence for acid-fast bacilli or Legionnaires' disease was found. Progressive bilateral infiltrates were noted with respiratory failure necessitating mechanical ventilation. Clindamycin and gentamicin were added to the therapy but he expired on the 11th hospital day.

On the day of death, respiratory secretions from one of the several bronchoscopies done during the admission produced a Gram-negative bacillus subsequently identified as *B. pseudomallei.* Postmortem exam revealed multiple abscesses in lung, liver, spleen, prostate and other organs. The well developed nature of the prostatic abscess suggested it as the primary focus for dissemination.

7.2 The Organism

7.2.1 The History of Melioidosis

The disease was first described in Rangoon, Burma (now Myanmar) by Whitmore and Krishnaswami in 1912 among homeless, debilitated morphine addicts. Autopsies performed on the remains of these individuals revealed a process reminiscent of glanders, an abscess-forming infection of horses and, quite rarely now, man. Microbiologically, the physicians from Her Majesty's Indian Health Service could distinguish the isolated organism from the glanders bacterium and others. The term melioidosis as related by White [3] was coined by Fletcher and Stanton from Kuala Lumpur, Malaysia, from the Greek words *melis* (a distemper of asses) and *eidos* (resemblance). Cases were subsequently described with isolation of the organism from clinical specimens and soil from many countries primarily in eastern Asia.

The infection was recognized in both Allied and Japanese soldiers during the Second World War and subsequently was recognized in northern Australia. Later, during the Vietnamese war of independence with France and, more so, the United States involvement there were many more cases described. Because of the infection's potential to produce potentially life-threatening reactivations several decades after exposure, the term "Vietnam time bomb" was used. It is likely that many of the acute and fatal cases in troops remained undiagnosed.

Also a disease of animals, melioidosis is not truly a zoonosis since it is not transmitted from animals to man but rather both acquire the infection from its soil reservoir. It may cause infection in many species and has become a significant veterinary pathogen in zoological gardens. As pointed out by White [3], the infamous *L'affaire du Jardin des Plantes* was said to have occurred after a panda donated in 1973 by Mao Tse-Tung to the French president Pompidou was the index case of melioidosis that significantly impacted on several French zoos as well as race and equestrian horses.

7.2.2 *Burkholderia pseudomallei*

The organism has gone through many name changes from *Loefflerella* or *Pfeifferella whitmori* and *Bacillus* or *P. pseudomallei* to, in 1992, its current designation. The genus is named for Walter Burkholder who first characterized *B. cepacia* as a phytopathogen responsible for a root rot of onions. *Burkholderia pseudomallei* is a motile, aerobic and nonspore-forming Gram-negative bacillus with a genome divided between two segments of DNA of about 4.1 and 3.2 megabases in length.

Although primarily an intracellular organism, it readily grows on most solid media resulting in prominently wrinkled (rugose) colonies that may manifest an earthy-like aroma. Selective media are available for isolation as well [4, 5]. Gram-stain of the bacillus can reveal the safety pin bipolar appearance often seen with *Y. pestis*. There are some *B. pseudomallei*–like organisms that are much less virulent. Formerly considered to be a separate biotype, these L-arabinoside assimilators are now classified as *B. thailandensis* and account for about a quarter of soil isolates in Thailand [6]. *B. thailandensis*, causing pneumonia and bacteremia, has been acquired in the United States [7]. Additionally, another similar organism, *B. oklahomensis* [8], has been isolated from soil and human sources in the US.

This is a hard-core survivalist organism is so nutritionally versatile that it can persist in triple-distilled water for long periods of time [3]. Among the virulence factors associated with *B. pseudomallei* is its polysaccharide capsule that is important in the formation of slime around microcolonies. This biofilm appears to protect the organism from antimicrobials by decreasing accessibility and helps resist phagocytosis. Other virulence factors include the cell wall lipopolysaccharide (LPS) and the ability of the organism to stimulate the host's inflammatory cytokine cascade.

7.3 Natural Infection

7.3.1 Epidemiology

The organism exists as an environmental saprophyte living in soil and surface water in endemic areas (Southeast Asia and northern, tropical Australia), particularly in rice paddies [9–11]. In endemic countries, the organism exists primarily in focal areas and not equally distributed throughout the landscape. Sporadic cases have been reported to have been acquired in parts of Africa and the Americas. The organism may exist in a viable, non-cultivable state in the environment, interacting with other organisms, particularly protozoa, which might explain its adaptation to an intracellular niche [12, 13]. Two recent outbreaks in Australia have also implicated potable water supplies rather than surface water as a potential source of the infection [14, 15].

Melioidosis is a disease of rainy season in the endemic areas [9, 16], mainly affecting people who have direct contact with soil and water. Many have an underlying predisposing condition such as diabetes (most common risk factor), renal disease, cirrhosis, thalassemia, alcohol dependence, immunosuppressive therapy, chronic obstructive lung disease, cystic fibrosis, and excess kava consumption [17–20]. Kava is an herbal member of the pepper family that can be associated with chronic liver disease. HIV infection, however, may not a clear risk factor for more severe disease [21]. Melioidosis may present at any age, but peaks in the fourth and fifth decades of life [14], affecting males more than women. In addition, although severe fulminating infection can and does occur in healthy individuals, severe disease and fatalities are much less common in those without risk factors.

In northeastern Thailand, melioidosis accounts for 18% of community-acquired septicemia [9] and in the Northern Territory of Australia it is the commonest cause of community-acquired septicemia [13, 14]. Most of the population in endemic areas of East Asia has antibodies to *B. pseudomallei*, but these antibodies have not been shown to be protective against future overt infection.

7.3.2 Modes of Transmission

Infection in humans is usually acquired by inoculation in an open wound or inhalation of aerosolized soil or water and not generally by ingestion. In hamsters, however, infection following ingestion has been reported to be possible but much less efficient than by other routes [22]. Although inhalation of aerosolized organisms causing pneumonia clearly occurs, pneumonia has also occurred following well documented skin injuries [23] suggesting that the lung involvement can be related to bacteremic spread as well.

Rarely, nosocomial transmission has been observed in patients and laboratory personnel [24, 25], hence this bacterium is considered a level 3 pathogen. Both neonatal and sexual person-to-person spreads have also been reported but (as well as animal-to-person spread) are quite uncommon [24–27]. The risk of transmission may be higher if the recipient has diabetes, cystic fibrosis or other diseases for which *B. pseudomallei* is more opportunistic [28, 29].

The incubation period after exposure can be as short as 1 day but averages about 9 days; however, because of "latency" (the mechanism of which is unclear) has been up to 63 years [30]. Recrudescent infections in veterans of Vietnam War have given rise to the nickname "Vietnamese Time Bomb" [31]. Despite of this risk of reactivation, documented American cases were fairly uncommon as compared to the individuals affected in Vietnam. An Australian study, in fact, suggested that only 3% of melioidosis infections were related to reactivation and 97% were acute disease [32].

7.4 Diagnosis

7.4.1 Clinical Presentation

Melioidosis presents mostly as a febrile illness, ranging from an acute fulminant septicemia to a chronic debilitating localized infection to an unknown subclinical infection. As virtually every organ can be affected, melioidosis has been termed a "great imitator" of many other infectious diseases [33].

The majority of infected patients are asymptomatic. In northeastern Thailand, 80% of children have antibodies to *B. pseudomallei* by 4 years of age without having developed recognized clinical disease [34]. Influenza-like illness can be associated with seroconversion and has reported from Australia [35].

The most commonly recognized presentation of melioidosis is pneumonia associated with high fever, significant muscle aches, chest pain and although the cough can be nonproductive, respiratory secretions can be purulent, significant in quantity and associated with on and off bright red blood. The lung infection can be rapidly fatal with bacteremia and shock or somewhat more indolent.

In addition to an acute pneumonitis, chronic pulmonary infection may also be caused by *B. pseudomallei,* either as a continuum for acute disease or reactivation years later. The presentation is quite similar to reactivation tuberculosis with upper lobe involvement associated with productive cough, weight loss and hemoptysis. Fever and pleuritic chest pain are also prominent complaints [36]. Histopathologically, the lung shows granulomatous changes with few bacilli seen in tissue sections [37].

Acute melioidosis septicemia is the most severe complication of the infection. It presents as a typical sepsis syndrome with hypotension, high cardiac output and low systemic vascular resistance. In many cases, a primary focus in the soft tissues or lung can be found. The syndrome, usually in patients with risk factor comorbidities, is characteristically associated with multiple abscesses involving the cutaneous tissues, the lung, the liver and spleen and a very high mortality rate of 80%–95%. With prompt optimal therapy, the case fatality rate can be decreased to 40%–50%.

In acute severe melioidosis, there is characteristically the rapid progression of respiratory failure that is due to acute respiratory distress syndrome and/or pneumonia. It has been suggested that the ARDS to melioidosis sepsis is more rapid in progression than with other bacteria and may be related to the intracellular interactions of the bacillus and the leukocyte [38]. Bacteremia without shock/hypotension has a substantially better prognosis.

Abscesses can be found in many organs. Two organs that are particularly relevant in disease are the prostate and the parotid gland. Acute prostatic abscess may cause urinary retention. Residual prostatic abscess appears to be a potential focus for reactivation infection or relapse and unlike other visceral collections unless the abscesses are large and accessible, ought to be definitively drained as needed. The purulent material obtained is yellow to tan in color and odorless. Parotitis is a common manifestation of melioidosis among pediatric cases in Thailand but not in Australia and may be associated with a peripheral seventh cranial nerve palsy. In focal melioidosis without bacteremia, the mortality rate is 4%–5%.

Neurologic involvement occurs in 4%–5% of cases in northern Australia (much less frequently in Thailand) and is noteworthy because, although brain abscesses can occur, the process is more likely to be a brainstem encephalitis with cerebellar signs, cranial nerve palsy (especially sixth and seventh) or flaccid paraparesis [39]. This complication of melioidosis has a 25% mortality rate and a substantial degree of neurological residua. The patients generally have a normal or almost normal degree of alertness. The CSF pleocytosis is usually mononuclear.

7.4.2 Clinical Presentation of Biowarfare Melioidosis

The pathogen, if used in biological warfare, would likely to be spread via an aerosol. Presumably, therefore, victims suffering from a biological attack that employed *B. pseudomallei* would present clinically with influenza-like illnesses associated in some cases with pneumonic disease. Such high concentration of the organism aerosolized as a dry powder would contaminate the environment and also give rise to the whole spectrum of disease ranging from skin/subcutaneous abscesses to fulminant septicemic pneumonia. Large enough respiratory inocula may be able to overcome the severe infection rarity in normal individuals. Indeed, in a mouse model for aerosol transmission of *B. pseudomallei*, higher mortality is associated higher inocula [40].

Since a whole variety of animals are susceptible to infection with melioidosis, parallel illnesses may be seen in rodents, primates, sheep, swine, horses, dolphins and birds. Melioidosis, therefore, would need to be considered with a scenario of a cluster of influenza-like illnesses in humans who may be exposed to an unknown biological weapon. This may be particularly relevant with a coexisting outbreak in animals.

Illness may begin abruptly, or with a vague prodrome of headache, anorexia, and myalgia. Fever (often over 39°C.), pleuritic chest pain, and cough will usually be present. It can progress to acute septicemic disease that may follow a terminal course with death within days as demonstrated by the first scenario.

Finding cases of melioidosis without a travel history in the Americas can bring up to the forefront the possibility of a bioterrorism event. Naturally acquired cases of *B. pseudomallei* have clearly been described from the Western Hemisphere [41] especially from Brazil and the Caribbean. A human outbreak has been described in Brazil [42] and an animal outbreak reported from Aruba [43]. Travel to South America has produced imported melioidosis in Europe [44]. Locally acquired cases have also been described from the Middle East and Africa [45].

7.4.3 Radiographic Diagnosis

Quite widely variable chest radiograph findings are described in melioidosis. Acute pneumonia can present with patchy, diffuse or discrete lobar or multilobar abnormalities with or without pleural fluid. Infiltrates may coalesce and cavitate as well. It has been pointed out [23], at first, the x-ray can show much more limited involvement than what might be expected based on constitutional complaints. This supports that contention that the pneumonia is a manifestation of a bacteremia. In chronic melioidosis, upper lobe involvement is common that mimics tuberculosis as streaky, fibrotic-looking lesions with nodularity and, often cavitation.

Because of the propensity for *B. pseudomallei* infection to cause abscesses, abdominal imaging should be done on all suspected cases to see if hepatic and/or splenic abscesses could be visualized. These abscesses may have a “swiss cheese” like appearance.

7.4.4 Laboratory Diagnosis

7.4.4.1 Microbiology

Laboratory diagnosis generally relies on the isolation and identification of *B. pseudomallei* in clinical samples, although serology may be useful in nonendemic areas. The organism is easily from cutaneous sites or the blood and throat cultures seem to be useful in those individuals who are not able to produce sputa [46]. Direct immunofluorescence of sputum or pus has been used to facilitate rapid diagnosis but is not as sensitive as culture [47]. A positive sputum culture may be an independent risk factor for mortality in patients with this disease [48].

Microscopy reveals bipolar, irregularly staining Gram-negative bacilli. Motile, obligately aerobic, nonspore-forming bacteria with dry wrinkled appearance on culture media appear after a few days of inoculation. Selective media such as Ashdown's media may be required to be able to identify the organism in respiratory culture as it may need 48–72 h to grow and is easily overgrown in the mixed culture of upper respiratory flora using nonselective media.

7.4.4.2 Serology

Serodiagnosis is generally not helpful in those individuals who are native to endemic areas since a substantial background of positivity exists in the population as a whole. Serologic assays that are available are the indirect hemagglutination test, which is easy to perform and low cost item with IgM titers of >1:40 [34] in nonendemic areas and 1:80 with increasing titers in endemic areas is suggestive of disease. The ELISA with the IgG antibody being 97% sensitive and specific, and the IgM is 74% sensitive and 99% specific [13]. Borderline or false negative serologic assays have been reported especially in acute septic episodes of *B. pseudomallei* [49]. Overall [3], however, the serological testing may help to rule out the infection in endemic areas but may be useful in a biowarfare scenario occurring in a nonendemic area.

A urinary melioidosis antigen test has been developed with a reported 81% sensitivity and 96% specificity [50]. A latex agglutination assay using a monoclonal antibody has been reported to be quite useful in patients with community-acquired melioidosis bacteremia in Thailand [51]. Polymerase chain reaction assays for rapid diagnosis have been developed and have been used for rapid diagnosis of the melioidosis bacterium in blood [52] and soil [53].

7.5 Therapeutic Interventions

The melioidosis bacillus is intrinsically insensitive to many antimicrobials. It should be noted that bioterrorism strains may be engineered to be even more resistant. *Burkholderia pseudomallei* is usually inhibited by tetracyclines, chloramphenicol, trimethoprim-sulfamethoxazole (SXT), antipseudomonal penicillins, carbapenems, ceftazidime and amoxicillin/clavulanate or ampicillin/sulbactam. Ceftriaxone and cefotaxime have good in vitro activity but poor efficacy [3] and cefepime did not appear, as well, to be equivalent to ceftazidime in a mouse model [54]. The unusual antimicrobial profile of resistance to colistin and polymyxin B and the aminoglycosides but sensitivity to amoxicillin/clavulanate is a useful tool to consider the organism.

Samuel and Ti [55] have reviewed the randomized and quasi-randomized trials comparing melioidosis treatment and found that the formerly standard therapy of chloramphenicol, doxycycline and SXT combination had a higher mortality rate than therapy with ceftazidime, imipenem/cilastatin or amoxicillin/clavulanate (or ampicillin/sulbactam). The betalactam-betalactamase inhibitor therapy, however, seemed to have a higher failure rate [56].

A more prolonged oral phase of treatment is used to decrease the risk of late relapse with total therapy of 20 weeks. During the oral therapy phase, the conventional standard regimen appears to be equivalent to any newer therapies. Table 7.1 lists current treatment recommendations [3, 58, 59].

Table 7.1 Treatment of *Burkholderia pseudomallei* Infection[a]

Initial Parenteral Therapy for Severe Infection (usual 14 days minimum)

Ceftazidime[b]40 mg/kg intravenous (iv) every 8 h (typical adult dose 2 g)

or

Imipenem/Cilastatin[c] 20 mg/kg iv every 6–8 h (typical adult dose 1 g)

(Note: IV amoxicillin/clavulanate or ampicillin/sulbactam can be used in a every 4-h dosing but is associated with a higher failure rate)

Followup Oral Therapy (to complete 20 weeks of treatment)

(Note: In mild, localized disease, oral therapy can be used for the entire 20 weeks)

Doxycycline 2 mg/kg orally (po) every 12 h (typical adult dose 100–200 mg)

and

Trimethoprim-Sulfamethoxazole (Fixed 1:5 Combination) (typical adult dose 2 double strength (trimethoprim 320/sulfamethoxazole 1600) po every 12 h

and[d]

Chloramphenicol 10 mg/kg po every 6 h for the first 8 weeks (typical adult dose 500–1000 mg)

or (especially in children or pregnant women)

Amoxicillin/Clavulanate (Fixed Combination 2:1) 10 mg/kg amoxicillin/5 mg/kg clavulanate po every 8 h (typical adult dose 1000 mg/500 mg)

and

Amoxicillin 10 mg/kg po every 8 h (typical adult dose 1000 mg)

[a] Dosing may require adjustments in renal or hepatic dysfunction

[b] Ceftriaxone and cefotaxime has good in vitro activity but a higher mortality rate and should not been used. No human data is found for cefepime

[c] Meropenem [57], 1 g or 25 mg/kg iv every 8 h) may be used in lieu of imipenem/cilastatin

[d] Reference [3] recommends chloramphenicol and reference [59] does not

Based on historical control data [13] and in the absence of any randomized, controlled studies, recombinant granulocyte colony stimulating factor (G-CSF) has been used empirically in cases of melioidosis presenting with shock. In a 2003 murine study, however, G-CSF and ceftazidime did not offer any survival advantage over ceftazidime alone [60] but retrospective clinical data suggests that the compound may contribute to decreased mortality [61].

7.6 Preventative Measures

7.6.1 Infection Control

The organism should be handled in Containment Level 3 facilities in the lab and patients should ideally be nursed in standard isolation in case of an epidemic, with strict isolation and quarantine until smallpox and plague is ruled out. The risk of person-to-person spread is quite low but described.

Despite the ability of this organism to survive in the environment, except for a highly localized contamination as might occur following a lab accident, environmental antibacterial disinfection is not generally suggested. Those exposed to a laboratory accident or clandestine release of a *B. pseudomallei* aerosol should remove their outer clothes and shower. Although there is little recent data, the organism is susceptible to a variety of disinfectants such as a 5-min exposure to 0.7% tincture of iodine or sodium hypochlorite (500 ppm chlorine) or 10-min exposure to 5% phenol [62].

Prevention of the infection in endemic-disease areas can be difficult since contact with contaminated soil is so common. Persons with diabetes and skin lesions should avoid contact with soil and standing water in these areas. Wearing boots during agricultural work can prevent infection through the feet and lower legs.

There is no data on the use and efficacy of prophylactic antibiotics in case of a biologic attack. In a rodent model, either doxycycline or ciprofloxacin, when administered before or at the same time as a intraperitoneal challenge, were able to increase the mean lethal dose of *B. pseudomallei* by as many as five logs but did not completely protect [63]. Because of this, either doxycycline 100 mg or ciprofloxacin 500 mg orally twice daily could be suggested for individuals who have been exposed to significant contamination. There is no reported efficacy in humans and those significantly exposed should be made aware of potential life-long risk. In human trials, fluoroquinolones, however, have been disappointing when used therapeutically [3].

7.6.2 Immunization

There is no commercially available vaccine for melioidosis prevention in man, although experimental vaccines are under development and have been used in animals. Using a conjugate of the flagellin and the LPS, it has been found that this vaccine produced IgG antibodies that protected diabetic rats from a challenge with heterologous *B. pseudomallei* [64]. Antibodies against the LPS II of the organisms seemed to correlate with human survival from melioidosis when examined retrospectively [65].

Since *B. thailandensis* is much less virulent that *B. pseudomallei*, Reckseidler et al. [66] used subtraction hybridization to analyze virulence factors. The capsular polysaccharide seemed to represent a major virulence determinant and in a mouse model capsular mutants in a mouse model did not seem to be protective for subsequent wild type challenge [67]. *B. pseudomallei* auxotrophic mutants are also attenuated and have been found to be protective in a mouse model [68]. Vaccines for melioidosis have recently been reviewed by Warawa and Woods [69].

References

1. Brundage, W. G., Thuss, C. J., and Walden, D. C. Four fatal cases of melioidosis in U. S. soldiers in Vietnam. *Am. J. Trop. Med. Hyg.* 17, 183–191, 1968.
2. Morrison, R. E., Lamb, A. S., Craig, D. B., and Johnson, W. M. Melioidosis: a reminder. *Am. J. Med.* 84, 965–967, 1988.
3. White, N. J. Melioidosis. *Lancet* 361, 1715–1722, 2003.
4. Ashdown, L. R. An improved screening technique for isolation of *Pseudomonas pseudomallei* from clinical specimens. *Pathology* 11, 293–297, 1979.
5. Howard, K. and Inglis, T. J. Novel selective medium for isolation of *Burkholderia pseudomallei*. *J. Clin. Microbiol.* 41, 3312–3316, 2003.
6. Smith, M. D., Angus, B. J., Wuthiekanun, V., and White, N. J. Arabinose assimilation defines a nonvirulent biotype of *Burkholderia pseudomallei*. *Infect. Immun.* 65, 4319–4321, 1997.
7. Glass, M. B., Gee, J. E., Steigerwalt, A. G., et al. Pneumonia and septicemia caused by *Burkholderia thailandensis* in the United States. *J. Clin. Microbiol.* 44, 4601–4604, 2006.
8. Glass, M. B., Steigerwalt, A. G., Jordan, J. G., et al. *Burkholderia oklahomensis sp. nov.*, a *Burkholderia pseudomallei*-like species formerly known as the Oklahoma strain of *Pseudomonas pseudomallei*. *Int. J. Syst. Evol. Microbiol.* 56, 2171–2176, 2006.
9. Chaowagul, W., White, N. J., Dance, D. A., et al. Melioidosis: a major cause of community-acquired septicemia in northeastern Thailand. *J. Infect. Dis.* 159, 890–899, 1989.
10. Wuthiekanun, V., Smith, M. D., Dance, D. A. B., and White, N. J. The isolation of *Pseudomonas pseudomallei* from soil in Northeastern Thailand. *Trans. R. Soc. Trop. Med. Hyg.* **89**, 41–43, 1995.
11. Strauss, J. M., Groves, M. G., Mariappan, M., et al. Melioidosis in Malaysia. II. Distribution of *Pseudomonas pseudomallei* in soil and surface water. *Am. J. Trop. Med. Hyg.* 18, 698–702, 1969.
12. Phetsouvanh, R., Phongmany S., Newton, P., et al. Melioidosis and Pandora's box in Lao People's Democratic Republic. *Clin. Infect. Dis.* **32**, 653–654, 2001.
13. Dance, D. A. Melioidosis. *Curr. Opin. Infect. Dis.* 15, 127–132, 2002.
14. Currie, B. J., Fisher, D. A., Howard, D. M., et al. Endemic melioidosis in tropical northern Australia: a 10-year prospective study and review of the literature. *Clin. Infect. Dis.* 31, 981–986, 2000.
15. Currie, B. J., Mayo, M., Anstey, N. M., et al. A cluster of melioidosis cases from an endemic region is clonal and is linked to the water supply using molecular typing of *Burkholderia pseudomallei* isolates. *Am. J. Trop. Med. Hyg.* 65, 177–179, 2001.

16. Leelarasamee, A. and Bovornkitti, S. Melioidosis: review and update. *Rev. Infect. Dis.* 11, 413–425, 1989.
17. Suputtamongkol, Y., Chaowagul, W., Chetchotisakd, P., et al. Risk factors for melioidosis and bacteremic melioidosis. *Clin. Infect. Dis.* **29,** 408–413, 1999.
18. Suputtanongkol, Y., Hall, A. J., Dance, D. A., et al. The epidemiology of meliodoisis in Ubon Ratchutani, northeast Thailand. *Int. J. Epidemiol.* 23, 1082–1090, 1994.
19. Heng, B. H., Goh, K. T., Yap, E. H., et al. Epidemiological surveillance of melioidosis in Singapore. *Ann. Acad. Med. Singap.* 27, 478–484, 1998.
20. Holland, D. J., Wesley, A., Drinkovic, D., and Currie, B. J. Cystic fibrosis and *Burkholderia pseudomallei* infection: an emerging problem? *Clin. Infect. Dis.* 35, 138–140, 2002.
21. Chierakul, W., Wuthiekunun, V., Chaowagul, W., et al. Disease severity and outcome of melioidosis in HIV-coinfected individuals. *Am. J. Trop. Med. Hyg.* 73, 1165–1166, 2005.
22. Miller, W. R., Pannel, L., Cravitz, L., et al. Studies on certain biological characteristics of *Malleomyces mallei* and *Malleomyces pseudomallei.* II. Virulence and infectivity of isolates. *J. Bacteriol.* 55, 127–135, 1948.
23. Currie, B. J., Fisher, D. A., Howard, D. M., et al. The epidemiology of meliodosis in Australia and Papua New Guinea. *Acta Trop.* 74, 121–127, 2000.
24. Ashdown, L. R. Nosocomial infection due to *Pseudomonas pseudomallei*: two cases and an epidemiologic study. *Rev. Infect. Dis.* 1, 891–894, 1979.
25. Schlech, W. F., Turchik, J. B., Westlake, R. E., et al. Laboratory-acquired infection with *Pseudomonas pseudomallei* (melioidosis). *N. Engl. J. Med.* 305, 1133–1135, 1981.
26. Abbink, F. C., Orendi, J. M., and de Beaufort, A. J. Mother-to-child transmission of *Burkholderia pseudomallei. N. Engl. J. Med.* 344, 1171–1172, 2001.
27. McCormick, J. B., Sexton, D. J., McMurray, J. G., et al. Human-to-human transmission of Pseudomonas pseudomallei. *Ann. Intern. Med.* 83, 512–513, 1975.
28. Kunakorn, M., Jayanetra, P., and Tanphaichitra, D. Man-to-man transmission of melioidosis. *Lancet* 337, 1290–1291, 1991.
29. Currie, B. J. Advances and remaining uncertainties in the epidemiology of *Burkholderia pseudomallei* and Melioidosis. *Trans. Roy. Soc. Trop. Med. Hyg.* 102, 225–227, 2008.
30. Ngauy, V., Lemeshev, Y., Sadkowski, L., and Crawford, G. Cutaneous melioidosis in a man who was taken prisoner of war by the Japanese during World War II. *J. Clin. Microbiol.,* 43, 97–972, 2005.
31. Currie, B. J., Fisher, D. A., Anstey, N. M., and Jacups, S. P. Melioidosis: acute and chronic disease, relapse and reactivation. *Trans. R. Soc. Trop. Med. Hyg.* 94, 301–304, 2000.
32. Goshorn, R. K. Recrudescent pulmonary melioidosis. A case report involving the so-called "Vietnamese time bomb." *Indiana Med.* 80, 247–249, 1987.
33. Poe, R. H., Vassalo, C. L., and Domm, B. M. Melioidosis: the remarkable imitator. *Am. Rev. Respir. Dis.* 104, 427–431, 1971.
34. Kanaphun, P., Thirawattasuk, N., Suputtamongkol, Y., et al., Serology and carriage of *Pseudomonas pseudomallei*: a prospective study in 1000 hospitalized children in northeastern Thailand. *J. Infect. Dis.* 167, 230–233, 1993.
35. Ashdown, L. R., Johnson, R. W., Koehler, J. M., and Cooney, C. A. Enzyme linked immunosorbent assay for the diagnosis of clinical and subclinical melioidosis. *J. Infect. Dis.* 160, 253–260, 1989.
36. Everett, E. D. and Nelson, R. A. Pulmonary melioidosis. Observations in thirty-nine cases. *Am. Rev. Resp. Dis.* 112, 331–340, 1975.
37. Piggott, J. A. and Hochholzer, L. Human melioidosis. A histopathologic study of acute and chronic melioidosis. *Arch. Pathol.* 90, 101–111, 1970.
38. Puthucheary, S. D., Vadivelu, J., Wong, K. T., and Ong, G. S. Y. Acute respiratory failure in melioidosis. *Singapore Med. J.* 42, 117–121, 2001.
39. Currie, B. J., Fisher, D. A., Howard, D. M., and Burrow, J. N. Neurological melioidosis. *Acta Trop.* 74, 145–151, 2000.

40. Jeddeloih, J. A., Fritz, D. L., Waag, D. M., et al. Biodefense-driven murine model of pneumonic melioidosis. *Infect. Immun.* 71, 584–587, 2003.
41. Inglis, T. J. J., Rolim, D. B., and Sousa, A. Q. Melioidosis in the Americas. *Am. J. Trop. Med. Hyg.* 75, 947–954, 2006.
42. Rolim, D. B., Vilar, D. C., Sousa, A. Q., et al. Melioidosis, northern Brazil. *Emerg. Infect. Dis.* 11, 1458–1460, 2005.
43. Sutmoller, P., Kraneveld, F. C., and van der Schaaf, D. Melioidosis (*Pseudomalleus*) in sheep, goats, and pigs on Aruba (Netherlands Antilles). *J. Am. Vet. Med. Assoc.* 130, 415–417, 1957.
44. Aardema, H., Luijnenburg, E. M., Salera, E. F., et al. A case of pulmonary melioidosis with fatal outcome imported from Brazil. *Epidemiol. Infect.* 133, 871–875, 2005.
45. Cheng, A. C. and Currie, B. J. Melioidosis: epidemiology, pathophysiology, and management. *Clin. Microbiol. Rev.* 18, 383–416, 2005.
46. Wuthiekanun, V., Suputtamongkol, Y., Simpson, A. J. H., et al. Value of throat culture in diagnosis of melioidosis. *J. Clin. Microbiol.* 39, 3801–3802, 2001.
47. Walsh, A. L., Smith, M. D., Wuthiekanun, V., et al. Immunofluorescence microscopy for the rapid diagnosis of melioidosis. *J. Clin. Pathol.* 47, 377–379, 1994.
48. Huis int' Veld, D., Wuthiekanun, V., Cheng, A. C., et al. The role and significance of sputum cultures in the diagnosis of melioidosis. *Am. J. Trop. Med. Hyg.* 73, 657–661, 2005.
49. Appassakij, H., Silpapojakul, K. R., Wansit, R., and Pornpatkul, M. Diagnostic value of the indirect hemaglutination test for melioidosis in an endemic area. *Am. J. Trop. Med. Hyg.* 42, 248–253, 1990.
50. Aucken, H., Suntharasamai, P., Rajchanuwong, A., and White, N. J. Detection of *P. pseudomallei* antigen in urine for the diagnosis of melioidosis. *Am. J. Trop. Med. Hyg.* 51, 627–633, 1994.
51. Ekpo, P., Rungpanich, J., Pongsunk, V., et al. Use of a protein-specific monoclonal antibody bound latex agglutination for rapid diagnosis of *Burkholderia pseudomallei* infections in patients with community-acquired septicemia. *Clin. Vaccine Immunol.* 14, 811–812, 2007.
52. Supraprom, C., Wang, D., Leeaquwat, C., et al. Development of real-time PCR assays and evaluation of their potential use for rapid detection of *Burkholderia pseudomallei* in clinical blood specimens. *J. Clin. Microbiol.* 45, 2894–2901, 2007.
53. Kaestri, M., Mayo, M., Harrington, G., et al. Sensitive and specific detection of *Burkholderia pseudomallei*, the causative agent of melioidosis, in the soil of tropical northern Australia. *Appl. Environ. Microbiol.* 73, 6891–6897, 2007.
54. Ulett, G. C., Hirst, R., Bowden, B., et al. A comparison of antibiotic regimens in the treatment of acute melioidosis in a mouse model. *J. Antimicrob. Chemother.* 51, 77–81, 2003.
55. Samuel, M. and Ti, T. Y. Interventions for treating melioidosis (Cochrane Review). In: *The Cochane Library*, Issue 4, 2003. Chichester, UK: John Wiley & Sons, Ltd.
56. Suputtamongkol, Y., Dance, D., Chaowagul, W., et al. Amoxycillin-clavulanic acid treatment of melioidosis, *Trans. R. Soc. Trop. Med. Hyg.* 85, 672–675, 1991.
57. Cheng, A. C., Fisher, D. A., Anstey, N. M., et al. Outcome of patients with melioidosis treated with meropenem. *Antimicrob. Agents Chemother.* 48, 1763–1765, 2004.
58. Short, B. H. Melioidosis: an important emerging infectious disease – a military problem? A. D. F. Health 3, 13–21, 2002 http://www.defence.gov.au/dpe/dhs/infocentre/publications/journals/NoIDs/Topics/topicindex.html Accessed 30 November 2003.
59. Health Protection Agency – Colindale. Glanders and melioidosis. Interim Guidelines for Actionb in the Event of a Deliberate Release. Version 2.2, issued 14 Aug 2003. <http://www.hpa.org.uk/infections/topics_az/deliberate_release/menu.htm> Accessed 1 December 2003.
60. Powell, K., Ulett, G., Hirst, R., and Norton, R. G-CSF immunotherapy for treatment of acute disseminated murtine melioidosis. *FEMS Microbiol. Lett.* 224, 315–318, 2003.

61. Cheng, A. C., Stephens, D. P., Anstey, N. M. and Currie, B. J. Adjunctive granulocyte colony-stimulating factor for treatment of septic shock due to melioidosis. *Clin. Infect. Dis*. 38, 32–37, 2004.
62. Russell, P., Eley, S. M., Ellis, J., et al. Comparison of efficacy of ciprofloxacin and doxycycline against experimental melioidosis and glanders. *J. Antimicrob. Chemother*. 45, 813–818, 2000.
63. Miller, W. R., Pannel, L., Cravitz, L., et al. Studies on certain biological characteristics of *Malleomyces mallei* and *Malleomyces pseudomallei*. I. Morphology, cultivation, viability and isolation of contaminated specimens. *J. Bacteriol*. 55, 115–126, 1948.
64. Brett, P. J. and Woods, D. E. Structural and immunological characterization of *Burkholderia pseudomallei* O-polysaccharide-flagellin protein conjugates. *Infect. Immun*. 64, 2824–2828, 1996.
65. Charuchaimontri, C., Suputtamongkol, Y., Nilakul, C., et al. Antilipopolysaccharide II: an antibody protective against fatal melioidosis. *Clin. Infect. Dis*. 29, 813–818, 1999.
66. Reckseidler, S. L., DeShazer, D., Sokol, P. A., and Woods, D. E. Detection of bacterial virulence genes by subtractive hybridization identification of capsular polysaccharide of *Burkholderia pseudomallei* as a major virulence determinant. *Infect. Immun*. 69, 34–44, 2001.
67. Atkins, T., Prior, R., Mack, K., et al. Characterisation of an acapsular mutant of *Burkholderia pseudomallei* identified by signature tagged mutagenesis. *J. Med. Microbiol*. 51, 539–547, 2002.
68. Atkins, T., Prior, R. G., Mack, K., et al. A mutant of *Burkholderia pseudomallei*, auxotrophic in the branched chain amino acid biosynthetic pathway, is attenuated and protective in a murine model of melioidosis. *Infect. Immun*. 70, 5290–5294, 2002.
69. Warawa, J. and Woods, D. E. Melioidosis vaccines. *Expert Rev. Vaccines* 1, 477–482, 2002.

Chapter 8
Epidemic Typhus Fever

Mohammad Mooty and Larry I. Lutwick

8.1 Clinical Scenarios

8.1.1 Imported Acute Epidemic Typhus [1]

A 38-year-old Red Cross nurse was hospitalized in Switzerland after 5 days of fever, chills and myalgias. Other than a fever to 39°C, the physical exam was unremarkable and no rash was observed. Laboratory evaluation was remarkable for thrombocytopenia only. Because of a history of having returned from working in a prison in Burundi, malaria was considered but blood smears for parasites were negative and blood and urine cultures unrevealing. Ciprofloxacin was begun but her condition rapidly deteriorated with stupor, dyspnea, hypotension and multiorgan failure developing. Death ensued on the fourth hospital day.

Histopathology from the autopsy revealed glial nodules in the brain suggestive of a rickettsial process and immunostaining confirmed a typhus group infection. An indirect fluorescent antibody (IFA) titer for *Rickettsia prowazekii* was found to be 1:2,048 and a PCR for a *R. prowazekii* DNA fragment coding for surface protein in the blood was positive.

8.1.2 Imported Latent Epidemic Typhus [2]

An immigrant from Poland who lived resided in the United States for 16 years was admitted to a medical facility with fever to 41°C and severe headache. An infectious disease consult, called on the fifth hospital day for persistent fever, found the patient to be seemingly indifferent to his surroundings without meningeal signs and a maculopapular rash on the back and abdomen was noted. Initial blood and urine cultures and cerebrospinal exam were negative

L.I. Lutwick
Infectious Diseases (IIIE), VA New York Harbor Health Care System, 800 Poly Place, Brooklyn, NY 11209, USA
e-mail: larry.lutwick@va.gov

L.I. Lutwick, S.M. Lutwick (eds.), *Beyond Anthrax*,
DOI: 10.1007/978-1-59745-326-4_8, © Springer Science+Business Media, LLC 2008

or unremarkable. A history of incarceration in the World War II German concentration camp at Belsen was obtained from family members.

On day 7 of his illness, because of a suspicion of recrudescent typhus, oral tetracycline was begun. The headache ceased within 24 h and the fever remitted within 48 h. An IFA titer for *R. prowazekii* was 1:8,192.

8.2 The Organism

8.2.1 The History of Epidemic Typhus

Many classical typhus sources including Osler [3] quote August Hirsch's seminal text, *Handbook of Geographical and Historical Pathology* [4], to best describe the significance of typhus in history:

The history of typhus is written in those dark pages of the world's story that tells of the grievous visitations of mankind by war, famine and misery of every kind. In every age, as far back as the historical inquirer can follow the disease as all, typhus is met with an association with the saddest misfortunes of the populace; and it is, therefore, a well-grounded surmise that the numerous pestilences of war and famine in ancient times and in the Middle Ages, which are known to us... had included typhus fever as a prominent figure among them.

There has always been some disagreement as to when epidemic typhus first entered Europe. It is believed to be responsible for the Athenian Epidemic (430–426 BC) during the Peloponnesian War, playing a major role in the fall of Greece [5]. The first reliable description is from the Spanish siege of Moorish Granada in 1489 [6]. Of the 20,000 Spanish soldiers who died by early 1490, 17,000 died from disease, mostly probably from typhus. The infection also probably played a substantial role in the defeat of Napoleon's invasion of Russia.

Typhus disseminates quickly among distressed, disorganized populations produced by wars, disasters or famines. During World War I, it ravaged the armies of the Eastern front causing Lenin to say, "either socialism will defeat the louse, or the louse will defeat socialism." During the 8-year period from 1917 to 1925, over 25 million cases of epidemic typhus occurred in Russia, causing an estimated 3 million deaths [7]. Stephenson notes, indeed, that among the great wars for which records are available only the American Civil War and the Franco-Prussian War of 1870 are thought to not have had typhus in a starring role [8].

During World War II, typhus erupted throughout Europe, North Africa and the Middle East. It became so important to the war effort that, in 1942, the United States established a special Typhus Commission by an executive order of President Franklin D. Roosevelt [8]. Its reputation as a military medical problem was cleverly utilized to protect residents of occupied areas from departure to concentration camps [9]. Using the blood Weil–Felix reaction to detect pockets of infection, the German army avoided the areas for exportation to the camps. Ingeniously, Dr. Eugene Lazowski and others saved more than 8,000 individuals by using formalin killed *Proteus* OX-19 organisms as an immunogen to create an artificial "epidemic area." Control efforts during and a war are exemplified by Foster [10] and Davis [11].

Not known to be native to the Western Hemisphere, *R. prowazekii* was introduced by the Spanish during the conquests of the sixteenth century. The United States and Canada, in North America, experienced epidemic typhus in the late 1840s during a great wave of Irish immigration caused by one of Mother Nature's biological warfare events, the potato famine caused by the fungus (*Phytophthora infestans*). Many of the cases were acquired and caused death on route [12], causing many of the ships to be called "coffin ships." In Canada, among the 75,000 immigrants from Ireland in 1847, 30,000 contracted typhus and 20,000 died [8]. In the late twentieth century, outbreaks of epidemic typhus continued to occur given opportunistic human conditions including more than 45,000 cases in the African country of Burundi associated with civil war [13].

8.2.2 The Pathogen: Rickettsia prowazekii

Epidemic typhus and the zoonosis Q fever have been placed among the category B bioterrorism diseases with illness from other rickettsiae in category C. Walker [14] argues, however, that because of high infectivity by a stable, small particle aerosol, a low level of immunity in most populations and the potential of substantial morbidity and mortality, epidemic typhus should be a category A agent. He believes that the other rickettsiae require consideration for an upgrade as well. Despite this, most of this chapter will focus on the epidemic typhus organism.

R. prowazekii is named to honor two early workers in rickettsiology, Howard Ricketts and Stanislaus Prowazek, who both died from typhus in the early part of the twentieth century. *R. prowazekii* is an obligate non-motile intracellular bacterium. The organism reproduces by binary fission resulting in pair morphology. Difficulty of staining with common methodologies is a striking feature, including failure to retain the stain by Gram's method. Giemsa's solution, a modification of Romanowsky's method, is the most satisfactory tool for visualization of the organisms in the cytoplasm of cells, which can also be readily visualized by immunohistological staining.

Rickettsiae appear to attach to host cell receptors via outer membrane proteins (omp) as adhesions, inducing focal cytoskeletal rearrangements to enter the cell. The entry, requiring rickettsial metabolic activity, is followed by rapid lysis of the cell's phagosomal membrane before phagolysosomal fusion, avoiding exposure to the lysosomal enzymatic process [15]. *R. prowazekii* produces an invasion protein, InvA, which after entering the cytoplasm, functions as a dinucleoside oligophosphatase hydrolyzing stress-induced compounds [16]. Target cells are primarily vascular endothelial cells of all organs. Spread is by hematogenous means. The typhus group rickettsiae spread from cell to cell by rupture of an infected cell but the spotted fever group appears, in part, to use actin-based motility to spread [17].

Host entry of rickettsia is via the skin and mucous membrane but potentially all the rickettsiae can enter through the respiratory tract mucosa. The latter site, via aerosol, can occur naturally for *R. prowazekii* via contaminated clothing. Aerosolization in epidemic typhus can also occur from a laboratory accident or from an intentional bioterrorism event.

The complete nucleic acid sequence of *R. prowazekii* has been reported by Andersson et al [18], consisting of about 1.11 megabase pairs and 834 protein-coding genes. Characterization of the functional profiles of the genes by this group suggested that the organism is more closely related to mitochondria than any other microbe studied. This includes similar methods of ATP production and the reliance on host cell proteins for the biosynthesis and regulation of amino acids and nucleosides. The epidemic typhus rickettsia contains the highest proportion of noncoding DNA found in microbial genomes, 24%. It has been suggested that these noncoding sequences of DNA that these genomic areas are remnants of degenerated DNA [19].

8.2.3 The Vector: *Pediculus humanus humanus*

Of the 3,000 or so species of lice that have been characterized, only three are strictly human parasites, the clothing or body louse, *P. humanus humanus*; the head louse, *P. humanus capitus*; and the crab or pubic louse, *Pthrius pubis*. The taxonomy of the clothing and head louse has been debated over the years and it is generally regarded that they are variants of the same species [20,21]. Human lice have been recognized as parasites of man for thousands of years [6], having been identified on Egyptian mummies and on Pompeii's conserved bodies [21]. The principal vector of *R. prowazekii* is the clothing louse. This observation, resulting in a Nobel prize, was made by Dr. Charles Nicolle [22]. Nicolle, while working as the director of the Pasteur Institute in Tunis, observed that it was the clothing of typhus-infected individuals that contained the infectivity and subsequently demonstrated in 1909 that body lice were the source of typhus using chimpanzees. This louse is also the vector for *Borrelia recurrentis*, the agent of louse-borne relapsing fever and *Bartonella quintana*, the agent of trench fever [23].

For interest, it should be pointed out that free living lice-like insects (*Psocoptera*) may infest humans. Sometimes referred book lice because they can feed on mildewed books as well as other decaying matter, they are not known to transmit diseases to man [24] but can be a major household allergen [25].

Although it has generally been taught that the human body louse is the sole vector of *R. prowazekii* and that man was the sole reservoir of infection, neither is actually true. Indeed, it was shown by Nicolle that *P. h. capitus* is a competent vector of epidemic typhus as well. This observation has been confirmed by other investigators [26] and Murray and Torrey [27] have demonstrated that virulent *R. prowazekii* were excreted by head lice beginning 6 days after exposure. Man has been found to have company as a reservoir for *R. prowazekii* as well. In 1975, it was demonstrated that infection occurred in flying squirrels in southeastern United States [28]. Subsequent studies revealed that the squirrel flea, *Orchopeas howardii*, may feed on humans and transmit *R. prowazekii* if its principal host, the flying squirrel (*Glaucomys volans*), is unavailable [29]. Alternatively, since the flea is quite host-specific, infectious feces may be aerosolized. A case of *R. prowazekii* without travel history was diagnosed in New Mexico [30] suggesting that other small mammals may be reservoirs as well.

The *P. humanus* lice are members of *Anoplura*, sucking lice, feeding on mammals to use blood as a source of nutrients and water. It is important to realize that these lice are under constant water stress because their cuticular lipid components are not able to prevent dehydration [21]. Consequently, the lice must consistently replace its water supply by feeding on its host's blood. In the native situation, for survival the louse must feed 5 or 6 times daily. The feeding is usually performed leisurely due to the small diameter of the louse proboscis that does not allow rapid ingestion against the high pressure gradient needed to suck in the viscous blood [21]. Lice may survive without a blood meal for about 3 days [20].

Using lice raised in the laboratory, the natural interaction of *R. prowazekii* and the louse has been studied. Louse populations are now raised using rabbits but initially human volunteers were utilized [31]. As summarized and confirmed by Raoult's laboratory [32], the louse acquires *R. prowazekii* after feeding on a bacteremic host. The rickettsiae enter and replicate in the gut endothelium with subsequent release of large numbers of organisms into the gut lumen and passage in louse feces. Unlike the interactions between most vectors and their transmitted human pathogens, the life expectancy of the louse is clearly shortened when infected by *R. prowazekii*. The louse's demise is related to the transmural, infection-related disruption of the gut releasing blood into the hemolymph and turning the louse red, with death occurring within hours. The life span of infected lice in the laboratory was found to be 14.5 ± 3 days as compared to 39 ± 1.7 days for uninfected lice [32]. Rickettsiae-harboring lice are found in the feces beginning on day 5 following exposure. Viable organisms could be cultured into the feces for at least 10 days after emission but no evidence of rickettsiae could be found in the eggs or subsequently hatched larvae of infected lice [32].

The feeding itself is facilitated by the injection into the host skin of a variety of biologically active substances including an anticoagulant and an anesthetic. These proteins elicit a host immune response after several weeks. The reaction produces itching, the onset of which is likely to be the first sign of infestation.

Heavily fed areas of the body such as the groin and flanks can become increasing pigmented, referred to as Vagabond's disease [33]. The female body louse attaches her eggs to clothing, not to the body or hair, often on the inner belts of underwear, pants or skirts [20]. When removed from the body, even in the absence of insecticides, the unwashed clothes will be absent of viable lice and eggs within 7 days. Raoult and Roux [33] cite Maunder [34] who hypothesized that religious Sabbath and Sunday ritual days of rest with a change of clothes could be attributed to a delousing cycle.

8.3 Natural Disease

8.3.1 Epidemiology

Epidemic typhus is a vector-borne disease with a complex epidemiology. Because lice live in clothing, weather, humidity, and lack of hygiene determine their prevalence. Consequently, *P. h. humanus* is more prevalent during the colder months and epidemic typhus is more frequently reported during the winter and early spring [35]. The permanent foci of the body louse occur in regions subject to cold weather, where inhabitants need to wear multiple layers of clothes, and in poverty-stricken communities whose inhabitants lack multiple sets of clothes. Such populations are most common in mountainous regions of countries in intertropical zones, including Ethiopia [36], Burundi, and Rwanda in Africa [13], Peru in South America, and Nepal and Tibet in central Asia [37]. The prevalence of body lice increases with altitude [38]. Infestation with lice is more frequent during wars, in trenches and in jail, where conditions are cramped, when cold is present, and where hygiene is limited. Large outbreaks of lice have been associated with the recent civil wars in Burundi [39]. Two years later, an outbreak of typhus occurred in jail in Burundi [40], and subsequently, a huge outbreak of typhus occurred in several refugee camps where nearly all inhabitants were louse-infested [13]. More recently, the disease has reemerged in the highlands of Algeria [41] and a case was more recently diagnosed in Marseilles, France [42].

8.3.2 Modes of Transmission

During a blood meal, the louse defecates highly infective feces at the site of its feeding. *Rickettsiae* present in louse feces may then be introduced into abraded or injured skin or mucus membranes by either scratching or hand contamination since skin irritation commonly occurs at the site of a louse bite. Lice feces may remain infectious for as long as 100 days and, as a result, human to human transmission can occur via the sharing of clothes or via transfer of the dust-like, rickettsia-laden feces from one human to another [35] with an incubation period of 1–2 weeks. In the absence of lice, person-to-person transmission ought not to occur.

The feces may be aerosolized and typical epidemic typhus has been clearly associated with previously infested clothing long after any viable lice or eggs would have remained. The mechanism of prolonged survival of *R. prowazekii* in louse feces is unclear. In examining the ultrastructure of *R. prowazekii* from various parts of the louse gut as well as the feces, no morphological differences were noted [43]. Louse feces do not appear to contain any unique protective substances and has been postulated [43] that an adaptive physiological change may account for the survival, which may be related to the mechanism of "latency" in Brill–Zinsser disease (see Sect. 8.4.1.2).

The sylvatic cycle of infection involving flying squirrels and their ectoparasites with secondary transmission to humans has been recognized in the United States [29]. In these conditions, transmission occurs only when human have direct contact with infected flying squirrels especially when the animals are nesting in the attics of homes during colder months. Using restriction endonuclease digestion, human and flying squirrel-associated epidemic typhus strains can be distinguished [44].

8.3.3 Pathogenesis

The precise mechanism by which *R. prowazekii* produces cellular injury is still uncertain. Oxidative stress injury to the host cell membrane occurs during rickettsial infection of endothelial cells, (at least with *R. rickettsii*) and antioxidant moieties such as α-lipoic acid in vitro can lessen injury in a cell culture model [45]. A rickettsia-produced phospholipase is also likely to be a virulence factor during infection [46]. A gene encoding for a phospholipase D has been identified in *R. prowazekii* [47] and antibody against this enzyme was found to decrease rickettsial cytotoxicity in cell culture.

R. prowazekii causes cellular injury in the absence of inflammatory responses with a widespread vasculitis contributing to increased vascular permeability, edema, and activation of humoral inflammatory and coagulation mechanisms. As illness advances, progressive endothelial damage leads to widespread vascular dysfunction. Mural and intimal thrombi in small vessels surrounded by inflammatory infiltrates may occur throughout the central nervous system, named typhus nodules.

In severe infection, plasma and protein permeability is enhanced from the intravascular compartment to the interstitium. In addition, microscopic and macroscopic foci of hemorrhage occur as a result of disrupted vessel injury [48]. Vasculitis can be generalized and virtually any organ can be affected [49].

8.4 Diagnosis

8.4.1 Clinical Presentation

R. prowazekii infection produces two distinct clinical syndromes. Primarily, typhus is an acute potentially severe infection occurring 7–14 days after exposure to infected lice or lice feces but the infection can occur as a recrudescent form called Brill–Zinsser disease that may occur 10–50 years after primary infection.

8.4.1.1 Acute R. prowazekii Infection

After an incubation period of 10–14 days, the symptoms often abruptly with a chill followed by fever but can be preceded by a few days of anorexia, malaise, nausea and significant headache. The fever curve reaches its peak by the end of the first week of illness and may reach 104–106°F. Although morning remissions of fever may occur early, they are not very significant during the second week, the end of which the fever often drops precipitously [3]. Other symptoms include conjunctivitis, severe headache, constipation, profound prostration and orthopnea (from cardiac dysfunction) become more prominent at the onset of the typhus rash. Symptoms are outlined in Table 8.1.

The rash begins around the fourth day of fever initially involving the axillae and flanks then spreading to the chest and back before involving the extremities, all over 2 or 3 days. The exathem often spares the face, is most prominent on the back, and can become almost measles-like. Difficult to see in dark-skinned individuals, the cutaneous eruption can involve the palms and soles and persists for a variable time, from days to weeks [20]. Osler [3] describes it as having dual elements: a fine, irregular, red subcuticular mottling and distinct papular rose spots that may evolve into petechiae. In severe disease, there is the development of cutaneous hemorrhage.

Table 8.1 Frequency of clinical symptoms associated with epidemic typhus

Parameter	Reference [13]	Reference [50]
Cases	102	60
Fever	100	100
Headache	100	100
Myalgias	100	70
Rash (any)	25	38
Purpuric eruption	10	33
Delirium or confusion	80	18
Coma	4	0
Nausea or vomiting	56	42
Cough	70	38
Diarrhea	12	7
Splenomegaly	8	13
Conjunctivitis	15	53

Potentially impacting on the aerosolization of organisms in a bioterrorism event is the presence of respiratory symptoms in natural occurring typhus. Stephenson [8] remarks that cough is extremely frequent and, although it may occur at the onset of symptoms, is most prominent at the time of the appearance of the rash. He refers to physicians who believe that some amount of pneumonia is always present in epidemic typhus but does not differentiate from rickettsial or secondary bacterial causes. Pulmonary involvement in scrub typhus (caused by *Orientia tsutsugamushi*) spread by infected mite bites) has been found to occur frequently and in part is due to an ARDS-like picture rather than a focal process [51]. Histopathologic studies of the lung in scrub typhus have shown neither vasculitis nor evidence of rickettisae in the lung tissue suggesting an immunologic mechanism [52]. Q fever, the rickettsial disease that is spread by aerosol without a vector, does cause pneumonia as its primary manifestation.

The symptom complex for which the illness typhus is named relates to the mental status changes accompanying the illness, developing towards the end of the first week. The term typhus is derived from a Greek word for cloud that relates to the cloudy mental status of the affected person. Typhoid (also referred to as abdominal typhus) has a similar neuropsychiatric picture that also can be seen in other infectious diseases. Often suggesting a poor prognosis, the state is referred to as coma vigil or the typhoid state [53]. Coma vigil, also referred to as muttering delirium, is a condition in the patient lies on his or her back with muscular twitching and tremulous hands picking at the bedclothes and at imaginary objects. Despite deceptively bright eyes and continual whispering, the individual is unconscious of the surroundings [3]. Alternative neuropsychiatric manifestations include restlessness and hallucinations. Some degree of confusion and disorientation may remain for weeks or months following the acute illness. Hearing loss may also be a residual symptom [54].

Patients with severe disease may develop gangrene of the distal extremities. Mortality (Table 8.2) generally occurs during the second week and, as reported by Osler [3], was 12%–20% in the preantimicrobial era. Case fatality rates were much lower in children but reached as high as 50% in older adults. Deaths are related in cardiac failure and vascular collapse and later deaths from secondary bacterial infections (Table 8.2). Adequate and prompt therapy can reduce the mortality substantially.

Table 8.2 Mortality rate: epidemic typhus Egypt 1943–1944 (adapted from [55])

Age (years)	Male mortality rate (%)	Female mortality rate (%)
16–20	9.6	8.7
21–25	15.2	10.4
26–30	25.5	13.7
31–35	30.8	18.8
36–40	33.6	25.4
41–48	47.0	32.6

8.4.1.2 Brill–Zinsser Disease

Recrudescent typhus or Brill–Zinsser disease can appear in patients who had totally recovered from epidemic typhus, years after the onset of the first infection [2,56]. For unclear reasons, immunological or otherwise, viable *R. prowazekii* retained in the body become activated. The disease is sporadic, occurs in the absence of infected lice and, for unknown reasons, clusters more commonly in the months of June and July [57]. In contrast to acute primary infection, Brill–Zinsser disease is generally milder with minimal mortality.

The disease is best described by Nathan Brill's 1910 report of 221 cases from New York City [57] and it is consistent with a typhus-like illness. Brill's original postulate ruled out typhoid by virtue of negative serological and blood culture confirmation and he felt that, in the absence of transmissibility, no mortality and the occurrence during warmer months, it was not typhus. Subsequently, Hans Zinsser utilized epidemiological and cultural means to suggest that Brill's disease was an imported form of classical epidemic typhus, recrudescent from an initial infection acquired in Europe [58]. Additionally, *R. prowazekii* was not only confirmed as obtainable for the blood of Brill–Zinsser patients but clothing lice fed on these patients became infected with the rickettsia [59].

8.4.1.3 Latency in Rickettsial Infections

Although the pathophysiology of persistent rickettsial presence in individuals infected months or decades previously is not well established, documentation of such isolations exists. Indeed, Price [60, 61] demonstrated that *R. prowazekii* could be isolated from abdominal lymph nodes of two Russians who migrated to the United States decades before. Isolation of the organism required initial incubation of minced lymph node in tissue culture, intraperitoneal inoculation into cotton rats and passage of a rat brain suspension into chicken embryo yolk sacs. Primary isolation was not accomplished, suggesting the organism was in a dormant state initially.

Similar observations have been made with several other rickettsiae. Smadel and colleagues isolated the scrub typhus rickettsia from lymph nodes obtained from individuals 1–2 years following acute infection [62]. Likewise, similar observations have been made in Rocky Mountain spotted fever (RMSF) [63]. That such strains may be of lower virulence is suggested by *R. prowazekii* isolated after long-term persistence in cotton rats was of lower antigenicity and virulence [64] and an attenuated strain of *Coxiella burnetii* used for vaccinating against Q fever was able to persist in mice [65].

8.4.1.4 Bioterrorism-Associated *R. prowazekii* Infection

The relatively stable, easily aerosolizable *R. prowazekii*-laden dust-like lice feces clearly represent a readily easily producible source of the agent of epidemic typhus. Both the Japanese during World War II [66] and the Soviet Union during the Cold War era of the 1970s [67] studied the agent in an airborne form. A disease of substantial morbidity and mortality if not recognized and treated quickly, in and of itself typhus is not felt to be transmissible from person-to-person. Substantial spread, however, can occur if the organism is introduced into a *P. h. humanus* infested population. A biologically weaponized *R. prowazekii* could be engineered to be manifest antimicrobial resistance and could produce mortality rates as reported with natural disease during World War II in Egypt [68].

Demonstrating potential infectivity of a rickettsial aerosol are the numerous laboratory-associated cases of infection. Although direct transcutaneous inoculation of the pathogen in the lab milieu occurs, many cases appear to be related to infectious aerosols of the rickettsia causing RMSF [69], murine typhus [70], scrub typhus [71] as well as *R. prowazekii* [72]. In the latter, a cumulative report of 3,921 cases of laboratory-associated infection collected over several decades and published in 1976, Pike cited a total of 573 cases of rickettsial infection (381 in the United States) with 56 cases of *R. prowazekii* infection (22 in the United States). In the analysis of the proven or probable cases, 217 of the rickettsial total (36%) were aerosol in nature and 230 (40%) were of unknown or unclear source.

Rickettsiae can be found in the lung after transcutaneous or aerosol exposure. In a histopathological study of 10 fatal cases of *R. rickettsii* [73], the distribution of the spotted fever organism by immunofluorescence coincided with vasculitis in the lung. Here, the location of the organisms suggested that person-to-person aerosol spread was unlikely, the same observation made epidemiologically. In epidemic typhus, however, a pathologic study from Egypt during World War II [74] found rickettsiae-like organisms primarily in the cytoplasm of leukocytes in alveolar and bronchial exudates. Besides demonstrating that pneumonia in typhus was at least partly due to the primary infection, the possibility of respiratory spread was brought up by the findings. The authors, however, cited earlier work that neither sputum, nasal washings, nor tracheal aspirates demonstrated the organism.

8.4.2 Laboratory Diagnosis

8.4.2.1 Laboratory Abnormalities

Thrombocytopenia, elevated serum aminotransferases, and increased bilirubin levels may occur in severe cases. The frequency with which these laboratory abnormalities occur is illustrated in Table 8.3. Electrocardiographic evidence of myocarditis and diffuse or focal pulmonary infiltrates on chest x-ray occur in minority of patients may occur in a small percentage of patients [55].

Table 8.3 Frequency of laboratory abnormalities associated with epidemic typhus

Parameter	Reference [50]
Cases	60
Thrombocytopenia	43
Increased aspartate aminotransferase level	63
Increased alanine aminotransferase level	35
Increased bilirubin level	20
Increased serum creatinine level	2
Hematuria	44
Proteinuria	28

8.4.2.2 Serology

Weil and Felix described the classical assay for rickettsial antibody detection in 1916 [75]. The methodology took advantage of heterophilic (cross-reacting) antigens of members of the genus *Rickettsia* and several species of the Gram negative bacillus *Proteus*. In the Weil–Felix test, bacteria of *Proteus vulgaris* OX-19 agglutinate with sera of the infected with the typhus group organisms as well as from RMSF. Cells of *P. vulgaris* OX-2, on the other hand, agglutinate with sera from individuals with spotted fever infection except RMSF. The OX-19 agglutination is seen in epidemic typhus but usually not in Brill–Zinsser recrudescent disease. *P. mirabilis* OX-K can be similarly used in the serological diagnosis of scrub typhus. Because of the both relatively poor sensitivity and specificity of this test including for epidemic typhus [76], more specific assays are needed for diagnosis.

Such specific serologic tests are the mainstay of diagnosis, since isolation of *R. prowazekii* is generally impractical and can be dangerous to laboratorians. Serologic tests include indirect fluorescence antibody (IFA) [77, 78], latex agglutination [79], complement fixation and enzyme-linked immunosorbent assay [78, 80]. A diagnosis of recent epidemic or murine typhus rickettsial infection can be established by demonstrating a fourfold or greater rise in titer of antibody in properly collected acute and convalescent serum samples. Titers are usually detectable during or after the second week.

Two of the serological tests are widely available for epidemic typhus: an IFA test and an immunoblot technique. These tests are available in most state health departments, the CDC, and a few specialized research laboratories. Neither of these can reliably differentiate between acute primary infections from Brill–Zinsser disease [81]. Additionally, epidemic and endemic typhus (due to *R. typhi*) cannot be differentiated by serology, unless Western immunoblot (WB) and/or cross-adsorption of sera are done [82].

The IFA is generally considered to be the gold standard for rickettsial serological diagnosis [78]. The WB assay has been found in Mediterranean spotted fever to be somewhat more sensitive that IFA for early antibody with the first antibody detected being against the lipopolysaccharide [83]. Latex agglutinins that are group specific are available for *R. prowazekii* and require minimal equipment [79]. Antibodies against outer membrane proteins (omp) may be useful for even earlier serological diagnosis. Using a recombinant omp of scrub typhus, an immunochromatographic assay was significantly better than IFA [84]. In the study, this assay was positive before IFA (by about a week) in 50 and the reverse in only seven.

8.4.2.3 Molecular

Molecular diagnostic assays are becoming increasingly common for the diagnosis of infectious diseases. Techniques using polymerase chain reaction (PCR) technology have been used to detect typhus in blood and to detect these organisms in their vector [13, 39, 85, 86]. DNA sequencing of PCR products provides a definitive method for the differentiation of closely related etiologic agents that are cross-reactive serologically and that cause infections with similar clinical presentations, as is the case with murine and epidemic typhus.

In a 2001 case report [30], typhus-specific 17 kDa gene assay that used a nested PCR protocol was found to increase sensitivity. This assay amplified the DNA of both *R. typhi* and *R. prowazekii.* Using nine nucleotide differences within the region of the 17 kDa gene amplified by the nested assay, it allowed identification of the infection as either endemic or epidemic. Subsequently, a real-time quantitative PCR assay, specific for *R. prowazekii,* showed it to be sensitive to 1–5 copies per sample and was useful in experimentally infected mice [87].

Biopsy of a skin rash can lead to a definitive diagnosis by demonstrating the characteristic changes of rickettsial vasculitis and the presence of rickettsiae in tissue by use of fluorescent antibody conjugates. The use of monoclonal antibodies has been utilized to improve the specificity of the assay and can differentiate epidemic from endemic typhus [88].

8.4.2.4 Culture

Due to the nature of the organism, culture is usually difficult to perform requiring 5–8-day-old embryonated eggs from flocks on antimicrobial-free diets or susceptible animals such as guinea pigs or mice in an isolated environment to provide protection to the laboratory worker. More recently, a centrifugation-shell vial system has been used to cultivate *R. prowazekii,* reported to be the first clinical isolation of the epidemic typhus fever rickettsia in 30 years. The small area of the cell containing coverslip enhanced the ratio of organisms to cells as well as detection [89]. Identification was then made by PCR amplification of specific genes.

8.5 Therapeutic Intervention

Rickettsial in vitro susceptibility has been evaluated in lice [90] and cells [91]. Tetracycline and chloramphenicol have been generally thought to be the agents to use in the treatment of epidemic typhus [92]. Doxycycline, 200 mg orally once, is the regimen of choice. Medical facilities are often diagnostically inadequate in areas where epidemic typhus is seen. An alternative for empiric treatment in the absence of confirmation of the diagnosis serologically would be the administration of chloramphenicol 500 mg orally or intravenously four times for 5 days. This regimen is highly effective in epidemic typhus and simultaneously covers the possibility of meningococcemia and typhoid fever. Doxycycline is, however, preferable for therapy of human *R. prowazekii* infection.

Most typhus-infected individuals treated with doxycycline or chloramphenicol improve markedly within 48 h following initiation of therapy. Failure to show a response within 48–72 h after starting empirical treatment is often considered to be clinical evidence that a rickettsial disease is not present. In a small study, a single 200 mg oral dose of doxycycline cured 35 of 37 patients, and 29 of 37 patients were afebrile 48 h after therapy was started [93]. Although antimicrobial resistance to the tetracyclines and/or chloramphenicol in the genus *Rickettsia* is rare, poor responsiveness of some northern Thailand strains of *R. tsutsugamushi* in human disease, murine models and cell culture have been described [94]. A biowarfare laboratory should be able to transform *R. prowazekii* into a tetracycline and/or chloramphenicol resistant form.

Other antimicrobial agents with evidence for activity [91] include fluoroquinolones such as ciprofloxacin, ofloxacin and levofloxacin, macrolides such as erythromycin and clarithromycin, and rifampin. Typhus group rickettsiae are more sensitive to the macrolides than the spotted fever group [91] although patients with recrudescent typhus have been reported not to respond to azithromycin [95]. Additionally, heterogeneity in rifampin resistance has been found in some subgroups of rickettsiae but not the typhus group [91].

Beta-lactams, aminoglycosides and sulfonamides are not active. Importantly, not only are sulfa drugs not active but the use of this class of antimicrobials for human rickettsial infection is harmful. The medications inhibit production of para-aminobenzoic acid, a compound that has a therapeutic effect in rickettsial infections including louse-borne typhus [96]. Indeed, more severe rickettsial infections and higher mortality rates have been reported after the use of this class of antimicrobials [97, 98].

Anecdotal case reports have appeared of a patient misdiagnosed as having typhoid who died from typhus after treatment with ciprofloxacin, despite in vitro efficacy [1] and of patients with the successful use of the fluoroquinolone in *R. typhi* infection [99, 100].

Supportive care, including fluids, vasopressors, oxygen, and even dialysis may be required in patients with severe illness. The prognosis is dependent upon several factors including age, underlying nutritional status, previous health of the patient, and the delay in initiation of therapy. In the preantibiotic era, the mortality rate was higher in older and male patients. In the modern era, mortality is uncommon if treatment is given. In a series of 60 treated patients, none of those treated died [101]. In another small study, two of nine patients died despite chloramphenicol therapy [39]. The death rate of untreated epidemic typhus is approximately 15%. This rate is reduced to 0.5% with a single 200 mg dose of doxycycline. Infections are rarely fatal in children; however, the mortality rate can be as high as 60% without treatment [102]. The prognosis of Brill–Zinsser disease is generally good, although rare fatalities have been reported [103].

8.6 Preventive Measures

8.6.1 Infection Control

Eradication of human infestation with lice will prevent natural transmission of epidemic typhus. People who live and work in close proximity to a louse-infested individual may secondarily acquire lice, even if they regularly wash their clothes and have good hygiene. Thus, all louse-infested persons and workers in close contact with infested persons may require long acting insecticides. Application of effective residual insecticide powder at appropriate intervals by hand or power blower to clothes and populations at risk is recommended. Spread of infection does not need contact with live, typhus-infected lice, as previous mentioned, since organism-laden feces can be aerosolized from clothing or bed sheets.

Insecticides that can be used include DDT, malathion, and lindane. Reports of resistance to one or more of these agents have appeared. The synthetic pyrethroid permethrin has been demonstrated to be effective and long-lasting when applied as a dust or spray on clothing and bedding [104]. Fabric treated with permethrin has been shown to retain toxicity to body lice even after 20 washings, offering long-term passive protection [105].

The use of chloramphenicol or tetracycline for prophylaxis may be highly effective in interrupting typhus outbreaks [91]. Some experts recommend the use of one 200 mg dose of doxycycline once weekly by travelers in which epidemic typhus is present. Prophylaxis is generally continued for 1 week after leaving such areas.

Afflicted patients should be reported to local health authority. Louse-infested susceptibles exposed to typhus fever should be quarantined for 15 days after application of insecticide with residual effect. Isolation is not required after proper delousing of patient, clothing, living quarters and household contacts. Lice tend to leave hot or cold bodies in search for a normothermic clothed body. If death from louse-borne typhus occurred, delousing the body and clothing by application of an insecticide is recommended [106].

All immediate contacts should be kept under surveillance for 2 weeks. Every effort should be made to trace the infection to the index case. Application of an insecticide with residual effect to all contacts will result in rapid control of typhus. Systematic application of residual insecticide to all people in the community is indicated in widespread infestations. Notification by governments to World Health Organization (WHO), and to adjacent disease free countries is indicated.

8.6.2 Immunization

The history of typhus vaccination is one of the most colorful in vaccinology. Both inactivated and live attenuated vaccines against *R. prowazekii* have been developed and tested. Woodward [107] stated that the earliest protective methodology for epidemic typhus was the eating of lice but it was and is of totally unclear efficacy. Weigl in Poland developed the first vaccine for *R. prowazekii* in lice [107], using a technique developed for the RMSF/*Dermacentor* tick model by Spencer and Parker. The vaccine required the intrarectal inoculation of the lice with viable rickettisae using the equivalent of a miniature enema and subsequent feeding of the lice on convalescent typhus individuals. The louse intestinal tract was then harvested and formalinized to produce an inactivated vaccine, which appeared to be protective, requiring 30–100 intestines for each human dose. The procedure was not only tedious but also resulted in infections and death of laboratory workers.

Woodward also described another early epidemic typhus vaccine and produced in a unique manner. Originally reported by Blanc and Baltazard from Morocco, the technique used murine typhus-infected guinea pigs as rickettsial donors placed in pits containing tens of thousands of hungry fleas. As a result, the donors died from exsanguination and the fleas became infected with *R. typhi*. The vaccine recipe then required the addition of white cotton rats to the pit. These rodents also died of blood loss and became brown colored from the flea fecal matter deposited in their coat. The rats were removed and rubbed over a mesh to collect the rickettsial-laden flea feces. This material was "reconstituted" with saline and ox bile prior to injection. Ox bile was used as "attenuation," which may have attenuated *R. typhi* as the organism caused a milder disease in most cases and could provide subsequent protection against *R. prowazekii* [107].

An attenuated *R. prowazekii*, referred to as the E (for España) or Madrid E strain, was developed in Spain in the early 1940s. The organism, isolated from a severe case of typhus, was passed 11 times in eggs prior to the decrease of virulence in guinea pigs [108]. This vaccine seemed to be able to prevent classical typhus but further development was limited [107] by moderate to severe reactions and concern about possible reversion to virulence. Interestingly, in terms of rickettsial replication and louse mortality, there is no different in virulence between the E and the Breinl (virulent) strain [109]. Comparing the genome of the E and Breinl strains, there are genomic variations in about 3% of the 834 protein-coding sequences of the attenuated strain [109] and 24 genes in E had decreased expression and one had increased expression as compared to the virulent strain.

A number of inactivated typhus vaccines have been evaluated including chicken egg (Cox) and rat lung (Durand) types. In a small study, Woodward reported [107] that both were reasonably well tolerated with little local or systemic toxicity and most recipients developed antibody. The inactivated vaccines provided some level of protection [107, 110] but incidence reduction was not conclusively demonstrated [111]. Vaccinees are more likely to have milder disease [68]. In the United States, Cox-type vaccine had been available in the past with the recommendation of two subcutaneous doses given at least a month apart with a booster given every 6–12 months as long as continued risk existed [112].

Genomic technology has begun being utilized in the production of DNA typhus vaccines. As an example, Coker et al [113] utilized the genome sequence of the E strain of *R. prowazekii* to identify genes that might be potential targets in immunoprotection to provide, in particular, cellular immune responses to the intracellular rickettsiae. These genes have been amplified and introduced into a cloning vector for further study. Using a spotted fever model, a DNA vaccine with outer membrane protein (omp) A and B genes was studied in mice [114]. Protection was achieved in this model with the use of a DNA vaccine prime followed by boosting with a recombinant omp. A cellular immune response was detected and protection occurred without any detectable antibody response. A murine typhus ompB was completely protective in mice and partially protective in guinea pigs against lethal doses of *R. typhi* [115, 116].

References

1. Zanetti, G., Francioli, P., Tugan, D., et al. Imported epidemic typhus. *Lancet* 352, 1709, 1998.
2. Lutwick, L. I. Brill-Zinsser disease. *Lancet* 357, 1198–1200, 2001.
3. Osler, W. The Principles and Practice of Medicine, 3rd edn. D. Appleton and Co., New York, 1899.
4. Hirsch, A. Handbook of Geographical and Historical Pathology. Translated by Creighton, C. New Syndenham Society, London, 1885.
5. Retief, F. P. and Cilliers, L. The epidemics of Athens, 430-426 BC. *S. Afr. Med. J.* 88, 50–3, 1998.
6. Zinsser, H. Rats, Lice and History. Little Brown, Boston, 1934.
7. Weiss, E. The role of rickettsioses in history. In: Biology of Rickettsial Diseases, vol. 1, Walker, D. H (ed). CRC Press, Boca Raton, pp.1, 1988.
8. Stephenson, C. S. Epidemic typhus fever and other rickettsial diseases of military importance. *N. Engl. J. Med.* 231, 407–413, 1944.
9. Lasowski, E. S. and Matulewicz, S. Serendipitous discovery of artificial positive Weil–Felix reaction used in "primitive immunological war". *ASM News* 43, 300–302, 1977.
10. Foster, G. M. Typhus disaster in the wake of war: the American-Polish relief expedition, 1919–1920. *Bull. Hist. Med.* 55, 221–232, 1981.
11. Davis, W. A. Typhus at Belsen. I. Control of the typhus epidemic. *Am. J. Hyg.* 46, 66–83, 1947.
12. Gelston, A. L. and Jones, T. C. Typhus fever: report of an epidemic in New York City in 1847. *J. Infect. Dis.* 136, 813–821, 1977.
13. Raoult, D., Ndihokubwayo, J. B., Tissot-Dupont, H., et al. Outbreak of epidemic typhus associated with trench fever in Burundi. *Lancet* 352, 353–358, 1998.
14. Walker, D. H. Principles of the malicious use of infectious agents to create terror. Reasons for concern for organisms of the genus *Rickettsia. Ann. N. Y. Acad. Sci.* 990, 739–742, 2003.
15. Walker, D. H., Valbuena, G. A., and Olano, J. P. Pathogenic mechanisms of diseases caused by *Rickettsia. Ann. N. Y. Acad. Sci.* 990, 1–11, 2003.

16. Gaywee, J., Xu, W., Radulovic, S., et al. The *Rickettsia prowazekii* invasion gene homolog (invA) encodes a nudix hydrolase active on adenosine (5′)-pentaphospho-(5′)-adenosine. *Mol. Cell. Proteomics* 1, 179–185, 2002.
17. Heinzen, R. A., Grieshaben, S. S., Van Kirk, L. S., et al. Dynamics of actin-based movement of *Rickettsia rickettsii* in Vero cells. *Infect. Immun.* 67, 4201–4207, 1999.
18. Andersson, S. G., Zomorodopour, A., Andersson, J. O. The genome sequence of *Rickettsia prowazekii* and the origin of mitochondria. *Nature* 396, 133–140, 1998.
19. Andersson, J. O. and Andersson, S. G. Pseudogenes, junk DNA, and the dynamics of rickettsial genomes. *Mol. Biol. Evol.* 18, 829–839, 2001.
20. Ko, C. J. and Elston, D. M. Pediculosis. *J. Am. Acad. Dermatol.* 50, 1–12, 2004
21. Burgess, I. F. Human lice and their management. *Adv. Parasitol.* 36, 271–342, 1995.
22. Gross L. How Charles Nicolle of the Pasteur Institute discovered that epidemic typhus is transmitted by lice: reminiscences from my years at the Pasteur Institute in Paris. *Proc. Natl. Acad. Sci. U.S.A.* 93, 10539–10540, 1996.
23. Fournier, P. E., Ndihokubwayo, J. B., Guidran, J., et al. Human pathogens in body and head louse. *Emerg. Infect. Dis.* 8, 1515–1518, 2002.
24. Elston, D. M. What's eating you? *Psocoptera* (Book lice, Psocids) *Cutis* 64, 307–308, 1999.
25. Patil, M. P., Niphadkar, P. V., and Bapat, M. M. *Psocoptera* spp. (book louse): a new major household allergen in Mumbai. *Ann. Allergy Asthma Immunol.* 87, 151–155, 2001.
26. Robinson, D., Leo, N., Prociv, P., and Barker, S. C. Potential role of head lice, *Pediculus humanus capitus*, a vector of *Rickettsia prowazekii. Parasitol. Res.* 90, 209–211, 2003.
27. Murray, E. S. and Torrey, S. B. Virulence of *Rickettsia prowazekii* for head lice. *Ann. N. Y. Acad. Sci.* 266, 25–34, 1975.
28. Bozeman, F. M., Masicllo, S. A., Williams, M. S., and Elisberg, B. L. Epidemic typhus isolated from flying squirrels. *Nature* 255, 545, 1975.
29. Sonenshine, D. E., Bozeman, F. M., Williams, M. S., et al. Epizootiology of epidemic typhus (*Rickettsia prowazekii*) in flying squirrels. *Am. J. Trop. Med. Hyg.* 27, 339–349, 1978.
30. Massung, R. F., Davis, L. E., Slater, K., et al. Epidemic typhus meningitis in the southwestern United States. *Clin. Infect. Dis.* 32, 979–982, 2001.
31. Culpepper, G. H. The rearing and maintenance of a laboratory colony of the body louse. *Am. J. Trop. Med. Hyg.* 24, 327–329, 1944.
32. Houhamdi, L., Fournier, P.-E., Fang, R., et al. An experimental model of human body louse infection with *Rickettsia prowazekii. J. Infect. Dis.* 186, 1639–1646, 2002.
33. Raoult, D. and Roux, V. The body louse as a vector of reemerging human diseases. *Clin. Infect. Dis.* 29, 888–911, 1999.
34. Maunder, J. W. The appreciation of lice. *Proc. R. Inst. Great Britain* 55, 1–31, 1983.
35. Patterson, K. D. Typhus and its control in Russia, 1870–1940. *Med Hist.* 37, 361–381, 1993.
36. Mumcuoglu, K. Y., Miller, J., Manor, O., et al. The prevalence of ectoparasites in Ethiopian immigrants. *Isr. J. Med. Sci.* 29, 371–373, 1993.
37. Fan, M. Y., Walker, D. H., Yu, S. R., and Liu, Q. H. Epidemiology and ecology of rickettsial diseases in the People's Republic of China. *Rev. Infect. Dis.* 9, 823–840, 1987.
38. Tesfayohannes, T. Prevalence of body lice in elementary school students in three Ethiopian towns at different attitudes. *Ethiop. Med. J.* 27, 201–207, 1989.
39. World Health Organization. A large outbreak of epidemic louse-borne typhus in Burundi. *Wkly. Epidemiol Rec.* 72, 152–153, 1997.
40. Raoult, D., Roux, V., Ndihokubwaho, J. B., et al. Jail fever (epidemic typhus) outbreak in Burundi. *Emerg. Infect. Dis.* 3, 357–360, 1997.
41. Mokrani, K., Fournier, P. E., Dalichaouche, M., et al. Reemerging threat of epidemic typhus in Algeria. *J. Clin. Microbiol.* 42, 3898–3900, 2004.

42. Badiaga, S., Brouqui, P., and Raoult, D. Autochthonous epidemic typhus associated with *Bartonella quintana* bacteremia in a homeless person. *Am. J. Trop. Med. Hyg.* 72, 638–639, 2005.
43. Silverman, D. J., Boese, J. L., and Wissman Jr., C. L. Ultrastructural studies of *Rickettsia prowazekii* from louse midgut cells to feces: search for "dormant" forms. *Infect. Immun.* 10, 257–263, 1974.
44. Regner, R. L., Yuan Fu, Z., and Spruill, C. L. Flying squirrel-associated *Rickettsia prowazekii* (epidemic typhus rickettsiae) characterized by a specific DNA fragment produced by restriction endonuclease digestion. *J. Clin. Microbiol.* 23, 189–191, 1986.
45. Eremeeva, M. E. and Silverman, D. J. Effects of the antioxidant α-lipoic acid on human umbilical vein endothelial cells infected with *Rickettsia rickettsii. Infect. Immun.* 66, 2290–2299, 1998.
46. Winkler, H. H. and Miller, E. T. Immediate cytotoxicity and phospholipase A: the role of phospholipase A in the interaction of *R. prowazekii* and L cells. In: Rickettsiae and Rickettsial Diseases, Burgdorfer, W. and Anacker, R. L. (eds). Academic Press, New York. pp.327, 1981.
47. Renesto, P., Dehoux, P., Gouin, E., et al. Identification and characterization of a phospholipase D-superfamily gene in rickettsiae. *J. Infect. Dis.* 188, 1276–1283, 2003.
48. Walker, D. H. Pathology and pathogenesis of the vasculotropic rickettsioses. In: Biology of Rickettsial Disease, Walker, D. H. (ed.), CRC Press, Boca Raton. pp.115–1138, 1988.
49. Wolbach, S., Todd, J., and Palfrey, F. The Etiology and Pathology of Typhus. Harvard University Press, Cambridge, MA, 1922.
50. Perine, P. L., Chandler, B. P., Krause, D. K., et al. A clinico-epidemiological study of epidemic typhus in Africa. *Clin. Infect. Dis.* 14, 1149–1158, 1992.
51. Tsay, R.-W. and Chang, F.-Y. Acute respiratory distress syndrome in scrub typhus. *Q. J. Med.* 95, 126–128, 2002.
52. Park, J. S., Jee, Y. K., Lee, K. Y., et al. Acute respiratory distress syndrome associated with scrub typhus: diffuse alveolar damage without pulmonary vasculitis. *J. Korean Med. Sci.* 15, 343–345, 2000.
53. Verghese, A. The "typhoid state" revisited. *Am. J. Med.* 79, 370–372, 1985.
54. Friedmann, I., Frohlich, A., and Wright A. Epidemic typhus fever and hearing loss: a histological study (Hall pike collection of temporal bone sections). *J. Laryngol. Otol.* 107, 275–283, 1993.
55. Diab, S. M., Araj, G. F., and Fenech, F. F. Cardiovascular and pulmonary complications of epidemic typhus. *Trop. Geogr. Med.* 41, 76–79, 1989.
56. Green, C., Fishbein, D., and Gleiberman, I. Brill-Zinsser: still with us. *JAMA* 264, 1811–1812, 1990.
57. Brill, N. E. An acute infectious disease of unknown origin. A clinical study based on 221 cases. *Am. J. Med. Sci.* 139, 484–502, 1910.
58. Zinsser, H. Varieties of typhus fever and the epidemiology of the American form of European typhus fever (Brill's disease). *Am. J. Hyg.* 20, 513–532, 1934.
59. Murray, E. S. and Snyder, J. C. Brill's disease. II. Etiology. *Am. J. Hyg.* 53, 22–32, 1951.
60. Price, W. H. Studies on the interepidemic survival of louse-borne epidemic typhus fever. *J. Bacteriol.* 69, 106–107, 1954.
61. Price, W. H., Emerson, H., Nagle, E., et al. Ecologic studies on the interepidemic survival of louse-borne epidemic typhus fever. *Am. J. Hyg.* 67, 155–178, 1958.
62. Smadel, J. E., Ley, H. L., Diercks, F. H., and Cameron, J. A. P. Persistence of *Rickettsia tsutsugamushi* in tissue of patients recovered from scrub typhus. *Am. J. Hyg.* 56, 294–302, 1952.
63. Parker, R. T., Menon, P. G., Merideth, A. M., et al. Persistence of Rickettsia rickettsii in a patient recovered from Rocky Mountain spotted fever. *J. Immunol.* 73, 383–386, 1954.
64. Ignatovich, V. F. Biological properties of *Rickettsia prowazekii* on long-term persistence in infected cotton rats. *Acta Virol.* 24, 144–148, 1980.

65. Freylikhman, O., Tokarerevich, N., Surorov, A., et al. *Coxiella burnetii* persistence in three generations of mice after application of live attenuated human M-44 vaccine against Q fever. *Ann. N. Y. Acad. Sci.* 990, 496–499, 2003.
66. Harris, S. Japanese biological warfare research in humans: a case study of microbiology and ethics. *Ann. N. Y. Acad. Sci.* 666, 21–49, 1992.
67. Alibek, K and Handelsman, S. Biohazard. Random House, New York, 1999.
68. Ecke, R. S., Gillaim, A. G., Snyder, J. C., et al. The effect of Cox-type vaccine on louse-borne typhus fever. *Am. J. Trop. Med.* 25, 447–462, 1945.
69. Johnson, J. E. and Kadull, P. J. Rocky Mountain spotted fever acquired in a laboratory. *N. Engl. J. Med.* 277, 842–847, 1967.
70. Centers of Disease Control. Laboratory-acquired endemic typhus – Maryland. *MMWR Morb. Mortal Wkly. Rep.* 27, 215–216, 1978.
71. Oh, M., Kim, N., Huh, M., et al. Scrub typhus pneumonitis acquired through the respiratory tract in a laboratory worker. *Infection* 29, 54–56, 2001.
72. Pike, R. M. Laboratory-associated infections: Summary and analysis of 3921 cases. *Health. Lab. Sci.* 13, 105–114, 1976.
73. Walker, D. H., Crawford, C. G., and Cain, B. G. Rickettsial infection of the pulmonary microcirculation: the basis for interstitial pneumonitis in Rocky Mountain spotted fever. *Hum. Pathol.* 11, 263–272, 1980.
74. Committee on Pathology, Division of Medical Sciences, National Research Council. Pathology of epidemic typhus. Report of fatal cases studied by United States of America Typhus Commission in Cairo, Egypt during 1943–1945. *Arch. Pathol.* 56, 397–435, 1953.
75. Weil, E. and Felix, A. Zur serologischen diagnose des fleckfiebers. *Wien. Klin. Wichenschr.* 29, 33–35, 1916.
76. Ormsbee, R., Peacock, M., Philip, E., et al. Serologic diagnosis of epidemic typhus fever. *Am J. Epidemiol.* 105, 261–271, 1977.
77. Newhouse, V. F., Shepard, C. C., Redus, M. D., et al. A comparison of the complement fixation, indirect fluorescent antibody and microagglutination tests for the serological diagnosis of rickettsial diseases. *Am. J. Trop. Med. Hyg.* 28, 387–395, 1979.
78. La Scola, B. and Raoult, D. Laboratory diagnosis of rickettsioses: current approaches to the diagnosis of old and new rickettsial diseases. *J. Clin. Microbiol.* 35, 2715–2727, 1997.
79. Hechemy, K. E., Osterman, J. V., Eisemann, C. S., et al. Detection of typhus antibody by latex agglutination. *J. Clin. Microbiol.* 13, 214–216, 1981.
80. Halle, S. and Dasch, G. A. Use of sensitive microplate enzyme-linked immunosorbent assay in a retrospective serological analysis of a laboratory population at risk to infection with typhus group rickettsiae. *J. Clin. Microbiol.* 12, 343–350, 1980.
81. Eremeeva, M. E., Balayeva, N. M., and Raoult, D. Serological response of patients suffering from primary and recrudescent typhus: Comparison of complement fixation reaction, Weil–Felix test, microimmunofluorescence, and immunoblotting. *Clin. Diagn. Lab. Immunol.* 1, 318–324, 1994.
82. La Scola, B., Rydkina, L., Ndihokobwayo, J. B., et al. Serological differentiation of murine typhus and epidemic typhus using cross-adsorption and Western blotting. *Clin. Diagn. Lab. Immunol.* 7, 612–616, 2000.
83. Teysselre, N. and Raoult, D. Comparison of Western immunoblotting and microimmunofluorescence for diagnosis of Mediterranean spotted fever. *J. Clin. Microbiol.* 30, 455–460, 1992.
84. Ching, W.-M., Rowland, D., Zhang, Z., et al. Early diagnosis of scrub typhus with a rapid flow assay using recombinant major outer membrane protein antigen (r56) of *Orientia tsutsugamushi. Clin. Diagn. Lab. Immunol.* 8, 409–414, 2001.
85. Eremeeva, M. E., Ignatovich, V. F., Dasch, G. A., et al. Genetic, biological, and serological differentiation of *Rickettsia prowazekii* and *Rickettsia typhi.* In: Rickettsia and Rickettsial Diseases, Kazar, J. and Toman, R. (eds). Publishing House of the Slovak Academy of Sciences, Veda, Bratislava. pp.43–50, 1996.

86. Carl, M., Tibbs, C. W., Dobson, M. E., et al. Diagnosis of acute typhus infection using the polymerase chain reaction. *J. Infect. Dis.* 161, 791–793, 1990.
87. Svraka, S., Rolain, J. M., Bechach, Y., et al. *Rickettsia prowazekii* and real-time polymerase chain reaction. *Emerg. Infect Dis.* 12, 428–432, 2006.
88. Fang, R., Houhamdi, L., and Raoult, D. Detection of *Rickettsia prowazekii* in body lice and their feces by using monoclonal antibodies. *J. Clin. Microbiol.* 40, 3358–3363, 2002.
89. Birg, M.-L., La Scola, B., Roux, V., et al. Isolation of *Rickettsia prowazekii* from blood by shell vial culture. *J. Clin. Microbiol.* 37, 3722–3724, 1999.
90. Boese, J. L., Wisseman, C. L. J., Walsh, W. T., and Fiset, P. Antibody and antibiotic action on *Rickettsia prowazekii* in body lice across the host-vector interface, with observation on strain virulence and retrieval mechanisms. *Am. J. Epidemiol.* 98, 262–282, 1973.
91. Rolain, J. M., Maurin, M., Vestris, G., and Raoult, D. In vitro susceptibilities of 27 rickettsiae to 13 antimicrobials. *Antimicrob. Agents Chemother.* 42, 1537–1541, 1998.
92. Krause, D. W., Perine, P. L., McDade, J. E., and Awoke, S. Treatment of louse-borne typhus fever with chloramphenicol, tetracycline, or doxycycline. *East Afr. Med. J.* 52, 421–427, 1975.
93. Huys, J., Kayihigi, J., Freyens, P., et al. Single-dose treatment of epidemic typhus with doxycycline. *Chemotherapy*18, 314–317, 1973.
94. Watt, G., Chouriyagune, C., Ruangweerayud, R., et al. Scrub typhus infections poorly responsive to antibiotics in northern Thailand. *Lancet* 348, 86–89, 1996.
95. Turcinov, D., Kuzman, I., and Herendic B. Failure of azithromycin in treatment of Brill-Zinsser disease. *Antimicrob. Agents Chemother.* 44, 1737–1738, 2000.
96. Yeomans, A., Snyder, J. C., Murray, E. S., et al. The therapeutic effect of para-aminobenzoic acid in louse borne typhus fever. *JAMA* 126, 349–356, 1944.
97. Steigman, A. J. Rocky Mountain spotted fever and the avoidance of sulfonamides. *J. Pediatr.* 91, 163–164, 1977.
98. Ruiz Beltrán, R. and Herrero Herrero, J. I. Deleterious effect of trimethoprim-sulfamethoxazole in Mediterranean spotted fever. *Antimicrob. Agents Chemother.* 36, 1342–1343, 1992.
99. Eaton, M., Cohen, M. T., Shlim, D. R., and Innes B. Ciprofloxacin treatment of typhus. *JAMA* 262, 772–773, 1989.
100. Strand, O. and Stromberg, A. Ciprofloxacin treatment of murine typhus. *Scand. J. Infect. Dis.* 22, 503–504, 1990.
101. Matossian, R. M., Thaddeus, J., and Garabedian, G. A. Outbreak of epidemic typhus in the northern region of Saudi Arabia. *Am. J. Trop. Med. Hyg.* 12, 82–90, 1963.
102. TYPHUS Clinical Reference, http://allhazards.state.wy.us. Accessed Feb 2004.
103. Murray, E. S., Baehr, G., Shwartzman, G., et al. Brill's disease. *JAMA* 142, 1059–1066, 1950.
104. Campbell, W. C. Insect infestations of man. In: Chemotherapy of Parasitic Diseases, Campbell, W. C. and Rew, R. S. (eds). Plenum Press, New York. pp.531–540, 1986.
105. Sholdt, L. L., Rogers Jr., E. J., Gerberg, E. J., and Schreck, C. E. Effectiveness of permethrin-treated military uniform fabric against human body lice. *Mil. Med.* 154, 90–93, 1989.
106. Notifiable Conditions, Washington State Department of Health, http://www.doh.wa.gov/Notify/guidelines/typhus.htm. Accessed Feb 2004.
107. Woodward, T. E. Rickettsial vaccines with emphasis on epidemic typhus: initial report of an old vaccine trial. *S. Afr. Med. J.* 11, 73–76, 1986.
108. Perez Gallardo, F. and Fox, J. P. Infection and immunization of laboratory animals with *Rickettsia prowazekii* of reduced pathogenicity, strain E. *Am. J. Hyg.* 48, 6–21, 1948.
109. Ge, H., Chuang, Y. Y., Zhao, S., et al. Comparative genomics of *Rickettsia prowazekii* Madrid E and Breinl strains. *J. Bacteriol.* 186, 556–565, 2004.
110. Weiss, K. and Walker, D. H. New and improved vaccines against rickettsia infections: Rocky mounted spotted fever, epidemic typhus, and scrub typhus. In: New Generation Vaccines, Woodrow, G. C. and Levine, M. M. (eds). Marcel Decker, New York. pp.357–374, 1990.

111. Wisseman, C. L. The present and future of immunization against the typhus fevers. In: Pan American Health Organization: First International Conference on Vaccines Against Viral and Rickettsial Diseases of Man. Pan American Health Organization, Washington, DC. pp.523–527, 1967.
112. Centers for Disease Control. Typhus vaccine. Recommendation on immunization practices. *Ann. Intern. Med.* 68, 785–786, 1968.
113. Coker, C., Majid, M., and Radulovic, S. Development of *Rickettsia prowazekii* DNA vaccine. Cloning strategies. *Ann. N. Y. Acad. Sci.* 990, 757–764, 2003.
114. Díaz-Montero, C. M., Feng, H.-M., Crocquet-Valdes, P. A., and Walker, D. H. Identification of protective components of two major outer membrane proteins of spotted fever group rickettsiae. *Am. J. Trop. Med. Hyg.* 65, 371–378, 2001.
115. Dasch, G. A., Bourgeois, A. L., and Rollwagen, F. M. The surface protein antigen of *Rickettsia typhi*: in vitro and in vivo immunogenicity and protective efficacy in mice. In: Raoult, D., and Brouqui, P., eds. Rickettsiae and Rickettsial Diseases at the Turn of the Third Millenium. Paris: Elsevier. pp.116–122, 1999.
116. Bourgeois, A. L. and Dasch, G. A. The species-specific surface protein antigen of *Rickettsia typhi*: immunogenicity and protective efficacy in guinea pigs. In: Rickettsiae and Rickettsial Diseases, Burgdorfer, W. and Anacker, R. L. (eds). Academic Press, New York. pp.71–80, 1981.

Chapter 9
Category B Biotoxins

Ricin, *Staphylococcus aureus* Enterotoxin B and *Clostridium perfringens* Epsilon Toxin

Larry I. Lutwick, Jeremy Gradon, and Jonathan Zellen

9.1 Ricin

9.1.1 Scenarios

9.1.1.1 The Assassination of Georgi Markov [1]

Mr. Markov was a novelist and playwright and political dissident in Bulgaria who left his country in 1969. By 1971, he was in the U.K. working for the Bulgarian service of the B.B.C., the German Deutsche Welle radio station and the U.S. associated Radio Free Europe expressing strongly anticommunist views.

On 7 September 1978, while waiting at a bus stop near Waterloo Bridge in London, he felt something hit his right thigh and turned around to see a man picking up an umbrella. Apologizing to Markov in a deep foreign accent, the man hailed a taxi and left. Shortly afterwards, at his London office, complaining of pain in the thigh, Markov observed a red, indurated area at the site of the pain. The following day, a weak and febrile Markov was admitted to a health care facility in a toxic looking state.

Upon hospital arrival, Mr. Markov was ill appearing, febrile, tachycardic and normotensive with a 6-cm. indurated, erythematous circular area with a 2-mm. puncture mark in the center in his thigh and tender lymphadenopathy in the right inguinal area. His white blood count was mildly elevated at 10.6 k/mm^3 and a radiograph did not reveal a foreign body in the thigh. He was placed on broad-spectrum antimicrobials. About 19 h after admission, Markov became hypotensive and hypothermic and his WBC had risen to 26.3 k. Within 2 days, anuria with renal failure, prominent vomiting with some hematemesis and a complete heart block developed. His WBC rose to 33.2 k and all cultures were unrevealing. He expired about 60 h after hospital admission.

L.I. Lutwick
Infectious Diseases (IIIE), VA New York Harbor Health Care System, 800 Poly Place, Brooklyn, NY 11209, USA
e-mail: larry.lutwick@gov

L.I. Lutwick, S.M. Lutwick (eds.), *Beyond Anthrax*,
DOI: 10.1007/978-1-59745-326-4_9, © Springer Science+Business Media, LLC 2008

The postmortem examination revealed congestive heart failure, hemorrhagic necrosis of the small bowel and right inguinal lymph nodes and scattered hemorrhages in the heart, particularly around the conduction system. A piece of the thigh lesion was excised. While preparing a piece of the thigh subcutaneous tissue for examination, a small 1.5 mm. pellet was exuded from the specimen that had two 0.3 mm holes at right angles in it. In evaluating the case, ricin poisoning was considered in the differential diagnosis but no direction evidence of ricin was found in Markov's body or the pellet so that the exact cause of death could not be determined. Of note, another Bulgarian defector, Vladimir Kostov, sustained a blow to the neck while in the Paris Metro 2 weeks before the Markov attack. He developed a milder version of Markov's illness, was hospitalized for 12 days before recovery and a pellet identical to Markov's was removed from him.

9.1.1.2 In the Mail and Elsewhere

A more recent demonstration of the continuing threat from ricin occurred on October 15, 2003, when threatening note and a sealed container that was subsequently found to contain ricin was discovered in an envelope at a postal facility in Greenville, South Carolina [2]. Accompanying the container was a note that said the author could make much more ricin and would "start dumping" large quantities of the poison if new federal trucking rules went in effect. The letter, signed "Fallen Angel," said the author was "a fleet owner of a tanker company [3]."

Investigations by federal and state authorities revealed no illness consistent with ricin exposure in any of the postal workers or in individuals residing in the surrounding areas. After closure during the investigation, the postal facility was reopened following all environmental samples being found to be negative for ricin and no illnesses were discovered.

The ease in producing ricin has made it relatively popular as a biothreat. In early 2004, a white powder found to contain ricin was found in a U.S. Senate mailroom [4]. Another circumstance in 2004 involved two women who planned to kill the husband of one of them having made a small amount of ricin from a recipe accessed on the Internet [5]. An episode that is particularly worrisome on a biowarfare level involved the arrest in January 2003 of six Middle Eastern men for producing ricin in their apartment in London, U.K. The individuals appeared to have previously attended terrorist training camps including an al-Qa'ida camp in Afghanistan and in Chechnya [6].

9.1.2 The Toxin

Ricin is found in castor beans from the plant *Ricinus communis* and is a residual product of the production of castor oil. The oil has applications as a purgative, an engine lubricant, and as a component of brake and hydraulic fluid. The industry is no longer active in the United States but the oil is produced in large quantities in other areas of the world. Importantly, the oil, if properly prepared, does not contain the toxin.

A fast-drying, non-yellowing oil, castor oil is also used in coating fabrics and other protective coverings, transparent typewriter and printing inks, and in textile dyeing (when converted into sulfonated castor oil or Turkey-Red Oil). The dehydrated oil is an excellent drying agent comparing favorably with tung oil and is used in paints and varnishes. Hydrogenated castor oil is utilized in the manufacture of waxes, polishes, carbon paper, candles and crayons.

Although native to Africa, the plant (belonging to the family of *Euphorbiacea*) is now grown all over the world. Any of the plants in the *Euphorbiacea* family is formally called a spurge, derived from the Old French word *espurgier*, to purge. Indeed, the *Euphorbiacea* name is derived from the name of a physician to King Juba II of Mauritania in 18 BC whose practice, as many healers of the day, was to purge individuals to treat their ills. Both derivations directly related to the castor bean's effect in diarrhea and emesis.

One million tons of castor beans are used each year for producing the oil. The waste mash from the oil production process can have as much as 5% ricin by weight and is readily and inexpensively isolated via a simple process in a low technology setting using materials easily obtainable. Ricin can be prepared in liquid or crystalline forms or as an aerosolizable, lyophilized powder. The toxin is stable and can also be poisonous in its native form in the beans. The toxin has also been obtained through the production of transgenic bacteria or plants [7, 8].

The plants are also exported worldwide for horticultural purposes [9]. The stalked leaves consist of usually eight radiating, pointed leaflets with slightly serrated edges. Many varieties are green, but some are reddish brown. The flowers are green and inconspicuous, but pink or red in the pigmented varieties. The soft-spined fruits containing attractively mottled seeds are distinctive features of the plant. It is grown as an ornamental in gardens and sometimes as a houseplant.

The 8–15-mm long brown, mottled seeds are available in the U.S. and elsewhere as they are used to make jewelry particularly outside the U.S. The genus name, *Ricinus*, is the Latin term relating to ticks, used since the seeds may be mistaken for an engorged tick. Necklaces, made from the attractive beans, can cause skin irritation at the contact point, an allergic manifestation, and rarely anaphylaxis. In areas around the globe, raw or roasted castor beans ingestion is not uncommon and the beans are used for a number of medicinal aims. Such utilization includes use as a cathartic, an emetic, and as a treatment for leprosy or syphilis [10].

It should be noted that other plant-derived protein synthesis inhibitors exist. One such toxin, abrin [11], is found in jequirity beans (also called precatory beans or rosary peas) produced by *Abrus precatorius* of the pea family. The beans are not uncommonly used for ornamental purposes such as prayer or rosary beads or in musical shakers such as maracas. The beans are bright red with a black spot.

Stillmark coined the term ricin in the 1880 s because the castor bean material agglutinated red blood cells [12]. The agglutinin properties, however, are not due to the toxin molecule itself but rather another coexisting protein. Ricin is a 66-kD globular protein with a toxic mode of action of inhibiting protein synthesis in eukaryotic cells. The mechanism is due to the enzymatic removal of a single adenine residue from (amino acid 4324) close to the 3′ end of 28S ribosomal RNA. The removal prevents elongation factor-2 from binding [13]. Structurally it is made up of two approximately equal molecular weight subunits, the A and B chains, linked by a disulfide bond. The B chain facilitates binding to cell surfaces and entry into the cell through binding to terminal galactose moieties of cellular membrane glycolipids and glycoproteins [10]. The time from exposure to toxic effects is due to the necessity of internalization and subsequent transportation via the Golgi apparatus into the cytoplasm.

Ricin can be used therapeutically in the production of agents targeting a particular cell or malignancy. As chimeric toxins, ricin can be bound to immunoglobulin or other molecule selecting preferentially the specific target cell and assist in the treatment of cancer or immunologically generated illnesses. As examples, the ricin toxin B chain has been produced as part of a fusion protein with granulocyte-macrophage colony stimulating factor receptor using transgenic models. After association with the active toxin A chain, the fusion protein is selectively toxic to acute myeloid leukemia cells [14]. Similarly, a ricin fusion toxin has been produced to attack cells with the cytokine interleukin-2 receptor [15]. Using a mutant ricin toxin, described as a potential vaccine below, may minimize endovascular damage associated with these potentially useful products. Additionally, the B chain has been used to facilitate antigen delivery in plant-based mucosal vaccines [16].

9.1.3 Ricin Disease

The clinical presentation of ricin poisoning depends on whether the exposure is injected, inhaled, or ingested. In mice, the dose found to be lethal to 50% (LD_{50}) of animals was found to be 3–5 μg/kg in inhalation or intravenous exposures and 20–25 μg/kg in intraperitoneal, subcutaneous or intragastric administration [10]. The time to death in the mice was 60 h for inhalation, 90 h for intravenous and 80–100 h for the other exposures. It is important to note that there is a variation of as much as two logarithms in the μg/kg dose of ricin between animals with the horse seeming to be the most sensitive and the frog and chicken the least [10]. The first symptoms of toxicity generally occur 6–12 h exposure but can occur as early as 3 h. This is longer than many of the chemical agents affecting the lung and more rapid than infectious agents.

9.1.3.1 Natural Disease

Naturally, ricin toxicity is usually related to a castor seed ingestion. Beans that are swallowed without chewing or otherwise damage to the husk do not cause toxicity. Symptoms, when they occur, may involve nausea, vomiting, diarrhea and cramping with an incubation time of one to four hours. The diarrhea may be profuse and bloody, leading to hypovolemic shock. The degree of gastrointestinal irritation can be severe, clinically similar to alkaline burns. In later stages of severe illness, cytotoxic effects may lead to significant, irreversible damage in the liver, kidneys, pancreas, adrenals and central nervous system [17].

Challoner and McCarron [17] reviewed the medical literature regarding castor seed ingestion. From case reports where enough clinical data was elaborated and symptoms did develop they found (Table 9.1) that gastrointestinal symptoms were indeed most common. In this review, the mortality associated with symptomatic castor bean ingestion was 3.4% with most deaths occurring in the literature prior to World War II. The number of castor seeds ingested that may cause death is somewhat variable. Variables that may impact include how much the husk of the seed is damaged during chewing, if the seeds are roasted prior to ingestion, and the ricin content of the seed.

Workers in or near castor bean processing plants exposed to castor bean dust can develop a hypersensitivity-like illness. The symptoms include nasal and throat congestion, eye irritation, hives, chest tightness and wheezing. Various sources describe incubation periods ranging from four to 24 h. The allergen does not appear to be ricin itself but other components of the bean. The development of respiratory symptoms after exposure in a setting with a link to castor beans, therefore, may not necessarily imply a deliberate biowarfare attack.

The plant pollen and components of the bean are efficient sensitizers and cause a significant degree of occupational allergies. This can occur not only those in or around bean processing factories but also in a variety of other

Table 9.1 Symptoms of castor bean intoxication

Symptom	Percent of those affected
Vomiting	84
Diarrhea	83
Dehydration	35
Shock	27
Abdominal pain	13
Others*	–

*(including laboratory tests) – leg cramps 6%, acrocyanosis 5%, miosis 3%, gastrointestinal bleeding 3%, hematuria 5%, hemolysis 3%, abnormal renal function tests 9%, abnormal liver function tests 5%

groups. These include merchant seamen and dock workers (who may been working only with green coffee bean sacks but sacks that may have previously stored castor beans or have been keep near bags that stored them) [18]; coffee industry workers, laboratory workers [19]; and those in the felt or upholstery industries (castor oil products can be used in the manufacture of felt) [20]. Since the castor bean plant is in the same *Euphorbiaceae* family of plants as the rubber tree *Hevea brasiliensis*, allergies to latex can be cross-reactive with castor beans [21].

9.1.3.2 Biowarfare Ricin Use

As a weapon of bioterrorism, ricin would most likely be dispersed as an aerosol although contamination of food or water supplies is also feasible. Although easily obtained, massive quantities of toxin are necessary to create a large-scale effect. Eight metric tons of ricin would have to be aerosolized compared to kilogram quantities of anthrax in order to cause 50% lethality over a 100-km^2 area [22]. Because signs and symptoms are non-specific, detection of an attack would require a high index of suspicion based on clinical and epidemiologic factors. The finding of a geographic cluster of patients with acute lung injury should arouse suspicion of an attack via an aerosolized agent, although the list of potential culprits is extensive and includes chemical as well as biologic agents. Ricin cases do not exhibit mediastinitis, as with anthrax, and they do not demonstrate any response to antibiotic therapy as would be expected with an infectious etiology. Pulmonary edema may develop 1–3 days after ricin exposure, in contrast to staphylococcal enterotoxin B or phosgene where time to development of pulmonary edema is twelve and six hours respectively.

There is limited data describing the outcome from an inhalation exposure. In the 1940 s, sublethal and accidental exposures were said to have occurred and were manifest 4–8 h after exposure with fever, cough, shortness of breath and nausea [23]. Studies in rodents suggest an inhaled ricin aerosol could lead to necrosis of the upper and lower airway, respiratory distress syndrome and respiratory failure. A lethal dose of intrapulmonary ricin also results in renal dysfunction in rodents. However, sublethal dosing did not result in extrapulmonary disease but can cause subsequent pulmonary fibrosis [24]. Chest x-ray would be expected to show bilateral infiltrates. In animal studies death occurred in 36–72 h and was dose dependent [10]. In primates [25], symptoms and time to death were also dose related and associated with alveolar flooding, fibropurulent pneumonia and necrotizing tracheitis. Death occurred 36–48 h after challenge following a 8–24-h preclinical period.

Exposures due to ingestion of purified ricin have not been reported. Due to poor absorption, lethality is less than with inhalation. The clinical presentation is most likely similar to that observed with castor bean ingestion.

9.1.3.3 Diagnosis of Ricin Exposure

In a biological attack, the diagnosis of ricin-induced disease is based on symptoms related to the route of delivery. Since aerosol transmission is presumed to be the route of choice in warfare, a cluster of severe respiratory disease linked to a finite area could suggest the diagnosis. Deliberate contamination of food or water with ricin would cause gastroenteritis, possibly very severe. Inoculation percutaneously, as seems to have occurred in the Markov incident, causes local inflammatory disease and a systemic illness with prominent leukocytosis indistinguishable from septic shock (but with negative cultures).

Specific confirmation of the diagnosis requires the detection of ricin in or on the victim or, in survivors since the toxin is quite immunogenic, rising anti-ricin antibodies developing by 2 weeks after the illness. Ricin is quickly metabolized. In rats, only 11% of an intravenously administered dose remains after 24 h with most of the toxin excreted in the urine as low molecular weight metabolites [26]. Additionally, regardless of the route of exposure, the toxin is rapidly tissue bound so that direct tissue immunohistological analysis may be preferable to body fluid testing. Franz and Jaax state that, after a ricin inhalation, the castor bean poison could be detectable from a nasal mucosal swab for at least 24 h after exposure [10]. ELISA using either polyclonal [27] or monoclonal [28] antibody can detect ricin. If assays could be developed to detect the low molecular weight metabolites of ricin, urine ricin testing could be valuable even after several days. Among the methods to detect ricin antibody is a biological system assaying the ability of a sample to protect a tissue culture line against ricin toxicity [29].

9.1.4 Therapeutic Measures

Therapy is primarily symptomatic and supportive and depends on the type of exposure. Patients with inhalation exposures may require mechanical ventilation and management of pulmonary edema. Ricin ingestion should be managed by gastric lavage and the use of cathartics. The large size of the ricin molecule seems to preclude the use of charcoal for gut decontamination [30, 31] although the procedure is recommended in most publications. Because exposures that involve ingestion may lead to significant gastrointestinal fluid loss from diarrhea and hemorrhage careful monitoring of volume status is crucial.

A variety of potential chemotherapeutic modalities have been studied using a cell culture model of protein synthesis inhibition [32]. In this model, the sugars galactose and lactose, a Golgi transport inhibitor brefeldin A and nucleoside derivatives including zidovudine (azidothymidine, AZT) had activity with protection up to 80% but not in a cell free translation assay [31] or in laboratory animals [10]. One report suggested that cholera toxin subunit B was able to partially protect tissue culture cells in vitro. The mechanism of inhibition was felt to be alterations in cellular membrane structure [33].

9.1.5 Preventive Measures

9.1.5.1 Environmental

Appropriate masking may be useful at the time of an aerosol attack. No clear data is available regarding the potential of secondary aerosols of ricin in the environment. The molecule, however, is inactivated on surfaces by hypochlorite solutions such as 0.5% sodium hypochlorite that can be used on skin after extensive washing with soap and water. The toxin is, however, not inactivated by low chlorine levels or by iodine. Although stable at ambient temperatures, it is detoxified by heat either 80°C for 10 min or 50°C at pH 7.8 for an hour [31]. There should be little concern regarding a toxic dermal exposure per se since, unless enhanced by solvents such as DMSO, absorption is insignificant.

9.1.5.2 Passive and Active Immunization

There are no currently available vaccines for ricin exposure. In 1995, it was noted that subcutaneously administered, formalin-inactivated ricin toxoid was immunogenic in rats [34], which pioneered the search for a vaccine. Challenge of the immunized animals with aerosolized ricin was found to protect against death but histopathologically significant pulmonary damage was found in the immunized animals. In order to deliver the immunogen to the target tissue for a ricin biowarfare attack, liposomally encapsulated toxoid administered intratracheally was found to be more antigenic than aqueous toxoid or toxoid mixed with alhydrogel and protection was found [35]. The whole toxin was more immunogenic in the model than the A chain alone [36]. The liposome/toxoid immunogen also protected against nonlethal lung damage [37].

Based on the pursuit of work done over the past decade, an oral formalin-inactivated ricin toxoid microencapsulated into biodegradable polymer (poly-DL-lactide-co-glycolide) microspheres has been found to be protective against an aerosolized ricin challenge in mice [38]. The vaccine was effective with two 3-consecutive-day series 4 weeks apart but not with shorter sequences or as a nonencapsulated aqueous toxoid. The microsphere vaccine was also protective when given subcutaneously. No data on the pulmonary pathology of the immunized survivors was reported. In a structure-based approach using the ricin A chain fold epitopes [39], the resultant immunogens manifested greater stability to thermal denaturation, much less toxicity as compared to native A chain and protected 100% of vaccinated animals challenged with supralethal aerosolized ricin doses. Most recently, a recombinant ricin A chain containing mutations at known toxic sites has been shown to be nontoxic and immunogenic in humans [40]. In rodents, immunization was protective against either gastric or aerosol ricin challenge [41].

Passive immunization against an aerosolized ricin exposure has also been studied. Aerosol administered polyclonal goat anti-ricin IgG was protective in a mouse model when ricin aerosol was administered 1 h later but some lung pathology occurred in survivors [42]. Polyclonal antibody was also protective when given intravenously [43]. Monoclonal antibody was also protective against ricin toxicity in vitro and in vivo when given before and after challenge. Pretreatment alone delayed the onset of toxicity and death [44].

9.2 Staphylococcal Enterotoxin B (SEB)

9.2.1 Scenario [45]

At least nine laboratory workers were exposed to aerosolized staphylococcal enterotoxin B following what was described as an accident in a lab. The ensuing illness was heralded by rigors and fever with reading as high as 106°F. The onset of the pyrexia averaged 12 h after the exposure (range 8–20 h) and the febrile period lasted from 12 to 76 h (mean duration 50 h). The fever was associated with myalgias and headache.

Respiratory symptoms began about the same time as the fever and myalgias as a nonproductive cough. Of the nine, five had inspiratory rales associated with dyspnea and three had dyspnea with but inspiratory and expiratory rales as well as orthopnea. One of these had "profound" shortness of breath for the first 12 h of symptoms and exertional dyspnea for 10 days. Chest x-rays obtained during this sublethal exposure revealed patchy pulmonary edema and interstitial edema. Chest pain, described as moderately intense, substernal and pleuritic also occurred with the respiratory symptoms lasting an average of 1 day (range 4 h to 4 days).

Vomiting and anorexia developed in most with a mean onset of 17 h (8–24-h range) with the anorexia lasting several days and the vomiting limited to a mean of 9 h (4–20-h range).

9.2.2 The Toxin

Staphylococcus aureus is one of the most commonly encountered bacteria in clinical medicine, familiar to all practicing clinicians. It appears as a Gram-positive coccus in grape-like clusters on staining and may be found as part of the normal flora of the nose and skin in humans as well as widely distributed in nature. Common reservoirs and disseminators of the organism are colonized or infected individuals, particularly if they have draining staphylococcal boils or lesions on their skin.

S. aureus naturally produces a number of enterotoxins [46]. These quite similar gastrointestinal toxins are responsible for the second most commonly reported type of food poisoning in the US. Of them, SEB is thought to have the best potential for use as a weapon. The ability to act as a superantigen is responsible for much of the symptoms of SEB intoxication. Superantigen mediated activation of a vast array of lymphocytes results in the release of large numbers of cytokines and the illness that ensues is largely cytokine-mediated. The arachidonic acid cascade is also activated with prostaglandins and leukotrienes becoming elevated [47]. Primates given an aerosolized non-lethal dose of SEB were found to have elevated cytokines, especially IL-2 and IL-6 [48]. Sequential production of cytokines has been described in an in vitro model where the same cell subpopulation produced IL-2, interferon-gamma and IL-10 with rapid, intermediate and slow kinetics, respectively [49]. Of note, IL-2 upregulates the interferon production and IL-10 downregulates it. The binding is to major histocompatibility complex class II molecules with each toxin having additional unique, stabilizing interactions to the cell membrane [50]. By amino acid sequence homology studies, SEB seems most close to the staphylococcal toxic shock syndrome toxin and SEB has been associated with some cases of toxic shock syndrome [51].

All the staphylococcal enterotoxins have similarities, in addition to super-antigenity, including causing emesis and gastroenteritis in primates, intermediate resistance to heat and pepsin digestion and tertiary structure similarities including an intramolecular disulfide bond [51]. Although most of the staphylococcal enterotoxins are resistant to proteolysis by pepsin, trypsin, papain and other enzymes, SEB is readily nicked by trypsin and the biological activity seems associated with the 17kD C-terminal fragment [52]. SEB has been shown to be a single 239 amino acid polypeptide [53] with a molecular weight of about 28 kDa. Recombinant toxin can be produced in transgenic bacteria [54] and an attenuated SEB as a vaccine candidate has been produced in *E. coli* as well [55].

The effect that superantigens such as SEB have on cytokine production may interact with aspects of infectious agent pathogenicity. Not only is inhaled SEB-induced toxicity in mice enhanced by lipopolysaccharide (LPS) [56] but also SEB potentiates LPS-induced toxicity in rats [57]. LPS is recognized by Toll-like receptors primarily targeting macrophages and dendritic cells and the super-antigen/LPS interaction is synergistic through interferon-gamma dependent pathways [58] although some antagonistic interactions are described as well. In a murine model, SEB pretreatment protected mice against lethal *Listeria monocytogenes* infection due to the enhancement of cytotoxic T cells [59]. In another mouse model [60], there was delayed viral clearance during primary viral infection but overall little effect on concurrent antiviral immunity although others report lethal synergism between influenza and SEB, which seemed to be mediated by tumor necrosis factor and interferon-gamma [61].

9.2.3 SEB Disease

9.2.3.1 Natural Disease

Staphylococcal food poisoning caused by the ingestion of preformed entero-toxin B (or one or more of the other enterotoxins of the organism) in food contaminated with toxin-producing strains of *S. aureus*. Enterotoxins A and D appear to be most frequently associated with the illness [52]. It has been the second most common cause of foodborne illness [62] and can be associated with retail-produced as well as home made foods. Those with a propensity to support toxin production are previously cooked or not adequately cooked, unrefrigerated or not rapidly cooled after preparation. Common vehicles include custard, dairy products, canned foods, potato salad and ice cream although many food including meats have also been implicated. Proteinaceous foods that are semi-preserved with salt or sugar such as cooked meats are not protected from *S. aureus* growth and are therefore at risk [52]. The food characteristically has a normal taste and appearance despite the presence of *S. aureus* and/or SEB.

Staphylococcal food poisoning presents with the acute onset of nausea, vomiting abdominal cramping and diarrhea usually within 4–6 h after ingestion. Following ingestion of the contaminated food there is an increased intestinal peristalsis due to sympathetic activation. The vomiting that occurs appears to be due to the effect of SEB on the local neural receptors in the gut, rather than a central neural effect, based on cross-circulation experiments performed in nonhuman primates [63]. Using SEB mutant toxins, it has been found that the emetic and T cell stimulatory activities of staphylococcal enterotoxins are not correlated [64]. Further studies of the emetic action of SEB may be accomplished using small animal models with ferrets or house shrews [65, 66].

The diarrhea, caused by more local effects on the intestines of the toxin, may contain blood. Diarrhea does not occur in the absence of vomiting [62]. The patient is usually afebrile in contrast to human aerosol exposure [45]. Hypotension may develop if fluid losses are of sufficient magnitude. Fatalities are uncommon but may occur in infants, the elderly and with large dose ingestions.

Although most individuals with staphylococcal food poisoning are afebrile, the presence or absence of fever is not felt to be a reliable diagnostic criterion [62]. In this large series of patients, however, subjective fever was reported in 16%, chills in 12% and sweats in 2%. In hospitalized patients, temperature readings were no higher than 38°C. Other features not found to be helpful in diagnosis were the presence of skin lesions in food handlers and large numbers of *S. aureus* in the food.

9.2.3.2 Biowarfare Disease

If the toxin is purified and released as an aerosol, it can also act as a pulmonary and systemic toxin in addition to deliberate contamination of food or water. The syndrome of inhalation of preformed staphylococcal enterotoxin B is not encountered in normal civilian clinical practice.

With effective aerosolization, it is likely that large numbers of persons would be affected. In addition, mixed pulmonary and gastrointestinal presentations are to be expected as some people will inhale and others ingest the released toxin. Severity of illness is related to initial host functional status and dose of toxin encountered. Overall, the use of SEB is not designed to be lethal but rather as an incapacitating agent that could be used against military and/or civilian populations.

Studies done in nonhuman primates were extensively used as a model for lethal inhaled SEB intoxication [44, 67] and are now used in SEB vaccination studies. Generally, self-limited gastrointestinal symptoms occurred within 24 h of exposure and remitted. About 48 h after the exposure, the primates have an acute onset of lethargy and dyspnea rapidly leading to death within hours. Postmortem exams of the monkeys revealed petechial hemorrhages of the intestines and lung and marked interstitial pulmonary edema. The alveolar spaces were found to be full of eosinophilic staining material and also manifested an acute purulent alveolitis. A mouse model has also been described for inhalation SEB disease that has similar pathological findings to primate intoxication [68]. A piglet model for systemic SEB intoxication is also reported [69].

In the 1960s, the United States studied the toxin as such a biological incapacitant. Low quantities of inhaled SEB (0.0004 μg/kg) could incapacitate and as many as 80% of personnel in the area of attack could be affected [70]. As illustrated in the first scenario, after an incubation period of 1–6 h following aerosol exposure, exposees would manifest high fever and chills, headache, myalgias, dry cough and periocular inflammation [70]. Most symptoms resolve within 7 days, fever within 4–5 days, but persistent cough and general unwellness may continue for three more weeks. Gastrointestinal symptoms, if the toxin is ingested after aerosolization, can also occur. It is felt that shock and death in humans after most aerosolization exposures would be rare unless that exposure was large [70]. A 2004 report from the US Army reported three laboratory workers who sustained inadvertent conjunctival exposure to SEB [71].

In addition, SEB was included in Project SHAD (Shipboard Hazard and Defense), which was part of the joint service chemical and biological warfare test program conducted in the 1960s. The testing, also known as Project 112 [72], was under the auspices of the Deseret Testing Center at Fort Douglas, Utah, and was to identify US warships' vulnerability to attacks with biological or chemical agents and to develop procedures to respond to such attacks while remaining in a war-fighting capability. Although many of the tests involved only simulants, some utilized actual agents. It is not clear that any results of the testing has been released but fact sheets describing some of the tests have been declassified by the Department of Defense. One such test in late 1968, DTC 68–50, involved the release of an aerosol containing SEB over a 40–50-km downwind grid encompassing a segment of Eniwetok Atoll (Marshall Islands) and an array of five Army tugboats [73].

9.2.3.3 Diagnosis

In natural foodborne outbreaks, the diagnosis of staphylococcal enterotoxin disease of any subtype is generally made clinically based on a short incubation, 24-h self-limited illness with little or no fever associated with prominent nausea and vomiting and some diarrhea.

Finding supportive evidence of the toxin requires testing directly for the relatively heat stable toxin. There are a variety of assays for the enterotoxins in food including the ELISA that can differentiate between the types of toxin and be performed rapidly [74]. In a biowarfare setting, rapid, portable settings for environmental as well as body fluid specimens such as blood, urine and respiratory secretions have been described. A variety of assay systems have been described [74–81].

9.2.4 Therapeutic Measures

Supportive care has been the major treatment for SEB toxin disease. For exposure in the gastrointestinal tract, adequate fluid and electrolyte should be maintained. Stools of affected patients are not thought to be toxic to others. Following respiratory exposure, cough and fever suppression can be utilized. In severe cases, mechanical ventilation may be required. Although cyclosporin A, that inhibits T cell cytokine production, does protect mice against lethal SEB intoxication, the compound was not protective against on 6 LD_{50} aerosolized SEB dose in rhesus monkeys [82]. Similarly, staphylococcal superantigen peptide antagonists were not effective in blocking the effects of SEB in a HLA class II transgenic mouse model [83].

Corticosteroids may have a role in the therapy of SEB-induced cytokine disease. Schramm and Thorlacius have observed [84] that, in mice, pretreatment with dexamethasone reduced the production of macrophage inflammatory protein 2 and neutrophil chemoattractant and reduced neutrophil recruitment by 82%. Catechin, a bioflavonoid in green tea, may also have a role in inhibiting the superantigen function of SEB [85]. Likewise, pirfenidone, a down-regulator of cytokine expression, decreased cytokine levels and increased survival in a mouse model [86].

The emetic response to SEB has been found in nonhuman primates to be completely blocked by H2 receptor antagonists and calcium channel blockers. The inhibition did not occur with H1 antihistamines or serotonin antagonists [87]. Additionally, cysteinyl leukotriene antagonists block the emetic response in monkeys [88] but indomethacin and aspirin do not.

9.2.5 Preventive Measures

9.2.5.1 Environmental

The water soluble toxin is quite resistant to temperature fluctuations, can withstand denaturation by boiling for several minutes, is stable in the environment and remains active for more than a year after freeze drying [89]. It should be noted that the amount of inactivation with heat is variable based on the medium containing the toxin, pH and toxin concentration [52]. In fact, it has been reported that toxin denatured by heat could be restored to activity by adjusting the pH to 11 (the toxins are stable up to pH 11) and then readjusted back to 7 [90]. Out of doors aerosolization can be effective since the toxin is relatively stable to gradation from ultraviolet light [70]. Appropriate masking may be useful at the time of the aerosol attack.

Aerosolization can contaminate water and food. The toxin is not thought to spread from person to person and the risk of secondary aerosols is thought to be low but may depend on how and in what the SEB is aerosolized. Dermal contact does not result in systemic disease and is not generally felt to be active by this route although intradermally administered SEB causes an immediate-type hypersensitivity reaction with degranulation of cutaneous mast cells [88]. Non-chlorinated water supplies are at risk. Contaminated articles can be decontaminated using 0.05% sodium hypochlorite (one tablespoon of household bleach in a gallon of water) [70]. Contact time should be 10–15 min.

9.2.5.2 Passive and Active Protection

Anti-SEB antibody raised in chickens immunized with holotoxin has been reported to be protective when passively infused into mice and rhesus monkeys [91]. The IgY antibody (purified from egg yolks) did prevent a cytokine response and prevented death when given just prior to or 4 hours after aerosol challenge with 5 LD_{50} of SEB. The authors suggest that such antibody might offer protection as both prophylaxis and treatment against aerosolized SEB.

There are no commercially available vaccines for SEB exposure. LeClaire and colleagues [91] reported fragments of SEB, despite being tolerated and immunogenic in mice even when given with LPS, did not prevent the T cell response to SEB challenge and were not protective. Protection did not occur with the fragments individually or injected together (encompassing the entire molecule) with adjuvant. Inactivated, formalin-treated SEB toxoid has been used as an immunogen. In one study [92], the toxoid was delivered in biodegradable microspheres made of poly(DL-lactide-co-glycolide) and protection of rhesus monkeys was demonstrated after a prime with intramuscular vaccine followed vaccine given intratracheally. The protection against SEB aerosol challenge correlated with antibody levels in the respiratory tract and serum. In another [93], the immunogen was inactivated SEB combined in outer membrane protein proteosome from *Neisseria meningitidis* and produced similar results in the nonhuman primate model.

Using recombinant mutant toxoid instead of natural formalin-treated product, Boles et al. [94] showed that the mutant was immunogenic and protective against aerosol challenge. The toxoid did not bind to the HLA class II binding sites or stimulate the release of cytokines. A recombinant SEB toxoid combined with cholera toxin, aerosolized or administered intraperitoneally, also protected against a lethal SEB aerosol but toxoid without adjuvant did not [95]. Such mutant toxins may serve as the backbone of possible vaccines for humans against life-threatening SEB disease.

9.3 *Clostridium Perfringens* Epsilon Toxin

9.3.1 Human C. Perfringens Toxin (non-ε) Scenario [96]

A large number of persons attended a roast beef luncheon given by the staff of a firehouse in rural Maryland. The food was prepared at a local school and the firehouse and was served family style. An outbreak of diarrhea and abdominal pain occurred with a mean incubation period of 13.4 h and mean duration of illness of 21.2 h. The roast beef was implicated as the vehicle as *C. perfringens* spores count in the stool of affected individuals was $>10^6$/g and the same serotype spore was found in the beef. A crude attack rate of 53.1% was reported.

9.3.2 The Toxin

The various serotypes of *C. perfringens* produce at least 12 different toxins [97]. Only types B and D produce the ε toxin which, probably based on its potential to produce a lethal toxemia from its initial intestinal location, has been designated as a category B biowarfare agent. The type D–derived toxin has been the target of most descriptive work.

Epsilon toxin is synthesized as a 32.5-kDa inactive polypeptide prototoxin that can be activated by intestinal proteases such as trypsin and chymotrypsin by cleavage of short peptide chains from both the N- and C-terminal ends. The *C. perfringens* lambda toxin, a metalloprotease cleaving almost the same size residues producing a 30.5-kDa ε toxin, also accomplishes the activation [98]. The prototoxin gene (etx) has been cloned and expressed in *E. coli* [99].

The toxin appears to function as a permease, enabling itself to enter the bloodstream by increased vascular permeability in the gut. From there, binding to vascular endothelial cells, ε toxin causes widespread osmotic alterations and vascular injury in the animal lung, brain, heart and kidney particularly. Several mosquitocidal toxins, Mtx2 and Mtx3, produced by another Gram positive rod, *Bacillus sphaericus*, appear to function similarly and are 20%–27% homologous to ε toxin [100].

Studies of toxin function in cell culture utilize Madine-Darby canine kidney (MDCK) cells, one of the few continuous cell lines susceptible to the toxin. Guinea pig and rabbit peritoneal macrophages are also susceptible [101] but not other cells from guinea pigs, rabbits, mice or sheep. The toxin causes MDCK cells to increase permeability through the production of a heptameric pore [102] after binding. The prototoxin binds to the cell but does not heptamerize. Similar effects were seen in rat synaptosomal cell membranes and the effect in MDCK cells could be diminished by cholesterol depletion [102]. The permeability change causes a rapid decrease in intracellular K^+ and increase in Cl^- and Na^+ leading to loss of cell viability [103].

Absorption of the toxin from the intestinal tract leads to toxemia and binding of the toxin to target cells. Binding, however, of active toxin does not necessarily result in severe injury. As an example, substantial accumulation of ε toxin in the kidney occurs after intravenous injection in the mouse. Unlike in the natural ovine model, severe kidney injury does not occur and preexisting bilateral nephrectomy increases murine fatality after toxin exposure [104].

Rodent models for ε toxin neurotoxicity has shown that, in addition to widespread permeability changes including effects at the blood-brain barrier [105], the hippocampus is directly affected by the toxin. This effect, independent of ischemic or edema effects, resulted in substantial damage of the pyramidal cell neurons. Excessive neural release of glutamate occurred [106, 107] which was thought to lead to the neural damage.

In a rat model, cardiovascular effects of the toxin were measured. In vivo, a rise in blood pressure was found without change in heart rate or electrocardiogram [108]. The effect was eliminated by pretreatment with specific antibody. In a rat isolated aorta system, arterial contraction was felt to be mediated through the nervous system [109].

9.3.3 Epsilon Toxin Disease

9.3.3.1 Natural Disease

Natural disease in humans due to *C. perfringens* infection and toxin elaboration includes foodborne enteritis and invasive clostridial infection causing gas gangrene. How much the ε toxin plays in these circumstances is not clear since a variety of toxins are elaborated. The foodborne enteritis is a not uncommon disease and is generally felt to be caused by in situ elaboration in the intestinal tract after ingestion of the vegetative cells [110]. In Europe and the US, meat and meat products are the principal foods associated with outbreaks. Type A *C. perfringens*, not a ε toxin producer, has been responsible for almost all cases of foodborne illness. This short-lived toxin illness (usually 24 h or less) presents with more diarrhea than SEB disease, minimal if any vomiting, usually no fever and with a longer incubation period, 8–20 h. *Clostridium perfringens* type C (also not a ε toxin producer) causes the potentially fatal necrotic enteritis in malnourished children living in New Guinea who ingest undercooked pig meat ("pig-bel").

Epsilon toxin causes a rapidly lethal, acute toxemia in sheep primarily but also in other herbivores such as goats and cattle. Eating habits appear to be particularly relevant as an introduction of a diet containing protein and energy-rich foods, as what occurs with fast growing young animals, is associated with increased susceptibility. The "overeating" disease may be caused by undigested, starch ladened food reaching the intestines where *C. perfringens* spores are more able to germinate and produce the prototoxin.

The toxin-produced increase in intestinal permeability with enteritis produces toxemia [111] causing pulmonary edema, pericardial effusions and swollen hyperemic kidneys ("pulpy kidney disease"). Central nervous system disease is reflected by nervousness in sheep and less commonly as seizures or loss of consciousness. Cattle and older sheep are more likely to demonstrate neurological signs and goats manifest more diarrhea. Cerebral edema in toxin-exposed animals appears to be a stimulus for the release of catecholamines and secondarily adenyl cyclase [112].

Although large doses of toxin in sheep result in a severe diffuse vasogenic cerebral edema with a rapid progression to death, with lower toxin doses or in a partially immune host more focal lesions with necrosis occur with a slower progression to death [113]. In calves and adult goats, subacute nonfatal cases occur. Intravenous injection of ε toxin in calves produces similar histopathological changes seen in sheep and goats after enteric exposure including acute pulmonary edema and cerebral edema [114].

9.3.3.2 Epsilon Biowarfare Disease

Published studies on human disease related to exposure to ε toxin as it may be used in biological warfare are not readily available. In vitro, only one human cell line is susceptible to ε toxin [115]. The dose for reducing cell culture viability by 50% is 280 μg/mL for the human renal leiomyoblastoma (G-402) cell line, 140 times higher and at a slower rate than for the standard nonhuman cell line MDCK. MDCK is the only other cell line susceptible to the toxin [116]. It should be noted that sheep, goat and cattle endothelial cell lines appear not to be responsive to ε toxin as well [117] yet the species are sensitive in vivo.

Delivered as an aerosol in adequate doses, it is thought that the ε toxin could initially cause pulmonary edema with the possibility of secondary kidney, cardiac and nervous system damage [111]. As with SEB, the ε toxin doses able to be delivered would result in debilitation of military or civilian populations rather than death. Although not specifically listed as an agent of biological warfare, *C. perfringens* α toxin, a potent phospholipase, when aerosolized causes severe, lethal pulmonary disease in animals due to a pulmonary capillary leak resulting in ARDS [118]. Absorbed α toxin could lead to intravascular hemolysis, thrombocytopenia and liver damage.

9.3.3.3 Diagnosis of Epsilon Disease

Radioimmunoassays have been developed for the detection of ε toxin in serum and intestinal contents [119]. Counterimmunoelectrophoresis and mouse neutralization tests have been used as well and have been compared with monoclonal antibody and polyclonal ELISAs in sheep and goats with marked inconsistency among the tests found [120]. This inconsistency was not noted between the mouse test and an ELISA in mice [119]. In animal intestinal infection/ε intoxication and likely in the human non-ε toxin-induced diarrhea, the genes for toxin production can be detected in the intestinal contents by PCR analysis [121]. Toxin can also be directly assayed in the stools of human diarrhea cases [122].

9.3.4 Therapeutic Interventions

In a mouse model, the lethal activity of the toxin [123] could be substantially diminished or eradicated by the prior administration of barbiturates and reserpine, respectively. Diazepam, apomorphine and gamma-butyrolactone also cause significant prolongation of the time to death when given prior to toxin exposure whereas atropine, diphenhydramine, chlorpheniramine and verapamil did not. The authors of this study suggested that drugs that directly or indirectly inhibit the release or block the receptors of dopamine may lessen the lethal effect of epsilon toxin. In a rat model for neurotoxicity, drugs that either inhibit glutamate release or function as a receptor antagonist also appear to diminish ε toxin neuroinjury [105, 106].

9.3.5 Preventive Measures

9.3.5.1 Environmental

Appropriate masking may be useful in an aerosol attack of ε toxin. It is not clear whether secondary aerosolization could occur from fomites. Little published information is found regarding the denaturation of the toxin but it is inactivated by autoclaving at 121°C for 1 hour [124]. Denaturation effectiveness by sodium hypochlorite with or without sodium hydroxide is not published [124]. Chemicals that have been shown to inactivate the toxin or prototoxin in vitro include iodination [125], tryptophan cleaving agents such as N-bromosuccinimide in urea [126] and modifiers of the amino groups of lysine residues such as 2,3-dimethylmaleic anhydride or 2,4,6-trinitrobenzenesulfonic acid [127].

9.3.5.2 Passive and Active Immunization

All published immunization studies available appear to be in nonprimates only. Epsilon toxin toxoid vaccines have been used in sheep to prevent lamb dysentery and pulpy kidney disease. These commercial vaccines are based on formalin-treated bacterial culture filtrates or whole cell cultures and have produced a high degree of protection. Before these vaccines were available, ε toxinemia produced more economic losses among both feedlot- and pasture-raised lambs than all other diseases combined [128]. Passive immunization can be used in conjunction with vaccine in a high-risk situation [129]. Enhancement of immunity using incomplete Freund's adjuvant instead of alum in goat kids produced higher antibody levels and protection against mild diarrhea that occurred after lethal challenge of commercially vaccinated animals [130].

Modern vaccine technologies have produced potential newer generation vaccines. An internal image anti-idiotype vaccine that raises a high titer of antibody directed against the active site of the toxin was protective both in tissue culture and in vivo studies [131]. Additionally, administration of a mutant ε toxin in which a proline was substituted for histidine at amino acid residue 106 resulted in induction of specific antibody and protection against a 1000 LD_{50} dose of wild type toxin in mice [132]. A liposomally-adjuvanted ε toxoid, however, was not immunogenic in goats [133].

References

1. Crompton, C. and Gall, D. Georgi Markov – death in a pellet. *Med. Leg. J.* 48, 51–62, 1980.
2. Schier, J. G., Patel, M. M., Belson, M. G., et al. Public health investigation after the discovery of ricin in a South Carolina post office. *Am. J. Public Health* 97, S152–S157, 2007.
3. CBS News.com. Feds plead for ricin leads. Available at <http://www.cbsnews.com/stories/2003/10/23/national/main579600.shtml> Accessed January 10, 2004.
4. CNN.com. Early tests show deadly ricin in Senate mailroom. Available at <http://www.cnn.com/2004/US/02/02/senate.hazardous/> Accessed February 3, 2004.
5. WHO TV News. Women accused in plot to poison husband with ricin. Available at <http://www.whotv.com/Global/story.asp?S = 1594218> Accessed January 10, 2004.
6. Bale, J. M. Ricin found in London: an al-Qa'ida connection? Monterey Institute of International Studies. CNS Reports. Available at <http://cns.miis.edu/pubs/reports/ricin.htm> Accessed October 23, 2003.
7. Robertus, J. D., Piatak, M., Ferris, R., and Houston, L. L. Crystallization of ricin A chain obtained from a cloned gene expressed in *Escherichia coli*. *J. Biol. Chem.* 262, 19–20, 1987.
8. Sehnke, P. C., Pedrosa, L., Paul, A. L., et al. Expression of active, processed ricin in transgenic tobacco. *J. Biol. Chem.* 269, 22473–22476, 1994.
9. Palmer, M. and Betz, J. M. Plants. In: *Goldfrank's Toxicologic Emergencies*, 7th edn. Goldfrank, L. R., Howland, M. A., Flomenbaum, N. E., et al. (eds). McGraw-Hill, New York, pp. 1150–1182, 2002.
10. Scarpa, A. and Guerci, A. Various uses of the castor oil plant (Ricinus communis) – a review. *J. Ethnopharmacol.* 5, 117–137, 1982.
11. Dickers, K. J., Bradberry, S. M., Rice, P., et al. Abrin poisoning. *Toxicol. Rev.* 22, 137–142, 2003.
12. Franz, D. R. and Jaax, N. K. Ricin toxin, In: *The Medical Aspects of Chemical and Biological Warfare*, Sidell, F.R., Takafuji, E.T., Franz, D.R. (eds), Bordon Institute, Washington, D.C., pp. 631–642, 1997.
13. Endo, Y., Mitsui, K., Motizuki, M., and Tsurugi, K. The mechanism of action of ricin and related toxic lectins on eukaryotic ribosomes. The site and the characteristics of the modification in 28 S ribosomal RNA caused by the toxins. *J. Biol. Chem.* 262, 5908–5912, 1987.
14. Burbage, C., Tagge, E. P., Harris, B., et al. Ricin fusion toxin targeted to the human granulocyte-macrocyte colony stimulating factor receptor is selectively toxic to acute myeloid leukemia cells. *Leuk. Res.* 21, 681–690, 1997.
15. Frankel, A. E., Burbage, C., Fu, T., et al. Characterization of a ricin fusion toxin targeted to the interleukin-2 receptor. *Protein Eng.* 9, 913–919, 1996.

16. Medina-Bolivar, F., Wright, R., Funk, V., et al. A non-toxic lectin for antigen delivery of plant-based mucosal vaccines. *Vaccine* 21, 997–1005, 2003.
17. Challoner, K. R. and McCarron, M. M. Castor bean intoxication. *Ann. Emerg. Med.* 19, 1177–1183, 1990.
18. Patussi, V., De Zotti, R., Riva, G., et al. Allergic manifestations due to castor beans: an undue risk for dock workers handling green coffee beans. *Med. Lav.* 81, 301–307, 1990.
19. Davison, A. G., Britton, M. G., Forrester, J. A., et al. Asthma in merchant seamen and laboratory workers caused by allergy to castor beans: analysis of allergens. *Clin. Allergy* 13, 553–561, 1983.
20. Topping, M. D., Tyrer, F. H., and Lowing, R. K. Castor bean allergy in the upholstery department of a furniture factory. *Br. J. Ind. Med.* 38, 293–296, 1981.
21. Palosuo, T., Panzani, R. C., Singh, A. B., et al. Allergen cross-reactivity between proteins of the latex from *Hevea brasiliensis*, seeds and pollen of *Ricinus communis*, and the pollen of *Mercurialis annua*, members of the Euphorbiaceae family. *Allergy Asthma Proc.* 23, 141–147, 2002.
22. Franz, D. R. Defense against toxin weapons: medical aspects of chemical and biological warfare. In: *Textbook of Military Medicine: Medical Aspects of Chemical and Biological Warfare*. Zajtchuk, B. G. R. and Bellamy, R. F. (eds). Office of the Surgeon General, Walter Reed Army Medical Center, Washington, DC, pp. 606, 1997.
23. Daniels, K. and Schier, J. Recognition, management and surveillance of ricin-associated illness. CDC Webcast. December 30, 2003. Available at <http://www.phppo.cdc.gov/phtn/webcast/ricin/tp_ricin_final_12-17-03.htm> Accessed on January 20, 2004.
24. Wong, J., Korcheva, V., Jacoby, D. B., and Majun, B. Intrapulmonary delivery of ricin at high dosage triggers a systemic inflammatory response and glomerular damage. *Am J. Pathol.* 170, 1497–1510, 2007.
25. Wilhelmsen, C. and Pitt, L. Lesions of acute inhalted lethal ricin intoxication in rhesus monkeys. *Vet. Pathol.* 33, 296–302, 1996.
26. Ramsden, C., Drayson, M., and Bell, E. The toxicity, distribution, and excretion of ricin holotoxin in rats. *Toxicology* 55, 161–171, 1989.
27. Poli, M. A., Rivera, V. R., Hewetson, J. F., and Merrill, C. A. Detection of ricin by colorimetric and chemiluminescence ELISA. *Toxicon* 32, 1371–1377, 1994.
28. Shyu, H. F., Chiao, D. J., Liu, H. W., and Tang, S. S. Monoclonal antibody-based enzyme immunoassay for detection of ricin. *Hybrid. Hybridomics* 21, 69–73, 2002.
29. Furukawa-Stoffer, T. L., Mah, D. C., Cheranogrodzky, J. W., and Weselake, R. J. A novel biological-based assay for the screening of neutralizing antibodies to ricin. *Hybridoma* 18, 505–511, 1999.
30. Burstein, J. L. Ricin as a biological weapon. Available at <http://www.mcph.org/BT/August%2020.03/Ricin%20JLB%20editsF.pdf> Accessed January 15, 2004.
31. U.S. Army Medical Research Institute of Infectious Diseases Ricin. Available at <http://www.nnh.org/BIOCASU/18/html> Accessed January 20, 2004.
32. Thompson, W. L., Scovill, J. P., and Pace, J. G. Drugs that show protective effects from ricin toxicity in in vitro protein synthesis assays. *Nat Toxins* 3, 369–377, 1995.
33. Delfini, C., Sargiacomo, M., Amici, C., et al. Cholera toxin B-subunit protects mammalian cells from ricin and abrin toxicity. *J. Cell. Biochem.* 20, 359–367, 1982.
34. Griffiths, G. D., Lindsay, C. D., Allenby, A. C., et al. Protection against inhalation toxicity of ricin and abrin by immunisation. *Hum. Exp. Toxicol.* 14, 155–162, 1995.
35. Griffiths, G. D., Bailey, S. C., Hambrook, J. L., et al. Liposomally-encapsulated ricin toxoid vaccine delivered intratracheally elicits a good immune response and protects against a lethal pulmonary dose of ricin toxin. *Vaccine* 15, 1933–1939, 1997.
36. Griffiths, G. D., Bailey, S. C., Hambrook, J. L., and Keyte, M. P. Local and systemic responses against ricin toxin promoted by toxoid or peptide vaccines alone or in liposomal formulations. *Vaccine* 16, 530–535, 1998.

37. Griffiths, G. D., Phillips, G. J., and Bailey, S. C. Comparison of the quality of protection elicited by toxoid and peptide liposomal vaccine formulations against ricin as assessed by markers of inflammation. *Vaccine* 17, 2562–2568, 1999.
38. Kende, M., Yan, C., Hewetson, J., et al. Oral immunization of mice with rice toxoid vaccine encapsulated in polymeric microspheres against aerosol challenge. *Vaccine* 20, 1681–1691, 2002.
39. Olson, M. A., Carra, J. H., Royas-Duncan, V., et al. Finding a new vaccine in the ricin protein fold. *Protein Eng. Des. Sel.* 17, 391–397, 2004.
40. Vitetta, E. S., Smallshaw, J. E., Coleman, E., et al. A pilot clinical trial of a recombinant ricin vaccine in normal humans. *Proc. Natl. Acad. Sci. U.S.A.* 103, 2268–2273, 2006.
41. Smallshaw, J. E., Richardson, J. A., and Vitetta, E. S. RiVax, a recombinant ricin subunit vaccine, protects mice against ricin delivery by gavage or aerosol. *Vaccine* 25, 7459–7469, 2007.
42. Poli, M. A., Rivera, V. R., Pitt, M. L., and Vogel, P. Aerosolized specific antibody protects mice from lung injury associated with aerosolized ricin exposure. *Toxicon* 34, 1037–1044, 1996.
43. Hewetson, J. F., Rivera, V. R., Creasia, D. A., et al. Protection of mice from inhaled ricin by vaccination with ricin or by passive treatment with heterologous antibody. *Vaccine* 11, 743–746, 1993.
44. Chanh, T. C., Romanowski, M. J., and Hewetson, J. F. Monoclonal antibody prophylaxis against the in vivo toxicity of ricin in mice. *Immunol. Invest.* 22, 63–72, 1993.
45. Ulrich, R. G., Sidell, S., Taylor, T. J., et al. Staphylococcal enterotoxin B and related pyrogenic toxins. In: *Medical Aspects of Chemical and Biological Warfare*, Sidell, F.R., Takafuji, E.T., Franz, D.R. (eds), Bordon Institute, Washington, D.C., pp. 621–630, 1997.
46. Marrack, P. and Kappler, J. The staphylococcal enterotoxins and their relatives. *Science* 248, 705–711, 1990.
47. Jett, M., Brinkley, W., Neill, R., et al. *Staphylococcus aureus* enterotoxin B challenge of monkeys: correlation of plasma levels of arachidonic acid cascade products with occurrence of illness. *Infect. Immun.* 58, 3494–3499, 1990.
48. Krakauer, T., Pitt, L., and Hunt, R. E. Detection of interleukin-6 and interleukin-2 in serum of rhesus monkeys exposed to a nonlethal dose of staphylococcal enterotoxin B. *Mil. Med.* 162, 612–615, 1997.
49. Assenmacher, M., Lohning, M., Scheffold, A., et al. Sequential production of IL-2, IFN-gamma and IL-10 by individual staphylococcal enterotoxin B-activated T helper lymphocytes. *Eur. J. Immunol.* 28, 1534–1543, 1998.
50. Ulrich, R. G., Bavari, S., and Olson, M. Staphylococcal enterotoxins A and B share a common structural motif for binding class II major histocompatibility complex molecules. *Nat. Struct. Biol.* 2, 554–560, 1995.
51. Dinges, M. M., Orwin, P. R., and Schlievert, P. M. Exotoxins of *Staphylococcus aureus*. *Clin. Microbiol. Rev.* 13, 16–34, 2000.
52. Tranter, H. S. Foodborne staphylococcal illness. *Lancet* 336, 1044–1046, 1990.
53. Huang, I. -H. and Bergdoll, M. G. The primary structure of staphylococcal enterotoxin B. III. The cyanogen bromide peptides of reduced and aminoethylated enterotoxin B, and the complete amino acid sequence. *J. Biol. Chem.* 245, 3518–3525, 1970.
54. Ranelli, D. M., Jones, C. L., Johns, M. B., et al. Molecular cloning of staphylococcal enterotoxin B gene in *Escherichia coli* and *Staphylococcus aureus*. *Proc. Natl. Acad. Sci. U. S.A.* 82, 5850–5854, 1985.
55. Coffman, J. D., Zhu, J., Roach, J. M., et al. Production and purification of a recombinant staphylococcal enterotoxin B vaccine candidate expressed in *Escherichia coli*. *Protein Expr. Purif.* 24, 302–312, 2002.
56. LeClaire, R. D., Hunt, R. E., Bavari, S., et al. Potentiation of inhaled staphylococcal B-induced toxicity by lipopolysaccharide in mice. *Toxicol. Pathol.* 24, 619–626, 1996.
57. Beno, D. W., Uhing, M. R., Goto, M., et al. Staphylococcal enterotoxin B potentiates LPS-induced hepatic dysfunction in chronically catheterized rats. *Am. J. Physiol. Gastrointest. Liver Physiol.* 280, G866–G872, 2001.

58. Dalpke, A. H. and Heeg, K. Synergistic and antagonistic interactions between LPS and superantigens. *J. Endotoxin Res.* 9, 51–54, 2003.
59. Okamoto, S., Kawabata, S., Nakagawa, I., and Hamada, S. Administration of superantigens protects mice from lethal *Listeria monocytogenes* infection by enhancing cytotoxic T cells. *Infect. Immun.* 69, 6633–6642, 2001.
60. Huang, C. C., Coppola, M. A., Nguyen, P., et al. Effect of Staphylococcus enterotoxin B on the concurrent CD8(+) T cell response to influenza virus infection. *Cell. Immunol.* 204, 1–10, 2000.
61. Zhang, W. J., Sarawar, S., Nguyen, P., et al. Lethal synergism between influenza infection and staphylococcal enterotoxin B in mice. *J. Immunol.* 157, 5049–5060, 1996.
62. Holmberg, S. D. and Blake, P. A. Staphylococcal food poisoning in the United States. New facts and old misconceptions. *JAMA* 251, 487–489, 1984.
63. Elwell, M. R., Liu, C. T., Spertzel, R. O., and Beisel, W. R. Mechanisms of oral staphylococcal enterotoxin B-induced emesis in the monkey. *Proc. Soc. Exp. Biol. Med.* 148, 424–427, 1975.
64. Harris, T. O., Grossman, D., Kappler, J. W., et al. Lack of complete correlation between emetic and T-cell-stimulatory activities of staphylococcal enterotoxins. *Infect. Immun.* 61, 3175–3183, 1993.
65. Wright, A., Andrews, P. L., and Titball, R. W. Induction of emetic, pyrexic, and behavioral effects of *Staphylococcus aureus* enterotoxin B in the ferret. *Infect. Immun.* 68, 2386–2389, 2000.
66. Hu, D. -L., Omoe, K., Shimoda, Y., et al. Induction of emetic response to staphylococcal enterotoxins in the house musk shrew (*Suncus murinus*). *Infect. Immun.* 71, 567–570, 2003.
67. Mattix, M. E., Hunt, R. E., Wilhelmsen, C. L., et al. Aerosolized staphylococcal enterotoxin B-induced pulmonary lesions in rhesus monkeys (*Macaca mulatta*). *Toxicol. Pathol.* 23, 262–268, 1995.
68. Savransky, V., Rostapshov, V., Pinelis, D., et al. Murine lethal toxic shock caused by intranasal administration of staphylococcal enterotoxin B. *Toxicol. Pathol.* 31, 373–378, 2003.
69. van Gessel, Y. A., Mani, S., Bi, S., et al. Functional piglet model for the clinical syndrome and postmortem findings induced by staphylococcal enterotoxin B. *Exp. Biol. Med.* 229, 1061–1071, 2004.
70. Office of the Surgeon General for the Army. Medical NBC aspects of staphylococcal enterotoxin B (SEB). Available at <http://www.cbiac.apgea.army.mil/products/seb_20010226.ppt> Accessed January 21, 2004.
71. Rusnak, J. M., Kortepeter, M., Ulrich, R., et al. Laboratory exposures to staphylococcal enterotoxin B. *Emerg. Infect. Dis.* 10, 1544–1549, 2004.
72. Subcommittee on Health of the Committee on Veterans' Affairs. House of Representatives. 117th Congress, Hearing: Military Operations Aspects of SHAD and Project 112, October 9, 2002, Serial 107-43, Washington, U.S. Government Printing Office, 2003.
73. Special Assistant to the Under Secretary of Defense (Personnel and Readiness) for Gulf War Illnesses, Medical Readiness and Military Deployments. Fact Sheet: Project Shipboard Hazard and Defense (SHAD), DTC Test 68–50.
74. Morisette, C., Goulet, J., and Lamoureux, G. Rapid and sensitive sandwich enzyme-linked immunosorbent assay for detection of staphylococcal enterotoxin B in cheese. *Appl. Environ. Microbiol.* 57, 836–842, 1991.
75. Scotte, U., Langfeldt, N., Peruski, A. H., and Mayer, H. Detection of staphylococcal enterotoxin B (SEB) by enzyme-linked immunosorbent assay and by hand-held assay. *Clin. Lab.* 48, 395–400, 2002.
76. Peruski, A. H., Johnson, L. H., and Peruski, L. F. Rapid and sensitive detection of biological warfare agents using time-resolved fluorescence assays. *J. Immunol. Methods* 263, 35–41, 2002.

77. Naimushin, A. N., Soelberg, S. D., Nguyen, D. K., et al. Detection of *Staphylococcus aureus* enterotoxin B at femtomolar levels with a miniature integrated two-channel surface plasmon resonance (SPR) sensor. *Biosens. Bioelectron.* 17, 573–584, 2002.
78. Tempelman, L. A., King, K. D., Anderson, G. P., and Ligler, F. S. Quantitating staphylococcal enterotoxin B in diverse media using a portable fiber-optic biosensor. *Anal. Biochem.* 233, 50–57, 1996.
79. Ewalt, K. L., Haigis, R. W., Rooney, R., et al. Detection of biological toxins on an active electronic microchip. *Anal. Biochem.* 289, 162–172, 2001.
80. Lin, H. C. and Tsai, W. C. Piezoelectric crystal immunosensor for the detection of staphylococcal enterotoxin B. *Biosens. Bioelectron.* 18, 1479–1483, 2003.
81. Kijek, T. M., Rossi, C. A., Moss, D., et al. Rapid and sensitive immunomagnetic-electrochemiluminescent detection of staphylococcal enterotoxin B. *J. Immunol. Methods* 236, 9–17, 2000.
82. Komisar, J. L., Weng, C. F., Oyejide, A., et al. Cellular and cytokine responses in the circulation and tissue reactions in the lung of rhesus monkeys (*Macaca mulatta*) pretreated with cyclosporin A and challenged with staphylococcal enterotoxin B. *Toxicol. Pathol.* 29, 369–378, 2001.
83. Rajagopalon, G., Sen, M. M., and David, C. S. In vitro and in vivo evaluation of staphylococcal superantigen peptide antagonists. *Infect. Immun.* 72, 6733–6737, 2004.
84. Schramm, R. and Thorlacius, H. Staphylococcal enterotoxin B-induced acute inflammation is inhibited by dexamenthasone: importance role of CXC chemokines and macrophage inflammatory protein 2. *Infect. Immun.* 71, 2542–2547, 2003.
85. Hisano, M., Yamaguchi, K., Inoue, Y., et al. Inhibitory effect of catechin against the superantigen staphylococcal enterotoxin B (SEB). *Arch. Dermatol. Res.* 295, 183–189, 2003.
86. Hale, M. L., Margolin, S. B., Krakauer, T., et al. Pirfenidone blocks in vitro and in vivo effects of staphylococcal enterotoxin B. *Infect. Immun.* 70, 2989–2984, 2002.
87. Scheuber, P. H., Denzlinger, C., Wilker, D., et al. Cysteinyl leukotrienes as mediators of staphylococcal enterotoxin B in the monkey. *Eur. J. Clin. Invest.* 17, 455–459, 1987.
88. Scheuber, P. H., Golecki, J. R., Kickhofen, B., et al. Skin reactivity of unsensitized monkeys upon challenge with staphylococcal enterotoxin B: a new approach for investigating the site of toxin action. *Infect. Immun.* 50, 869–876, 1985.
89. Williams, J. CBRNE – staphylococcal enterotoxin B. Available at <http://emedicine.com/emerg/topic888.htm> Accessed January 21, 2004.
90. Schwabe, M., Notermans, S., Boot, R., et al. Inactivation of staphylococcal enterotoxins by heat and reactivation by high pH treatment. *Int. J. Food Microbiol.* 10, 33–42, 1990.
91. LeClaire, R. D., Hunt, R. E., and Bavari, S. Protection against bacterial superantigen enterotoxin B by passive vaccination. *Infect. Immun.* 70, 2278–2281, 2002.
92. Tseng, J., Komisar, J. L., Trout, R. N., et al. Humoral immunity to aerosolized staphylococcal enterotoxin B (SEB), a superantigen, in monkeys vaccinated with SEB toxoid-containing microspheres. *Infect. Immun.* 63, 2880–2885, 1995.
93. Lowell, G. H., Colleton, C., Frost, D., et al. Immunogenicity and efficacy against lethal aerosol staphylococcal enterotoxin B challenge in monkeys by intramuscular and respiratory delivery of proteosome-toxoid vaccines. *Infect. Immun.* 64, 4686–4693, 1996.
94. Boles, J. W., Pitt, M. L., LeClaire, R. D., et al. Generation of protective immunity by inactivated recombinant staphylococcal enterotoxin B vaccine in nonhuman primates and identification of correlates of immunity. *Clin. Immunol.* 108, 51–59, 2003.
95. Stiles, B. G., Garza, A. R., Ulrich, R. G., and Boles, J. W. Mucosal vaccination with recombinationally attenuated staphylococcal enterotoxin B and protection in a murine model. *Infect. Immun.* 69, 2031–2036, 2001.
96. Gross, T. P., Kamara, L. B., Hatheway, C. L., et al. *Clostridium perfringens* food poisoning: use of serotyping in a outbreak setting. *J. Clin. Microbiol.* 27, 660–663, 1989.

97. Smedley, J. G., Fisher, D. J., Sayeed, S., et al. The enteric toxins of *Clostridium perfringens*. *Rev. Physiol. Biochem. Pharmacol.* 152, 183–204, 2004.
98. Minami, J., Katayama, S., Matsushita, O., et al. Lambda-toxin of *Clostridium perfringens* activates the precursor of epsilon-toxin by releasing its N- and C-terminal peptides. *Microbiol. Immunol.* 41, 527–535, 1997.
99. Hunter, S. E., Clarke, I. N., Kelly, D. C., and Titball, R. W. Cloning and nucleotide sequencing of the *Clostridium perfringens* epsilon-toxin gene and its expression in *Escherichia coli*. *Infect. Immun.* 60, 102–110, 1992.
100. Liu, J. W., Poter, A. G., Wee, B. Y. and Thanabulu, T. New gene from nine *Bacillus sphaericus* strains encoded highly conserved mosquitocidal toxins. *Appl. Environ. Microbiol.* 62, 2174–2176, 1996.
101. Buxton, D. In-vitro effects of *Clostridium welchii* type-D epsilon toxin on guinea-pig, mouse, rabbit and sheep cells. *J. Med. Microbiol.* 11, 299–302, 1978.
102. Miyata, S., Minami, J., Tamai, E., et al. *Clostridium perfringens* epsilon-toxin forms a heptameric pore with the detergent-insoluble microdomains of Madin-Darby canine kidney cells and rat synaptosomes. *J. Biol. Chem.* 277, 39463–39468, 2002
103. Petit, L., Maier, E., Gibert, M., et al. *Clostridium perfringens* epsilon toxin induces a rapid change of cell membrane permeability to ions and forms channels in artificial lipid bilayers. *J. Biol. Chem.* 276, 15736–15740, 2001.
104. Tamai, E., Ishida, T., Miyata, S., et al. Accumulation of *Clostridium perfringens* epsilon-toxin in the mouse kidney and its possible biological significance. *Infect. Immun.* 71, 5371–5375, 2003.
105. Worthington, R. W. and Mulders, M. S. Effect of *Clostridium perfringens* epsilon toxin on the blood brain barrier of mice. *Onderstepoort J. Vet. Res.* 42, 25–27, 1975,
106. Miyamoto, O., Minami, J., Toyoshima, T., et al. Neurotoxicity of *Clostridium perfringens* epsilon-toxin for the rat hippocampus via the glutamatergic system. *Infect. Immun.* 66, 2501–2508, 1998.
107. Miyamoto, O., Sumitani, K., Nakamura, T., et al. *Clostridium perfringens* epsilon toxin causes excessive release of glutamate in the mouse hippocampus. *FEMS Microbiol. Lett.* 189, 109–113, 2000.
108. Sakurai, J., Nagahama, M., and Fujii, Y. Effect of *Clostridium perfringens* epsilon toxin on the cardiovascular system of rats. *Infect. Immun.* 42, 1183–1186, 1983.
109. Nagahama, M., Iida, H., and Sakurai, J. Effect of *Clostridium perfringens* epsilon toxin on rat isolated aorta. *Microbiol. Immunol.* 37, 447–450, 1993.
110. Centers for Disease Control and Prevention. *Clostridium perfringens* gastroenteritis associated with corned beef served at St. Patrick's Day meals – Ohio and Virginia, 1993. *MMWR Morb. Mortal. Wkly. Rep.* 43, 137–138, 143–144, 1994.
111. Greenfield, R. A., Brown, B. R., Hutchins, J. B., et al. Microbiological, biological and chemical weapons of warfare and terrorism. *Am. J. Med. Sci.* 323, 326–340, 2002.
112. Worthington, R. W., Bertschinger, H. J., and Mulders, M. S. Catecholamine and cyclic nucleoside response of sheep to the injection of *Clostridium welchii (perfringens)* type D epsilon toxin. *J. Med. Microbiol.* 12, 497–501, 1979.
113. Finnie, J. W. Pathogenesis of brain damage produced in sheep by *Clostridium perfringens* type D epsilon toxin: a review. *Aust. Vet. J.* 81, 219–221, 2003.
114. Uzal, F. A., Kelly, W. R., Morris, W. E., and Assis, R. A. Effects of intravenous injection of *Clostridium perfringens* type D epsilon toxin in calves. *J. Comp. Pathol.* 126, 71–75, 2002.
115. Shortt, S. J., Titball, R. W., and Lindsay, C. D. An assessment of the in vitro toxicology of *Clostridium perfringens* type D epsilon-toxin in human and animal cells. *Hum. Exp. Toxicol.* 19, 108–116, 2000.
116. Beal, D. R., Titball, R. W., and Lindsay, C. D. The development of tolerance to *Clostridium perfringens* type D epsilon-toxin in MDCK and G-402 cells. *Hum. Exp. Toxicol.* 22, 595–605, 2003.

117. Uzal, F. A., Rolfe, B. E., Smith, N. J., et al. Resistance of ovine, caprine and bovine endothelial cells to *Clostridium perfringens* type D epsilon toxin in vitro. *Vet. Res. Commun.* 23, 275–284, 1999.
118. Headquarters, Departments of the Army, the Navy and the Air Force, and Commandant, Marine Corps. *Clostridium perfringens* toxins. Treatment of Biological Warfare Agent Casualities. Available at <http://www.vnh.org/FM8284/Chapter4/4-15.html> Accessed January 28, 2004.
119. Naylor, R. D., Martin, P. K., and Sharpe, R. T. Detection of *Clostridium perfringens* epsilon toxin by ELISA. *Res. Vet. Sci.* 42, 255–256, 1987.
120. Uzal, F. A., Kelly, W. R., Thomas, R., et al. Comparison of four techniques for the detection of *Clostridium perfringens* type D epsilon toxin in intestinal contents and other body fluids of sheep and goats. *J. Vet. Diagn. Invest.* 15, 94–99, 2003.
121. Uzal, F. A., Plumb, J. J., Blackall, L. L., et al. Detection by polymerase chain reaction of *Clostridium perfringens* epsilon toxin in faeces and in gastrointestinal contents of goats. *Lett. Appl. Microbiol.* 23, 13–17, 1996.
122. Arcieri, R., Dionisi, A. M., Caprioli, A., et al. Direct detection of *Clostridium perfringens* enterotoxin in patients' stools during an outbreak of food poisoning. *FEMS Immunol. Med. Microbiol.* 23, 45–48, 1999.
123. Nagahama, M. and Sakurai, J. Effect of drugs acting on the central nervous system on the lethality of *Clostridium perfringens* epsilon toxin. *Toxicon* 31, 427–435, 1993.
124. University of Florida. Toxins of biological origins. Available at <http://www.ehs.ufl.edu/Bio/toxin.htm> Accessed January 29, 2004.
125. Parreira, M. P., Aurélio, R., Campos, P. C., et al. Studies on the immunogenicity and stability of the epsilon prototoxin of *Clostridium perfringens* type D detoxified by controlled iodination. *J. Venom. Anim. Toxins* 9, 514, 2003.
126. Kumar, A., Kumar, S., Sarma Dagger, P. V., et al. Differential conformational environment of tryptophan in epsilon native prototoxin and active toxin from *Clostridium perfringens* type D. *J. Biochem. Mol. Biol. Biophys.* 6, 147–150, 2002.
127. Sakurai, J. and Nagahama, M. Amino groups in *Clostridium perfringens* epsilon prototoxin and epsilon toxin. *Microb. Pathog.* 1, 417–423, 1986.
128. Jenson, R. *Diseases of Sheep*, Lea and Febiger, Philadelphia, PA, 1974.
129. Odendaal, M., Visser, J., Bergh, N., et al. The effect of passive immunization on active immunity against *Clostridium perfringens* type D in lambs. *Onderstepoort J. Vet. Res.* 56, 251–255, 1989.
130. Uzal, F. A. and Kelly, W. R. Protection of goats against experimental enterotoxaemia by vaccination with *Clostridium perfringens* type D epsilon toxoid. *Vet. Rec.* 142, 722–725, 1998.
131. Percival, D. A., Shuttleworth, A. D., Williamson, E. D., and Kelly, D. C. Anti-idiotypic antibody induced protection against *Clostridium perfringens* type D. *Infect. Immun.* 58, 2487–2492, 1990.
132. Oyston, P. C. F., Payne, D. W., Harvard, H. L., et al. Production of a non-toxic site-directed mutant of *Clostridium perfringens* ε-toxin which induces protective immunity in mice. *Microbiology* 144, 333–341, 1998.
133. Uzal, F. A., Wong, J. P., Kelly, W. R., and Priest, J. Antibody response in goats vaccinated with liposomal-adjuvanted *Clostridium perfringens* type D epsilon toxoid. *Vet. Res. Commun.* 23, 143–150, 1999.

Chapter 10
Intentional Terrorist Contamination of Food and Water

Jeremy Sobel and John C. Watson

Abstract Sabotage of food and water by terrorists and criminals has occurred in the United States, though rarely. Recently, the threat of intentional contamination with ricin of community drinking water occurred in the United States. A multiplicity of suitable biological and chemical agents exists and the vast contemporary food supply is vulnerable as are community drinking water systems. Prevention requires enhancement of food and water security. An outbreak caused by sabotage of food or water would be detected and handled by the existing public health system in close collaboration with law enforcement and other local, state, and federal agencies. Therefore, minimization of casualties requires a robust standing public health infrastructure capable of detecting, investigating and controlling all foodborne and waterborne disease outbreaks, intentional and unintentional, and providing appropriate medical resources.

Key words Bioterrorism · terrorism · food · water · drinking water · epidemiology · public health · detection · response

10.1 Introduction

The sabotage of water, food, or beverage by contamination with the intention to assassinate individuals, incapacitate armies or demoralize populations has been practiced since antiquity. The vast and complex food supplies and water systems of nations are vulnerable to deliberate contamination [1, 2]. Contamination of water, food, or beverage with biological or chemical agents may serve the objectives of terrorists who seek to create panic, threaten civil order, or cause economic losses. Sabotage of crops or livestock may result in similar consequences.

J. Sobel
Foodborne and Diarrheal Diseases Branch, Centers for Disease Control and Prevention, MS-A38, 1600 Clifton Road, Atlanta, GA 30333, USA
e-mail: jsobel@cdc.gov

L.I. Lutwick, S.M. Lutwick (eds.), *Beyond Anthrax*,
DOI: 10.1007/978-1-59745-326-4_10,

Over 76 million foodborne illnesses are estimated to occur in the United States yearly [3] and over 1,000 outbreaks of foodborne disease are reported to the Centers for Disease Control and Prevention (CDC) each year. During 1999–2000, almost 100 outbreaks of disease associated with drinking or recreational water and affecting more than 4,000 persons were reported to the CDC [4]. Although these represent but a fraction of the actual events of foodborne and waterborne illness, the public health system and the food safety and water quality regulatory apparatus that have evolved over the past century generally are effective at protecting the public from very frequent and large outbreaks of illness caused by contaminated food and water. Specific epidemiological, laboratory, and legal approaches have been developed to detect, investigate and control these events [5, 6]. The same personnel who handle naturally occurring foodborne disease and waterborne disease in the course of their routine duties would almost certainly be the first to respond to an act of bioterrorism involving food or water [1]. However, in the case both of water and food, the personnel responsible for ensuring that community water is safe to drink and food is safe to eat are often from different parts of a health department (e.g., Environmental Health vs. Communicable Disease Control), or even from different departments within the government (e.g., Department of Health vs. Department of Environmental Quality vs. Department of Agriculture), than those responsible for investigating naturally occurring waterborne illness.

This chapter will focus on public health and human illness aspects of sabotage of water, foods, and other packaged beverages. The reader is referred to other sources on the topic of food and water security, which entails protecting the food and water supply from deliberate contamination in the first place [7, 8].

10.2 Vulnerability of the Food Supply

International and governmental authorities have recognized the threat of terrorism to the food supply [7, 9–11]. Biological contamination of food by terrorists and criminals has occurred in the US and elsewhere in recent decades [12–14]. The modern food supply comprises thousands of classes of foods, domestically produced or imported. Ever-more centralized production and processing and wide distribution of products has resulted in unintentional foodborne disease outbreaks that increasingly occur over large, dispersed geographic areas, a situation that may delay recognition of an outbreak and complicate identification of the contaminated food [15, 16]. Deliberate contamination of foods could produce a similar situation. Improved public health surveillance using molecular subtyping greatly increases capacity to detect and respond to such outbreaks [17].

The potential consequences of an attack on the food supply can be inferred from examples of large unintentional foodborne disease outbreaks. In 1985, over 170,000 persons in the United States were infected with *Salmonella* serotype Typhimurium resistant to nine antimicrobial agents by consuming contaminated pasteurized milk from a dairy plant in Illinois [18]. In 1994 about 224,000 persons in the United States were infected with *Salmonella* serotype Enteritidis from contaminated ice cream distributed in numerous states [19]. In 1996, over 7,000 children in Sakai City, Japan, were infected with *Escherichia coli* O157:H7 from contaminated radish sprouts served in school lunches. This outbreak resulted in broad-reaching psychological trauma, including suicide [20]. However, as the mailings of *Bacillus* anthracis-containing envelopes in the United States have demonstrated, even limited dissemination of biological agents using simple means and causing relatively few illnesses can produce considerable public anxiety and challenge the public health system; and contamination with no cases of illness can produce severe economic loss [21, 22].

Absolute protection of the food supply is impossible. Prevention falls under the rubric of food security and entails physical protection of the food supply along the "farm to table" continuum, including all stages of production, processing, transport, storage and retail [7, 8]. This challenge rests principally with food safety regulatory agencies, industry, and law enforcement. Approaches include identification of high-risk foods and critical control points at which contamination could be carried out in the complex web of production and commerce and executing appropriate control measures. Should an attack occur, preparedness entails maximizing capacity to detect and investigate the consequent outbreak with the objective of identifying the contaminated food and removing it from circulation, advising the public, managing associated illness, apprehending the perpetrators, and seizing the biological threat agents [1, 2].

10.3 Vulnerability of the Water Supply

Public community drinking water systems in the United States serve approximately 273 million persons [23]. Community surface water systems, in which the water source may include reservoirs, lakes, or flowing streams, serve about 187 million persons, including most communities with populations of more than 100,000 persons. An additional 86 million persons are served by community ground water systems in which water is drawn from underground aquifers that may be deep, confined, and highly protected or shallow and subject to contamination from surface water. Public water systems have three principal components: (1) a water source which may be surface or underground, (2) a "treatment facility" that can range from a sophisticated filtration, decontamination, and disinfection plant to a simple pumping station, and (3) a distribution system to carry the "treated" water to the public through a complex network of pipes and storage facilities.

Although sewage overflow, chemical runoff, and agricultural and industrial waste are examples of common unintentional sources of water contamination, world events have increased awareness of the potential for intentional contamination of water with biological, chemical, and radiologic agents [2]. The threat of intentional contamination with ricin of community drinking water occurred recently in the U.S. [24]. The large outbreak of cryptosporidiosis in Milwaukee in 1993 illustrates the impact on public health that can result from unintentional contamination of a community water system. An estimated 403,000 cases of illness and at least 54 deaths occurred during this outbreak [25–27]. Likewise, during May 2000, more than 2,300 cases of illness and seven deaths occurred in Walkerton, Ontario as a result of contamination of the community drinking water system with *E. coli* O157:H7 [28]. As noted above regarding food contamination, intentional contamination of even a small portion of a public water system resulting in relatively few illnesses could have major psychologic and economic consequences.

Vulnerability of water systems to terrorism can vary considerably and is influenced, among other things, by the type of water source and treatment processes and by characteristics of the distribution system [2]. Contamination of water can occur at any location, including the source, during treatment, or within the pipes and storage structures comprising the distribution system [29, 30]. A potential misconception is that because of the effect of dilution, a very large quantity of biological agent is necessary to contaminate a water system. This may be true if the point of contamination is a large lake or reservoir. However, a quantity of agent small enough for a terrorist to conceal and carry easily on his person could be sufficient to contaminate distal parts of a water distribution system. Another misconception is that filtration will provide adequate protection against contamination. Depending on the filtration method and skill of the filter operator, filters can effectively remove most microbial contaminants, as well as some chemicals. However, conventional filtration, as well as more advanced filtration methods may not remove biotoxins and most chemicals unless the treatment process has been specifically designed with these objectives in mind. Although filtration is required for treatment of surface water, some large cities with high quality source water have not installed filters. Moreover, any contaminant injected after the filtration process will not be removed.

10.4 Potential Threat Agents for Food and Water

The list of pathogens, chemicals, and toxins that can cause disease by ingestion is extensive [29, 31]. It is important to keep in mind that laboratory-based diagnosis and surveillance systems are geared to well known agents that are commonly recognized to cause disease in natural settings.

The CDC strategic plan for Bioterrorism Preparedness and Response includes a list of critical biological agents for public health preparedness [31, 31a, 32]. The highest priority category of agents includes the naturally occurring foodborne toxin, *Clostridium botulinum* neurotoxin, which produces a flaccid paralysis that can result in death from respiratory arrest if untreated, and *Bacillus anthracis*, ingestion of which uncommonly causes a high-mortality gastrointestinal illness in the developing world [31, 33–35].

The category of second most critical biological agents for public health preparedness consists of organisms that are moderately easy to disseminate, cause moderate morbidity and low mortality, and require specific enhancement of diagnostic and surveillance capacities [32]. This category includes several foodborne and waterborne pathogens (Table 10.1). With proper therapy, these organisms generally are rarely lethal. Beyond this list are a variety of foodborne and waterborne pathogens that could potentially be used, including viral and parasitic agents such as hepatitis A and *Cryptosporidium*. Additionally, various biological agents that have been weaponized may rarely cause unintentional disease following ingestion, and their full potential for malicious contamination of food and water is not fully known. These include *Bacillus anthracis*, *Yersinia pestis*, *Francisella tularensis*, and others. Outbreaks or cases of foodborne transmission of these agents have been reported [36–39].

In general, agents of greatest concern for water terrorism share certain characteristics. These agents would cause morbidity and/or mortality principally upon ingestion. However, unlike foodborne agents, waterborne agents also may pose a risk from inhalation of aerosolized droplets or from contact with skin. Agents of greatest concern generally have a low infectious or toxic oral dose. Waterborne agents of concern also would be easy to produce or obtain in large quantities, store for long periods of time, and be difficult to detect in water. Suitable waterborne agents are likely to be reasonably stable in water and resistant to chlorine and/or other disinfectants used in community drinking water systems. A common misconception is that chlorine disinfection of community water systems is effective against all waterborne agents and is universally practiced. Some biological agents of concern for waterborne terrorism are known to be resistant to chlorine levels present in drinking water. In addition, as many as 26 million persons in the United States live in areas, including several large cities, that are served by community water systems that do not disinfect their drinking water. Water utilities, public health agencies, and other local, state, and federal organizations are working together to address potential vulnerabilities that have been identified.

Assorted chemical agents could be used to contaminate water, foods, and packaged beverages. Many are available in the form of pesticides, cleaning compounds or industrial solvents. The CDC list includes blood agents such as cyanide; heavy metals including arsenic, lead and mercury; and corrosive industrial chemicals and toxins [31]. Naturally occurring biological toxins and synthetic chemicals have been weaponized for aerosolized battlefield use. These and similar substances, including aflatoxins, T-2 mycotoxins, saxitoxin, tetrodotoxin, and ricin, also could produce illness by ingestion [8, 40].

Table 10.1 Some potential foodborne and/or waterborne biological terrorist agents and select characteristics

Agent	Availability/source	Clinical syndrome(s) following ingestion
Botulinum toxin	Organism ubiquitous in environment; cultures require anaerobic conditions	Descending paralysis, respiratory compromise
Salmonella serotypes (excluding *S.* typhi)	Clinical and research labs, culture collections, poultry, environmental sources	Acute diarrheal illness, 1%–3% chronic sequelae
Salmonella typhi	Clinical and research labs	Acute febrile illness, protracted recovery, 10% relapse, 1% intestinal rupture [9]
Shigella spp.	Clinical and research labs	Acute diarrhea, often bloody
Shigella dysenteriae Type 1	Clinical and research labs	Dysentery, seizures
E. coli O157:H7	Clinical and research labs, bovine sources, farms	Acute bloody diarrhea, 5% hemolytic – uremic syndrome, longer-term complications
Vibrio cholerae	Clinical and research labs	Acute life-threatening dehydrating diarrhea
Cryptosporidium spp.	Clinical and research labs; water contaminated with human or animal feces	Asymptomatic; diarrhea, may be profuse and watery, with or without abdominal cramping; malaise, weakness, fatigue, anorexia, nausea, vomiting may accompany diarrhea
Bacillus anthracis	Contaminated soil, water, meat; processed animal skins/hides; research labs	Oropharyngeal syndrome: oropharyngeal ulcer, sore throat, dysphagia, submental swelling/edema, cervical lymphadenopathy, fever, sepsis, death Abdominal syndrome: nausea, vomiting, anorexia, fever, abdominal pain, hematemesis, bloody diarrhea, sepsis, death
Burkholderia pseudomallei	Contaminated soil and water; clinical and research labs	Acute localized suppurative disease: mucopurulent, blood-streaked nasal discharge associated with septal and turbinate nodules/ulcerations, lymphangitis/lymphadenopathy Systemic disease/fulminant septicemia: fever, rigors, sweats, myalgia, rash, liver/spleen abscesses, jaundice, diarrhea, pulmonary lesions/pneumonia, arthritis, osteomyelitis, meningitis, shock

Table 10.1 (continued)

Agent	Availability/source	Clinical syndrome(s) following ingestion
Francisella tularensis	Clinical and research labs; contaminated water and food; rabbits	Oropharyngeal: severe throat pain, exudative/ulcerative pharyngitis and/or tonsillitis, pharyngeal membrane, regional lymphadenopathy with or without abscess Typhoidal: fever, chills, headache, myalgias, pharyngitis, anorexia, nausea, vomiting, diarrhea (rarely bloody), abdominal pain, cough, dehydration, lymphadenopathy, meningismus
Yersinia pestis	Clinical and research labs; contaminated water, moist soil and grains; rodents/rabbits; tissues of infected animals; fleas; pets	Pharyngeal: (asymptomatic pharyngeal carriage possible), pharyngitis, anterior cervical lymphadenopathy, cervical buboes, peritonsillar abscesses; septicemia; fulminant pneumonia; gastrointestinal symptoms with nausea, vomiting, diarrhea, and abdominal pain

10.5 Detecting an Attack on Food or Water

Deliberate contamination of food or water may or may not be accompanied by a threat or statement by the perpetrator. Detection of a covert incident may be quite difficult, particularly when the biological, chemical, or radiological agent does not cause an obvious change in the appearance or physical properties of the contaminated food or water [41–43]. The potential for hoaxes is well recognized and outlandish claims might accompany a small-scale contamination. As with any outbreak involving food or water, early recognition and investigation is vital if the food or water has wide distribution. Prevention of continued exposure leading to additional cases may depend on identifying and recalling the yet-unconsumed food product or of preventing ingestion and potentially other exposure (e.g. respiratory, cutaneous) to the contaminated water. Epidemiologic investigation of the vehicle of transmission for common foodborne pathogens should not be limited initially only to food; water should also be considered and investigated as a potential vehicle so as to avoid unnecessary delay in the event that food eventually is ruled out as the cause of the outbreak. A health department should not delay in contacting the local drinking water utility very early in an investigation. The water utility can provide important information about water quality parameters, recent consumer complaints about taste, odor, or appearance, or other possible recent unusual occurrences related to the drinking water. Utilities also can provide water distribution system maps and information about customers that can prove useful in identifying areas of risk as well as additional cases of illness.

Prompt suspicion of the terroristic nature of an event will help direct the criminal investigation and bring into play the full array of federal, state, and local resources available to counter bioterroristic attacks [10]. Because an act of terrorism is a criminal event, patient interviews as well as clinical specimens and environmental samples (e.g. food, water, etc.) become potential evidence for future court proceedings. As such, they can be subject to a "chain of custody" in which their location and disposition can be accounted for at all times. If a terrorism event is suspected, the Federal Bureau of Investigation assumes a leadership role in the criminal investigation and response. As a result, public health officials, health care providers, the FBI, and other key responders must be able to work closely together to carry out both the public health and criminal investigation and response [44].

A covert attack involving food or water most likely would be recognized by epidemiologic investigation of an apparent outbreak of illness. As occurred in 2001 with the deliberate distribution of *Bacillus anthracis* spores via the postal system, the discovery of a terrorist attack with a biological or chemical agent may occur in a clinician's office, hospital emergency room, or outpatient clinic [40]. Practicing health care providers must understand their key role as front-line responders who must be alert to the presence and significance of clusters of patients with similar clinical symptoms and signs that may signal possible contamination of food or water and report these immediately to public health authorities [31, 45, 46]. Such reporting remains among the most rapid current modes of detection, and training clinicians to rapidly report suspicious syndromes and disease clusters is a cornerstone of preparedness for biological terrorism and epidemics.

An outbreak resulting from intentional contamination of food may or may not exhibit a wide geographic dispersion (e.g. multistate), whereas an outbreak due to contamination of water, other than bottled water, more likely will be limited to the area served by a particular water system. Where cases are widely geographically dispersed, laboratory-based surveillance systems may detect increases in illnesses. For foodborne diseases, the Public Health Laboratory Information System (PHLIS) electronically collects data on foodborne enteric pathogens, many of them on CDC's biological agents list [47]. Computerized algorithms such as the *Salmonella* Outbreak Detection Algorithm (SODA) analyze disease trends for increases in the incidence of specific serotypes compared to historical baselines [48, 49]. A national molecular subtyping network, PulseNet, performs pulsed-field gel electrophoresis "finger printing" on isolates of select foodborne bacterial pathogens from patients, foods and farm animals and has detected many common-source outbreaks that occurred over widespread geographic areas without the focal increase in case counts required by less sensitive systems [50–52].

In recent years, syndromic surveillance systems have been developed in several metropolitan areas [53, 54]. These systems attempt to monitor electronically in near-real time the rates of specific syndromes such as diarrhea, flu-like illnesses, pneumonia, or neurological symptoms from emergency medical services calls, emergency room admissions, discharge diagnoses, and other patient contact indicators. Some "enhanced surveillance" systems also monitor behavioral patterns such as the purchase of over-the-counter medications or school and work absenteeism. A unique surveillance system exists for botulism. A clinician suspecting a case must contact the state public health department in order to obtain the specific therapy, botulinum antitoxin, which is available in the United States only from CDC [33, 55]. Health departments and water utilities are being encouraged to develop stronger working relationships and to routinely share appropriate information from disease reports and daily water quality parameters (e.g. chlorine residual, pH, turbidity, coliforms, esthetics such as odor, taste, color, etc.) in order to be able to more rapidly identify illness potentially caused by water contamination.

10.6 Recognition of a Foodborne or Waterborne Disease Event as a Terrorist or a Criminal Act

Unusual relationships between person, time and place of the outbreak, or unusual or implausible combinations of pathogens and infection vehicles (e.g. water or specific foods) can provide epidemiologic clues to a deliberate, covert act of contamination (Table 10.2) [40, 56, 57]. Recognition of such clues by astute, well-informed clinicians and public health personnel who maintain a high index of suspicion may lead to more rapid identification of a terrorist event by guiding clinical and environmental laboratory testing and epidemiologic investigation to look for uncommon causes (e.g. *Brucella* sp., *Yersinia pestis*, ricin toxin, *Francisella tularensis*, *Burkholderia mallei*, and *B. pseudomallei*, *Bacillus anthracis*) of common clinical syndromes (e.g. flu-like illness, pharyngitis, gastroenteritis and diarrhea, rash and skin lesions, cough and respiratory difficulty). However, such features also may occur in an unintentional outbreak or may be absent in a deliberate contamination event. Therefore, epidemiologic features alone cannot prove a terroristic act; rather, they inform the investigators and may prompt consultation with law enforcement agencies that may confirm or refute the possibility of malicious contamination.

The adequacy of a response to a terrorist event involving contamination of food or water will depend on public health officials' capacity to respond to any foodborne and waterborne disease outbreak. Hence a cornerstone of preparedness is improving the public health infrastructure for detecting and responding to unintentional outbreaks by: (1) ensuring robust public health

Table 10.2 Epidemiologic clues suggesting a possible terrorism related outbreak

- A large epidemic with a similar disease or syndrome, particularly affecting a discrete population.
- Many cases of unexplained disease or death.
- Severe and/or frequent disease manifestations in previously healthy individuals.
- More severe disease than expected for a particular pathogen, or failure to respond to standard therapy.
- An unusual route of exposure or symptom complex for a particular pathogen, such as gastrointestinal illness rather than inhalational or cutaneous.
- Cases of disease occurring in an unusual geographic location and/or at an unexpected time of year and/or in an unusual age group and/or an unusual population and/or with a zoonotic impact.
- Cases of a disease normally transmitted by vector that is not present in the local area.
- A single case of disease caused by a very uncommon agent (e.g. smallpox).
- Similar genetic type for a pathogen/agent isolated from distinct sources at different locations or times.
- Unusual strains or variants of a pathogen and/or unusual antibiotic resistance patterns.
- Simultaneous and/or serial epidemics of different diseases in the same population.
- Adapted from: Distinguishing between natural and intentional disease outbreaks. In: *USAMRIID's Medical Management of Biological Casualties Handbook*. Kortepeter, M (lead ed). Operational Medicine Division, US Army Medical Research Institute of Infectious Diseases (USAMRIID), Fort Detrick, MD, 2001, pp. 11–14.

surveillance, (2) improving laboratory diagnostic capacity for patient, food product, and environmental water samples, (3) increasing trained staff for rapid epidemiologic investigations, and (4) enhancing effective communications. Preparedness for such a situation additionally requires the capacity to respond to and meet the extraordinary demands placed upon emergency services and medical resources.

10.7 Diagnosis of the Agent in Suspected Foodborne and Waterborne Terrorism

A key factor in rapid diagnosis of the etiologic agent during an investigation of an outbreak of unexplained foodborne and waterborne disease is ordering the appropriate clinical and environmental diagnostic laboratory tests as part of the basic public health response. This requires that clinicians, as well as infection control practitioners and public health officials investigating a potential outbreak, have some familiarity with the more serious agents and their clinical presentations, that they be attuned to epidemiologic clues that could indicate an intentional contamination of food or water, that they not be hampered in ordering diagnostic tests by cost concerns, and that they know how to contact public health sector consultants and do so rapidly when needed.

Most foodborne and waterborne pathogens on CDC's Strategic Plan for Bioterrorism Preparedness and Response [31, 32] are detectable in clinical specimens by using the routine staining, culture, serologic, and/or rapid diagnostic procedures available in state public health laboratories. Public health laboratories have protocols for evaluating outbreaks of gastroenteritis. Botulism is diagnosed in some state and municipal laboratories and at CDC. Identification of biotoxins requires testing of appropriate samples in specialized laboratories. CDC, in collaboration with the state public health laboratories, has developed the national Laboratory Response Network (LRN) specializing in the diagnosis of biological agents of terrorism [58]. Selected public health, military, veterinary, and commercial laboratories comprise the LRN, which provides standardized diagnostic protocols and reagents, makes rapid initial diagnoses, and refers specimens for confirmatory testing to appropriate specialty laboratories such as those of CDC and the Department of Defense (DoD). The LRN provides surge capacity to handle the increased numbers of diagnostic samples that would be anticipated during a bioterrorism event. For example, during the anthrax mailings investigations of 2001, more than 120,000 environmental and clinical samples were collected and analyzed.

Collection and analysis of samples of potentially contaminated food and water can be quite challenging. Food samples already may have been discarded and contaminated water already may have been flushed from the distribution system before contamination is suspected or illness is detected or investigated. In the case of community drinking water systems, hydraulic flow patterns throughout the distribution system change continuously based on water use demands within the system. These constantly changing flow patterns present a challenge when trying to determine where to draw water samples for analysis. In addition, because of the effect of dilution, a large volume of potentially contaminated water (e.g. 10 liters or more per sample) must be collected and concentrated before it is possible to detect a biological agent or biotoxin by polymerase chain reaction (PCR), immunodiagnosis, or culture. Much current research is directed towards developing and evaluating rapid and field deployable methods both for concentrating large volume samples of drinking water and for simultaneously identifying multiple biological and chemical contaminants in the concentrated samples. Such rapid water sampling and pathogen extraction and identification methods are necessary in order to determine, in the presence of a threat, whether and with what agent water has been contaminated, to assess the extent of an actual contamination and who is or may be at risk, and to determine if and when water is again safe to drink.

10.8 Response

In the United States, county, municipal, and in some cases state health departments typically are the first to be informed of disease outbreaks and to investigate and respond to them. State public health laboratories and some municipal laboratories play a primary role in diagnosing the etiology of an outbreak. Diffuse outbreaks with cases distributed over a wide geographic area without apparent clustering, such as occurs in a multistate outbreak, may be recognized first as a result of national laboratory-based surveillance systems. In such circumstances, CDC may play a coordinating role. The public health objectives of an investigation are to define the size and extent of the outbreak, its etiology, the food, water or other vehicle, to halt the outbreak by controlling that source, and to learn how to prevent future similar outbreaks.

A suspected terrorist event involving potential or actual intentional contamination of food or water requires a coordinated response by agencies representing public health, law enforcement, emergency response, health care, water utility, and others. The initial response occurs at the local level, but state and federal resources also will become involved. Any terrorist threat or action against the food or water supply is considered a criminal incident and must be reported to law enforcement authorities. During the response to a foodborne or waterborne terrorist incident, the goals of the public health investigation combine public health goals with the goals of the law enforcement investigation: to protect the public and public safety, to stop the spread of disease and prevent a criminal act, to protect public health personnel and law enforcement personnel, to identify and prevent the spread of the biological, chemical, or radiologic agent, and to identify, apprehend, and prosecute the perpetrators [59].

The objectives of the public health investigation of an outbreak of foodborne or waterborne disease would not change greatly if intentional contamination is suspected. However, the "mechanics" of the epidemiologic investigation would be affected by the need for coordination with law enforcement personnel, such as the FBI and state and local police, carrying out the criminal investigation. Because of the possibility that the perpetrator may strike again, the investigation must move quickly even if the outbreak appears to be over and be an all out" effort. Identification of the etiologic agent, vehicle of transmission, and manner of contamination remain the most important aspects of an investigation, followed by timely implementation of control measures, including removal of the contaminated food from circulation, recommendations for boiling or other restrictions on the use of water, and properly treating exposed persons [5]. The familiar components of the investigation include formulation of case definitions, case finding, pooling and evaluation of data on potential exposures in different geographic locations, rapid development of standardized data-collection instruments and execution of case-control studies to identify specific foods or other potential risk factors, collection of laboratory and environmental samples, transport and processing, collating information from tracebacks, coordination with law enforcement, food safety and water quality regulatory agencies, water utilities, and agencies involved in emergency medical response, and standardization of recommendations for treatment, prophylaxis, and other preventive measures. CDC and federal food regulatory agencies, FDA and USDA, routinely collaborate on tracebacks of contaminated foods implicated in many of the more than 1,000 foodborne disease outbreaks reported annually in the US, and this norm would be followed in a bioterrorism event. Similar cooperation between CDC and the US Environmental Protection Agency, and the drinking water industry is the norm for waterborne outbreaks, and would be as well in a bioterrorism event involving water.

A sophisticated bioterrorist attack on the food or water supply has the potential to produce many casualties. In the United States, the medical components of the response to such an event is part of overall bioterrorism response preparedness and have been described elsewhere [60]. Adequate stocks of antimicrobial drugs, antitoxins, other medications, and ventilators and other medical equipment are maintained in stockpiles and can be delivered rapidly. A biological terror attack targeting a food or beverage distributed over a wide geographic area could pose the challenge of needing to assure adequate medical supplies and personnel in many locations simultaneously. The effectiveness of the medical response will depend on timely epidemiologic surveillance data collected by public health investigators to direct the appropriate medical resources to the casualties and their caretakers.

A bioterrorist attack involving a community drinking water system might not only cause medical casualties, but also could affect a community's access to water for drinking, bathing and personal hygiene, cooking and preparing foods, fighting fires, and other health care, manufacturing, and industrial uses. An intentional contamination of a community's food and water supply could undermine public confidence in the safety of these universal commodities and the government's ability to ensure that they remain safe for public consumption and use. Public health and other government authorities must be well prepared to respond rapidly to address the public's questions and fears, to provide authoritative recommendations and guidance to the public about how to safeguard their health and deal with other consequences of the event, and to provide adequate safe alternative sources of food and water as necessary. Clinicians and other health care providers must be prepared to not only treat ill and exposed victims but to also address the questions and concerns of their patients by providing them timely and accurate information.

10.9 Communications

Swift communication among health care providers, public health officials at various levels, and government agencies is an absolute requirement for a rapid, appropriate and effective response to any outbreak related to the food or water supply. Communication patterns similar to those used in coordination of multistate outbreak investigations will likely be effective for incidents of intentional contamination of food or water [5]. Clinicians, clinical laboratory staff, and coroners who identify suspected cases or clusters of illness must have lists of appropriate local contacts in order to notify the public health sector of their findings. Local health departments should notify state public health departments even as they begin their investigation locally. There are standing modalities used routinely to inform public health officials at the state and federal level of ongoing outbreaks and to coordinate multistate investigations.

In the case of an intentional contamination of food, the communication systems would function much as they do in regular outbreaks. Depending on the food affected, the FDA or USDA's regulatory authorities would be engaged rapidly during a bioterrorist event linked to food. Communication between public health officials and food industries would be coordinated with the appropriate regulatory agency that can request a recall of contaminated food from the market. For incidents involving intentional contamination of a water system, close communication between public health officials, local water utilities, and environmental protection agencies is imperative to try to rapidly identify potential geographic areas of the drinking water system that may be at risk and to decide the best courses of action to prevent and reduce casualties. Authorities must be able to decide whether a community's water supply is safe to use, under what conditions it may be used, and what remedial actions may be necessary to assure it's current and/or continued safety. In addition, for any terrorist act against food or water, close communication among public health, water utility, environmental protection, law enforcement, emergency response, and other agencies at the local, state, and federal levels will be required. These channels of communication should be developed well before the occurrence of a terrorist threat or attack in order to be able to function optimally during an actual crisis.

Intense media coverage of a bioterrorist event is to be expected. Skill and experience are required to transmit accurate information through the media about the nature and extent of the event, the suspected or implicated foods or parts of the water system, and the measures to take to prevent exposure or the consequences of exposure. The accuracy, timeliness and consistency of the information provided may in part determine the success of control measures. It is imperative that medical, public health, water utility, law enforcement, and other local, state, and federal government representatives provide consistent, non-contradictory information and recommendations. Failure to do so reduces public confidence, creates confusion, and ultimately places parts of the public at greater risk of illness and possibly death.

10.10 Conclusions

Sabotage of food and water by terrorists and criminals has occurred in the United States, though rarely. In addition, a recent threat to intentionally contaminate a community drinking water system with ricin has been under investigation. Several possible biological and chemical agents exist and the vast contemporary food supply and community drinking water systems are vulnerable. Reducing the risk of intentional contamination requires enhancement of food and water security. Because an outbreak caused by sabotage of food or water would most likely be detected and handled by the existing public health system in close collaboration with law enforcement, water utility, and other local, state, and federal agencies, minimization of casualties requires a robust standing public health infrastructure capable of detecting, investigation and controlling all foodborne and waterborne disease outbreaks, intentional and unintentional, as well as the presence of well-established and maintained collaboration, cooperation, and communication among all parties who responsibility would be to detect and respond to such a terrorist event.

References

1. Sobel J., Khan A.S, Swerdlow D.S. The threat of a biological terrorist attack on the United States food supply: the CDC perspective. *Lancet* 359, 874–880, 2002.
2. Khan A.S., Swerdlow D.L., Juranek D.D. Precautions against biological and chemical terrorism directed at food and water supplies. *Public Health Rep* 116, 3–14, 2001.
3. Mead P., S., Slutsker L., Dietz V., et al. Food-related illness and death in the United States. *Emerg Infect Dis* 5, 607–625, 1999.
4. Lee S.H., Levy D.A., Craun G.F., Beach M.J., Calderon R.L. Surveillance for waterborne-disease outbreaks – United States, 1999–2000. *MMWR* 51, 1–47, 2002.
5. Sobel J., Griffin P.M., Slutsker L., Swerdlow D.L., Tauxe R.V. Investigation of multistate foodborne disease outbreaks. *Public Health Rep* 117, 8–19, 2002.
6. Waterborne Disease Subcommittee of the Committee on Communicable Diseases Affecting Man (Bryan F.L., Chairman). *Procedures to Investigate Waterborne* Illness (2nd edn). International Association of Milk, Food and Environmental Sanitarians, Inc., Des Moines, IA, 1996.
7. WHO. *Terrorist Threats to Food, Guidelines for Establishing and Strengthening Prevention and Response Systems*. World Health Organization, Geneva, 2002.
8. Lee R.V., Harbison R.D., Draughon F.A. Food as a weapon. *Food Prot Trends* 23, 664–674, 2003.
9. WHO. *Health Aspects of Chemical and Biological Weapons. Report of a WHO Group of Consultants. Annex 5, Sabotage of Water Supplies*. World Health Organization, Geneva, 1970.
10. U.S. General Accounting Office. *Food safety: agencies should further test plans for responding to deliberate contamination*. Washington, D.C., 1999, GAO/RCED-00-3.
11. US Food and Drug Administration. *Risk assessment for food terrorism and other food safety concerns*, 2003. Accessed at: www.cfsan.fda.gov/~dms/rabtact.html on October 13, 2003.
12. Torok T., Tauxe R.V., Wise R.P., et al. A large community outbreak of *Salmonella* caused by intentional contamination of restaurant salad bars. *JAMA* 278, 389–395, 1997.
13. Kolavic S.A., Kimura A., Simons S.L., et al. An outbreak of *Shigella dysenteriae* type 2 among laboratory workers due to intentional food contamination. *JAMA* 278, 396–398, 1997.
14. Phills J.A., Harrold A.J., Whiteman G.V., Perelmutter L. Pulmonary infiltrates, asthma, and eosinophilia due to *Ascaris suum* infestation in man. *N Engl J Med* 286, 965–970, 1972.

15. Hedberg C.W., MacDonald K.L., Osterholm M.T. Changing epidemiology of foodborne disease: a Minnesota perspective. *Clin Infect Dis* 18, 671–682, 1994.
16. Sobel J., Swerdlow D.L., Parsonnet J. Is there anything safe to eat? In: Remington J.S., Schwartz M.N. (eds). *Current Clinical Topics in Infectious Diseases*, Vol. 21. Blackwell Scientific Publications, Boston, 2001, pg. 114–134.
17. Ribot E.M., Fitzgerald C., Kubota K., Swaminathan B., Barrett T.J. Rapid pulsed-field gel electrophoresis protocol for subtyping of *Campylobacter jejuni*. *J Clin Microbiol* 39, 1889–1894, 2001.
18. Ryan C.A., Nickels M.K., Hargrett-Bean N.T., et al. Massive outbreak of antimicrobial-resistant salmonellosis traced to pasteurized milk. *JAMA* 258, 3269–3274, 1987.
19. Hennessy T.W., Hedberg C.W., Slutsker L., et al. A national outbreak of *Salmonella enteritidis* infections from ice cream. *N Engl J Med* 334, 1281–1286, 1996.
20. Mermin J.H., Griffin P.M. Invited commentary: public health crisis in crisis: outbreaks of *Escherichia coli* O157:H7 in Japan. *Am J Epidemiol* 150, 797–803, 1999.
21. Centers for Disease Control and Prevention. Update: investigation of bioterrorism-related anthrax and interim guidelines for clinical evaluation of persons with possible anthrax. *MMWR* 50, 941–948, 2001.
22. Grigg B., Modeland V. The cyanide scare. A tale of two grapes. *FDA Consum* 7–11, 1989.
23. US Environmental Protection Agency. *Factoids: Drinking Water and Ground Water Statistics for 2003*. US Environmental Protection Agency, Office of Ground Water and Drinking Water (4606 M)/EPA 816-K-03-001/www.epa.gov/safewater; 2004. Accessed at: http://www.epa.gov/safewater/data/pdfs/factoids_2003.pdf on May 3, 2004.
24. Centers for Disease Control and Prevention. Investigation of a ricin-containing envelope at a postal facility – South Carolina, 2003. *MMWR* 52, 1129–1131, 2003.
25. MacKenzie W.R., Hoxie N.J., Proctor M.E., et al. A massive outbreak in Milwaukee of *Cryptosporidium* infection transmitted through the public water supply. *N Engl J Med* 331, 161–167, 1994.
26. Kaminski J.C. *Cryptosporidium* and the public water supply [letter]. *N Engl J Med* 331, 1529–1530, 1994.
27. Goldstein S.T, Juranek D.J., Ravenholt O., et al. Cryptosporidiosis: an outbreak associated with drinking water despite state-of-the-art treatment. *Ann Intern Med* 124, 459–468, 1996.
28. Krewski D., Balbus J., Butler-Jones D., et al. Managing health risks from drinking water – a report to the Walkerton inquiry. *J Toxicol Environ Health* 65, 1591–1617, 2002.
29. Deininger R.A. *The Threat of Chemical and Biological Agents to the Public Drinking water supply systems*. Water Pipeline Database, Science Applications International Corporation. 2000, MacLean, VA.
30. Meinhardt P.L. Section 2: Understanding the Threat of Water Terrorism. In: *Physician Preparedness for Acts of Water Terrorism*. 2003, Accessed at: http://www.waterhealthconnection.org/bt/chapter2.asp on May 3, 2004.
31. Centers for Disease Control and Prevention. Biological and chemical terrorism: strategic Plan for preparedness and response. Recommendations of the CDC Strategic Planning Workgroup. *MMWR* 49, 1–14, 2000.
31a. Burrows W.D., Renner S.E. Biological warfare agents as threats to potable water. *Environ Health Perspect* 107, 974–984, 1999.
32. Centers for Disease Control and Prevention. *Emergency preparedness and response: bioterrorism agents/diseases by category*, 2004. Accessed at: http://www.bt.cdc.gov/agent/agentlist-category.asp on May 3, 2004.
33. Shapiro R., Hatheway C., Swedlow D. Botulism in the United States: a clinical and epidemiologic review. *Ann Intern Med* 129, 221–228, 1998.
34. Hatheway C.L. Toxigenic clostridia. *Clin Microbiol Rev* 3, 66–98, 1990.

35. Sirisanthana T., Brown A.E. Anthrax of the gastrointestinal tract. *Emerg Infect Dis.* 8, 649–651, 2002.
36. Erickson M.C., Kornacki J.L. *Bacillus anthracis:* current knowledge in relation to contamination in food. *J Food Prot* 66, 691–699, 2003.
37. Butler T., Fu Y.S., Furman L., Almeida C., Almeida A. Experimental *Yersinia pestis* infection in rodents after intragastric inoculation and ingestion of bacteria. *Infect Immun* 36, 1160–1167, 1982.
38. Reintjes R., Dedushaj I., Gjini A., et al. Tularemia outbreak investigation in Kosovo: a case control and environmental studies. *Emerg Infect Dis* 8, 69–73, 2002.
39. Tarnvik A., Berglund L. (2003) Tularemia. *Eur Respir J* 21, 361–373.
40. Franz D.R., Jaax N.K. Ricin toxin. In: Sidell FR, Takafuji ET, Franz DR (eds). *Medical Aspects of Chemical and Biological Warfare*. Borden Institute, Walter Reed Army Medical Center, Washington, DC, pg. 631–642.
41. Meinhardt P.L. Section 4: detection and diagnosis of waterborne terrorism. In: *Physician Preparedness for Acts of Water Terrorism*. Accessed at: http://www.waterhealthconnection.org/bt/chapter2.asp on May 3, 2004.
42. Linstren D.C. *Nuclear, Biological, and Chemical (NBC) Contamination to Army Field Water Supplies*. Report 2438, ADB109393, U.S. Army Belvoir Research, Development and Engineering Center, Fort Belvoir, VA, 1987.
43. NATO. *NATO Handbook on the Medical Aspects of NBC Defensive Operations*. AMedP-6, 1996. Accessed at http://www.fas.org/nuke/guide/usa/doctrine/dod/fm8-9/toc.htm on May 17, 2004.
44. Institute of Medicine Committee on Research and Development Needs for Improving Civilian Medical Response to Chemical and Biological Terrorism Incidents. *Chemical and Biological Terrorism. Research and Development to Improve Civilian Medical Response*. National Academy Press, Washington, DC, 1999.
45. Meinhardt P.L. Section 1: purpose of physician readiness guide for acts of water terrorism, 2003. In: *Physician Preparedness for Acts of Water Terrorism*, 2003. Accessed at: http://www.waterhealthconnection.org/bt/chapter2.asp on May 3, 2004.
46. Gerberding J.L., Hughes J.M., Koplan J.P. Bioterrorism preparedness and response: clinicians and public health agencies as essential partners. *JAMA* 287, 898–899, 2002.
47. Bean M.H., Martin S.M., Bradford H. PHLIS: an electronic system for reporting public health data from remote sites. *Am J Public Health* 82, 1273–1276, 1992.
48. Hutwagner L.C., Maloney E.K., Bean N.H, Slutsker L., Martin S.M. (1997) Using laboratory-based surveillance data for prevention: an algorithm for detecting *Salmonella* outbreaks. *Emerg Infect Dis* 3, 395–400, 1997.
49. Mahon B., Ponka A., Hall W., et al. An international outbreak of *Salmonella* infections caused by alfalfa sprouts grown from contaminated seed. *J Infect Dis* 175. 876–882, 1997.
50. Stephenson J. New approaches for detecting and curtailing foodborne microbial infections. *JAMA* 277, 1337–1340, 1997.
51. Swaminathan B., Barrett T.J., Hunter S.B., Tauxe R.V. PulseNet: the molecular subtyping network for foodborne bacterial disease surveillance, United States. *Emerg Infect Dis.* 7, 382–389, 2001.
52. Sivapalasingam S., Kimura A., Ying M., et al. *A multistate outbreak of Salmonella newport infections linked to mango consumption, November-December 1999*. Latebreaker Abstract. 49th Annual Epidemic Intelligence Service (EIS) Conference, Centers for Disease Control and Prevention, Atlanta, GA, 2002.
53. Greenko J., Mostashari F., Fine A., Layton M. Clinical evaluation of the emergency medical services (EMS) ambulance dispatch-based syndromic surveillance system, New York City. *J Urban Health* 80, i50–i56, 2003.
54. Pavlin J.A. Investigation of disease outbreaks detected by "syndromic" surveillance systems. *J Urban Health* 80, i107–i114, 2003.

55. Centers for Disease Control and Prevention. *Botulism in the United States, 1899–1996. Handbook for Epidemiologists, Clinicians, and Laboratory Workers*. Centers for Disease Control and Prevention, Atlanta, GA, 1998.
56. Treadwell T.A., Koo D., Kuker K., Khan A.S. Epidemiologic clues to bioterrorism. *Public Health Rep* 118, 92–98, 2003.
57. Kortepeter M. *USAMRIID's Medical Management of Biological Casualties Handbook*, 4th edn. Fort Detrick, MD, 2001.
58. Heatherley S.S. The laboratory response network for bioterrorism. *Clin Lab Sci* 15, 177–179, 2002.
59. U.S. Department of Justice. *Criminal and Epidemiological Investigation Handbook*, 2003 edition. U.S. Department of Justice, Federal Bureau of Investigation, U.S. Army Soldier Biological Chemical Command.
60. Khan A.S., Morse S., Lillibridge S. Public-health preparedness for biological terrorism in the USA. *Lancet* 356, 1179–1182, 2000.
61. Chin J (ed). *Control of Communicable Diseases Manual*, 17th edn. American Public Health Association, Washington, DC, 2000.
62. Mead P.S., Griffin P.M. *Escherichia coli* O157:H7. *Lancet* 352, 1207–1212, 1998.
63. Griffin P.M., Bell B.P., Cieslak P.R., et al. Large outbreak of *Escherichia coli* O157:H7 infections in the western United States: the big picture. In: Karmali M.A., Golglio A.G. (eds). *Recent advances in verocytotoxin-producing Escherichia coli infections*. Elsevier Science B.V., New York, NY, 1994, pp. 7–12.
64. Bennish M.L. Cholera: pathophysiology, clinical features, and treatment. In: Wachsmuth I.K., Blake P.A., Olsvik O. (eds). *Vibrio cholerae and cholera, molecular to global perspectives*. ASM Press, Washington, DC, 1994, pp. 229–256.
65. Friedlander A.M. Anthrax. In: Sidell F.R., Takafuji E.T., Franz D.R. (eds). *Medical aspects of chemical and biological warfare*. Borden Institute, Walter Reed Army Medical Center, Washington, DC, 1997, pg. 467–478.

Resources

Centers for Disease Control and Prevention. *Emergency preparedness and response, 2003*. Accessed at: http://www.bt.cdc.gov/index.asp on May 3, 2004.

Meinhardt P.L. (2000) Recognizing waterborne disease and the health effects of water pollution: a physician on-line reference. Accessed at: http://www.waterhealthconnection.org/index.asp on May 3, 2004.

Meinhardt P.L. (2003) *Physician preparedness for acts of water terrorism*. Accessed at: http://www.waterhealthconnection.org/bt/index.asp on May 3, 2004.

WHO. (2002) *Terrorist threats to food, guidelines for establishing and strengthening prevention and response systems*. World Health Organization, Geneva.

Sidell F.R., Takafuji E.T., Franz D.R. (eds). (1997) *Medical aspects of chemical and biological warfare*. Borden Institute, Walter Reed Army Medical Center, Washington, DC.

Chapter 11
Public Health Infrastructure

Isaac B. Weisfuse

11.1 Lessons Learned

The events of September 11, 2001, along with the subsequent anthrax attacks, fundamentally altered public health in the United States by giving it vast new responsibilities. Departments of Health (DOHs) must now organize themselves and their communities to respond to terrorist attacks of weapons of mass destruction and in particular to agents of bioterrorism (BT). Issues ranging from organizational structure, workforce training, relationships to other governmental entities and the public are being re-thought during this transition period to meet the new needs. All of this must be done while still maintaining the traditional mission of protecting the public's health. This chapter provides a brief overview of the scope of the challenges facing public health.

The "lessons learned" from several exercises and events illustrate some of the current gaps in preparedness. For example during TOPOFF, a federal drill involving an outbreak of *Yersinia pestis*, in Denver, Colorado [1], difficulties included:

- flawed decision making processes,
- limited public health resources,
- lack of knowledge about incident command systems (ICS),
- logistical issues in distributing prophylactic antimicrobial agents,
- overwhelmed hospitals,
- decisions on personal protective equipment, and
- reaching decisions about disease containment.

The World Trade Center disaster, although not a BT event revealed many of these same problems [2], as well as others:

I.B. Weisfuse
Division of Disease Control, New York City Department of Health and Mental Hygiene, 125 Worth Street, Room 326, CN #22, New York, NY 10013, USA
e-mail: iweisfus@health.nyc.gov

L.I. Lutwick, S.M. Lutwick (eds.), *Beyond Anthrax*,
DOI: 10.1007/978-1-59745-326-4_11,

- communication difficulties,
- the need to provide guidance and oversight over work-site safety,
- environmental risk communication controversies,
- difficulty in mobilizing local public health resources,
- difficulty in coordinating federal resources, and
- the need for mental health services for public health staff.

Issues evident during the anthrax attacks included:

- lack of identification of postal workers at risk,
- inadequate communication to the public and health-care providers,
- lack of standards for environmental assessment,
- lack of surge capacity for public health laboratories, and
- challenges in coordinating multijurisdictional investigations.

Other needs documented in a recent survey of state health departments [3] include increased need for planning time, new surveillance systems, and hiring of qualified staff.

11.2 Funding for BT Preparedness

Public health in the United States is seriously underfinanced, especially in comparison to the medical care system. Despite this, meeting the challenges of BT must occur at all levels of public health from large state and urban health departments to small county health departments with few resources. The threat must be addressed at the same time that public health is struggling to meet demands of a host of emerging public health issues such as the obesity and diabetes epidemics and communicable disease problems that require additional attention and resources such as HIV/AIDS or SARS. The United States Federal Government has been instrumental in providing resources to public health after 2001. During 2002, $918 million was provided for this purpose through the Centers for Disease Control and Prevention, with the same amount allocated for 2003–04. In addition, through the Health and Human Services Administration (HRSA), additional funds were provided to health departments for hospital preparedness.

11.3 Organizational Issues

DOHs have developed a deliberative consensus driven decision making process, and do not tend to have rigid hierarchies. As such, they must adapt to using incident command systems. An ICS requires a clear chain of command to promote rapid decision making with distinct roles for responders and needs a modular approach to managing emergencies that allows for expansion and contraction of activities. It also facilitates the interaction between responders and agencies by using standard terminology and roles. Public health agencies have only recently adopted ICS, with the resultant need to alter decision-making processes during crisis. ICS is needed not only within but between public health agencies as well. Federal personnel, such as CDC epidemic intelligence services officers, need to know how their activities will integrate with the state or local response plan and be able to adhere to ICS principles and structures.

Surge capacity, the ability to quickly obtain additional resources (principally personnel) to respond to an emergency, is an important aspect of preparedness. During the 2001 anthrax crises, nearly all public health laboratories reported requiring additional trained personnel, regardless of the presence or absence of actual anthrax cases in their jurisdiction. Several strategies may be employed to meet this need. An internal surge capacity plan involves informing and educating personnel and their unions of the need, providing training and drill experiences to allow personnel to feel comfortable in unfamiliar roles, and periodically providing updates and reminders to personnel. If possible, personnel should only perform their routine tasks, however they may be performed at different hours, work locations, and under the guidance of different supervisors during an emergency.

An additional strategy, most suitable for small health departments under the guidance of their state health departments, is the development of "mutual aid" agreements with surrounding jurisdictions. These agreements can provide personnel for such services as epidemiologic investigations and clinical services. This strategy is well recognized for other emergency responders such as fire departments and emergency medical service units. Finally, the Federal Government may provide critical surge capacity during emergencies through the deployment of CDC personnel, disaster medical assistance teams (DMAT), or disaster mortuary assistance teams (DMORT), although these resources are usually not immediately available.

Good emergency preparedness also requires developing working relationships with partners prior to an event. Many of these partners are dealt with routinely such as local or state emergency managers, hospital emergency preparedness staff, or CDC's Division of Quarantine. Some other nonhealthcare links are also required. These nontraditional partners may include fire and police departments, emergency medical service organizations, the local joint terrorism taskforce, local FBI, transportation authorities, veterinarians and medical distributors. The integration of the emergency response will be enhanced by these relationships.

11.4 Surveillance

Public Health Surveillance: "The ongoing, systematic collection, analysis, and interpretation of outcome-specific data for use in the planning, implementation, and evaluation of public health practice [4]"

Surveillance is a critical component of BT preparedness. The traditional form practiced by health departments is case surveillance, requiring the reporting of suspicious cases of a legally defined reportable event to the local or state health department by providers and laboratories. All of the anthrax cases diagnosed in 2001 were reported through traditional case surveillance. Case surveillance relies on several factors including the ability of the medical provider to recognize the signs and symptoms of the particular BT agent, and the knowledge of the need as well as how to report the case immediately to public health authorities.

Routine reporting of public health events has been historically poor [5] and barriers to reporting must be identified and overcome. Greater recognition of the crucial role of surveillance and public health may now overcome some of these barriers. Recognition of the signs and symptoms of BT agents may be difficult. For example, almost all western physicians have not seen a case of smallpox. Public health authorities need to work closely with medical schools, residency programs, hospitals, and state and local medical societies to provide information to clinicians on the signs and symptoms of bioterrorism agents. A number of excellent products have already been created, including a poster to evaluate patients with smallpox (Fig. 11.1), as well as pocket cards for physicians on a variety of terrorism events, including BT, nuclear and chemical attacks.

Syndromic surveillance systems are designed to quickly identify the prodromes and early presentations of BT related agents [6], and have become a

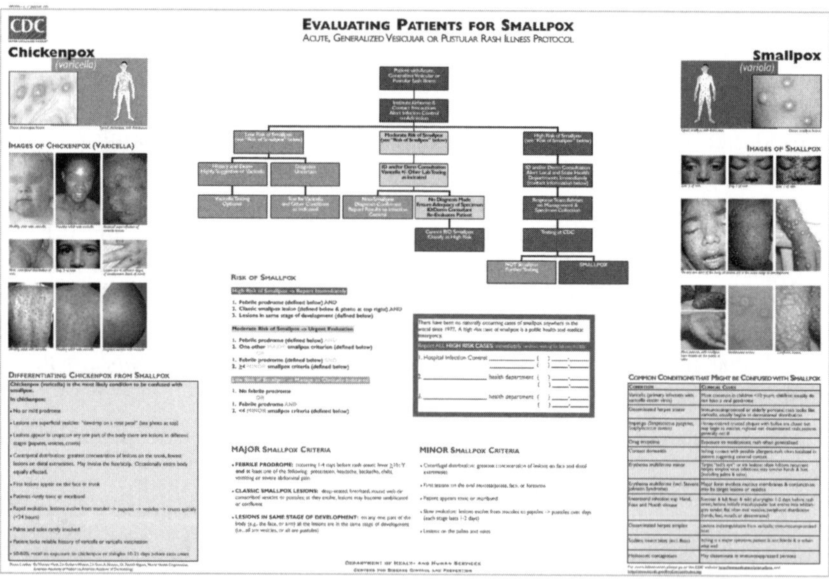

Fig. 11.1 Evaluating patients for smallpox – an example of physician education materials

standard of public health's response to bioterrorism. Many BT agents initially present clinically with nonspecific signs and symptoms, often as an influenza-like illness. Syndromic surveillance offers the possibility of identifying the dissemination of a BT agent in a population prior to the diagnosis and reporting of a patient with clinically manifest signs and symptoms of a particular agent, decreasing perhaps by several days (depending on the agent) the lag time for outbreak detection. An early warning may allow for more time to organize a public health and criminal investigatory response.

Syndromic surveillance relies on computerized information systems that can be shared with and analyzed by public health agencies on routine basis. Examples of systems include requests for ambulance service, visits to hospital emergency departments, purchases of pharmaceuticals from large distributors, outpatient clinical visits and school or large employee absenteeism or sick visits. Not all of these information systems are available or even needed in every jurisdiction. In addition to automated systems that can identify and locate increases in these syndromes, is the development of public health system interventions to clarify the nature of these "signals." These interventions may range from requesting to enhance diagnostic workups from physicians (such as use of rapid influenza testing) to obtaining clinical follow up information from patients themselves.

A new kind of surveillance system being introduced in the United States is biodetection. Originally developed for military use, these biodetection systems attempt to identify the earliest possible release of BT agents by collecting air samples at strategic locations in a municipality. For example, in the recently deployed Biowatch project, 20 cities are collecting air samples, using existing EPA monitors. Filter paper samples from these monitors are then tested routinely by public health laboratories for a variety of BT pathogens. The evolving technology of this strategy will include on site testing for BT agents.

The advent of such systems provides a new set of challenges for public health authorities. For each one, a robust public health and public safety consequence management plan must be created. These plans must answer basic questions:

- what is the testing algorithm for samples?
- at what stage is the public informed of a positive sample?
- who is informed of a positive sample?
- if there was a BT agent release, what was the dispersion area?
- who is at risk?
- what recommendations are made in terms of evacuation, clean-up, re-occupancy decontamination, and post-exposure prophylaxis?

Ideally, these and other concerns should be addressed at the local level prior to the deployment of any such system. Again, public health authorities must work with many other disciplines to create the consequence management plans.

11.5 Communication

Crisis communication is an integral part of any public health response. Several kinds of communication must be planned. These include internal communication to inform and mobilize agency staff, communication to the general public and communication to the provider community. Communication to staff is important to notify them of the crisis, provide updated information on their roles and the agency's in the response, and to provide a conduit for more mundane information and activities that may be influenced by the response (i.e., paycheck distribution and work site locations). In small agencies this may not be a problem, but in large state or city department's of health, communication with staff may be more difficult.

In New York City, there are several redundant strategies for communicating with staff. Each staff is given an employee wallet card that outlines the incident management system of the agency, providing a space for the contact information for their supervisor to learn more about deployment issues. Additionally, a pre-arranged call in number is listed that is only activated in an emergency so that staff can obtain the most up to date information about the agency's emergency response. Alternatively, telecommunication systems that automatically alert them may be employed. Finally, staff is instructed to refer to the agency's website if computer access is available. Copies of contact information for all staff are kept securely in the agency's main as well as backup emergency operations centers. During blackouts and other telephone disruptions when these methods are compromised, key personnel are given 800 MHz radios to communicate with each other. Simple radio announcements or newspaper announcements may be necessary to communicate with staff.

Communication with the public is critical to inform them of the latest information regarding the outbreak and to provide information to help them protect and reduce anxiety for themselves, their families and their communities. This issue was one of the most widely criticized aspects of the anthrax crisis during 2001. Polling data has shown that local medical or public health officials are credible voices regarding crises. Ideally a cadre of spokespersons, including those not affiliated with government, should be identified in advance of an event. Mechanisms need to be established to communicate with them during an event. Public health spokespersons will need to work alongside political and law enforcement leadership during times of emergencies. To the extent that is possible, fact sheets, press releases and frequently asked questions should be developed anticipating possible scenarios so they can be quickly available for use. The content of the announcements should follow the tenets of risk communication [7], which advocates for acknowledging the uncertainty of the situation, telling people what to expect and to acknowledge deficiencies in the response. It is important to recognize that the public wants to know what they can do to protect themselves and others and this information should routinely be a part of any public outreach during a crisis. Finally, public hotlines may be organized to provide further answers to the public.

Provider communication is still another important aspect of meeting the demands of a BT attack. Providers need to know the signs and symptoms of the BT agent in question are, how to report cases, laboratory diagnostic options and available treatments. Additionally, they need to understand what personal protective equipment or infection control precautions need to be taken and how to counsel patients on a myriad of issues. The most effective method to communicate with providers in the setting of an emergency is through a secure Internet website. Some of the Health Alert Network (HAN) systems notify registered providers when a new alert is available, and post these alerts on their website. Alternatives or supplements to website alerts are broadcast fax systems (with preloaded fax numbers of providers), provider hotlines, letters and grand round speakers. Creating and using these systems prior to emergency will allow providers to quickly get relevant information during a crisis.

11.6 Workforce Development and Needs

The public health workforce must meet the new challenges that BT preparedness requires. Foremost among the needs are the availability of qualified personnel (especially laboratorians and epidemiologists) to hire for BT readiness under a pay scale maintained by governmental agencies. Furthermore, education of the current workforce is important since this group has had no formal training in emergency preparedness. Competency standards for all public health workers on bioterrorism and emergency preparedness have been created [8]. These provide standards for preparedness and planning, response and mitigation, and recovery and evaluation for a variety of different public health staff. Innovative methods for delivering training for busy staff in accordance with principles of adult learning need to be prioritized. The Centers for Disease Control have funded 30 schools of public health to serve as Centers for Public Health Preparedness whose goal is to assist health departments with these training needs. Emergency preparedness and bioterrorism training should be integrated into schools of public health, schools of medicine, and other health professional training as well as in residency programs so that the future public health workforce is prepared to further this work.

Other needs of the public health workforce also require addressing. Worker safety must to be a component of every health department's plans including information, training and monitoring of the use of appropriate personal protective equipment. During 2001, public health departments worked 24 h a day for weeks, leading to exhaustion of responding personnel. In the case of the World Trade Center attack, public health workers were at the rescue site and subjected to the same kind of emotional turmoil that faced many New Yorkers. It is very important to address the mental health needs of the workforce before, during and after a crisis is necessary. Finally, all public health workers should create in advance a personal emergency plan that describes how issues such as childcare can be taken care of while they need to work. Planning ahead can allow the workforce to report to work when required.

11.7 Laboratory Services

Laboratory diagnosis of a BT pathogen is a key step in the identification and control of an outbreak caused by bioterrorism agents. Lab diagnosis will establish or confirm the presence of an outbreak, provide information on drug susceptibility, and may help in determining the origin of the agent in question. During 2001, public health laboratories were overwhelmed by the anthrax attacks, which resulted in the submission of 70,000 samples for suspected anthrax [9]. Identified gaps [10] included lack of qualified staff, inadequate facilities, a need for biosecurity upgrades, and lack of integrated management information systems. To address these issues, public health laboratories received $146 million in the first year of the CDC funding. Of this amount, about 25% were used to hire personnel and another 25% spent on equipment [11]. The need to create linkages amongst laboratories to quickly diagnose agents of bioterrorism has resulted in the creation of the Laboratory Response Network (LRN). The LRN consists of three levels:

Sentinel – Clinical and private laboratories
Reference – Public health laboratories
National – Federal laboratories

Each of these levels must work together and have specific roles and responsibilities. Sentinel labs (such as hospital based facilities) are considered the lab equivalent of "first responders," performing standard bacterial testing to isolate and rule out potential BT agents. They need to have pre-established relationships with reference labs, and must be able to ship suspect specimens safely, using chain of custody protocols. Reference laboratories receive reagents from the CDC for diagnostic testing of suspicious specimens. They are able to perform testing for anthrax, plague, tularemia, brucellosis, melioidosis, botulism and smallpox. National labs can confirm the diagnosis of reference laboratories as well as do molecular typing, viral cultures and genome sequencing when appropriate.

11.8 Environmental Issues and Bioterrorism

Once the epidemiology and strategies for control of the outbreak are established, environmental concerns will quickly become a focus of concern. Public health will need to answer questions related to the environment around the events such as:

- what are the areas where contamination occurred?
- how does one disinfect for the particular agent in question? and
- what kind of standards should dictate the level of clean-up required and for re-occupancy of residences or business establishments?

In addition, environmental expertise in determining the level of personal protective equipment needed for a particular agent is required. This is important not only for the public health practitioners but also for persons performing environmental sampling. Finally, monitoring clean-up efforts, solid and liquid waste disposal of contaminated material from the clean-up and long-term effects from exposure to materials used in the clean-up may be necessary.

Another need, discussed above, relates to the interpretation of the results from environmental biosurveillance. Should a positive sample be obtained on an outdoor monitor, environmental expertise will be required to help determine the distribution of the agent. Sampling is needed in geographic zones around the monitor and an analysis of wind currents and other environmental conditions that may effect spread of an airborne organism or toxin is necessary.

11.9 Medical and Hospital Preparedness

The roles and responsibilities of physicians and other health-care workers, as well as clinics and hospitals, have changed under the threat of bioterrorism. Medical providers are likely to be the initial identifier of a BT outbreak and, as such, play a critical role in protection of the public. All physicians need to take steps to prepare themselves, their workplaces and their practices for the potential of BT (Table 11.1).

Suspicious clusters of disease may take several forms including diseases not endemic in the medical practice area, an unusual age distribution for the disease or simultaneous outbreaks in human and animal populations. As mentioned previously, a HAN can provide information to health-care practitioners.

Table 11.1 Physician Preparedness for and Roles during BT events

Learn clinical signs and symptoms of BT agents
• Learn characteristics of suspicious clusters of diseases
• Know how to report potential cases/clusters to the local/state DOH
• Register with a local/state Health Alert Network, and become knowledgeable about other sources of authoritative information
• Identify and consider volunteer opportunities, such as offered by Medical Reserve Corps, or American Red Cross
• Identify steps to limit spread of infectious agents within the work setting
• Provide routine care to patients with appropriate counseling during the outbreak
• Understand emergency responsibilities at affiliated hospitals
• Create and maintain a family emergency plan for oneself and encourage employees to do the same

Physicians should check the web sites of their state or local health department to determine if there is a HAN in their jurisdiction as well as to find out how to register. In the absence of a HAN, the CDC and state health department's web sites routinely have useful information on BT and health alerts. In the midst of an outbreak, it is probable that elective physician visits and hospitalizations will be curtailed. The demand for physician counseling, however, is likely to increase either through sick visits to offices and hospitals or by the "worried well" over the phone, highlighting the importance of appropriate counseling including addressing mental health needs.

Medical Reserve Corps [12] are organizations to encourage health-care workers to assist at Points of Distribution Sites (PODS) (see below) when they are activated. Although PODS are not places where routine medical care is to be delivered, medical expertise is needed to triage sick individuals to hospitals as appropriate, administer injections (lay vaccinators will likely be used as well) and to provide counseling to those with complicated medical histories. Similarly, the American Red Cross and emergency management organizations work with mental health counselors to provide on site crisis counseling for a large variety of situations.

11.10 Delivery of Prophylaxis

Providing antimicrobial prophylaxis or appropriate vaccination to at risk individuals could significantly reduce morbidity and mortality due to release of some BT agents. Public health authorities will decide who is eligible for prophylaxis based on available epidemiologic, laboratory and law enforcement information. Specific recommendations for antimicrobials need to take into account known or suspected drug susceptibilities as well as the characteristics of the person(s) at risk such as pregnancy, children or allergies. Similarly, the decision to recommend vaccination following a release will depend on epidemiologic characteristics of both the outbreak and the characteristics of the exposed individuals such as persons with compromised immune systems and the live, attenuated smallpox vaccine. In the case of agents with capable of transmitting from person to person, such as smallpox and plague, aggressive and rapid contact tracing by public health would be needed to identify those in most need of prophylaxis, trying to limit spread of disease.

The Strategic National Stockpile (SNS) [13], is a repository of critical materials needed during emergencies including antimicrobial agents, respirators and life support medications maintained by the Department of Homeland Security. A state's governor must request the SNS from the Director of CDC. Initial, first response, National Pharmaceutical Stockpile "push packs" of critical supplies are located across the United States and can be delivered within 12 h to any location after the decision is made to deploy. These all-hazard push packs weigh 50 t and require seven semi-trucks or a wide body jumbo jet for transportation. A vendor managed inventory program that can deliver more supplies within 24–36 h backs up the push packs. Health departments are required to develop plans to receive, store and distribute the supplies. This requires identification or development of appropriate warehouse facilities and inventory control systems.

Although some SNS assets would go directly to hospitals, others would be sent to prophylaxis dispensing clinics referred to as Points of Distribution Sites (PODS). At risk individuals would be directed to report to these sites to obtain appropriate prophylaxis. Depending on the size of the population at risk, sites could be an individual clinic or, in the event of a large exposure, non-medical sites would be needed. Health department staff, along with lay volunteers and the medical community, would be needed to work at the sites. In many jurisdictions, hospitals would not be the sites of PODS, as they would be needed to take care of those affected by the bioterrorism event. Experience in New York City from 2001 [14] showed that formalized treatment algorithms, as well as adequate physical layout and clear staff roles and responsibilities, are key elements of a successful site.

Successful preparation for a PODS includes identification of volunteers, site selection, adequate operational solutions for rapidly outfitting and maintaining site equipment and furniture and creation of medical charts, consents, and patient fact sheets. Clear communication with those at risk is important and should utilize redundant mechanisms. For a large population, messages in newspapers, television and radio may be needed to inform and instruct people on where to go for prophylaxis and what to expect. Hotlines may be needed to reiterate these messages, answer specific questions and to provide mental health counseling. Finally, a plan needs to be developed for outreach to vulnerable populations who have issues of poor access to medical care such as the homeless and the housebound elderly.

11.11 Crisis Management

During a crisis, key policy and procedure plans need to be quickly operationalized. Notification protocols should be executed to provide information to political leadership, public health authorities and emergency management organizations at federal, state and local levels. Surveillance and epidemiologic activities, such as contact notification, may need to be significantly enhanced. In the setting of a smallpox outbreak, initial vaccination efforts should focus on first responders in hospitals, public health, emergency medical services and possibly law enforcement. Staff call up and deployment should commence with contact of medical reserve corps and volunteer lists possibly needed. Decisions also need to be made as to the extent of "routine" activities that will be maintained during the crisis.

Many of these actions may be done in the context of an emergency operations center (EOC). The EOC acts as the locus of situation assessments and decision making needed for the crisis. In New York City, the Office of Emergency Management will activate the citywide EOC, consisting of public and private agencies or institutions that contribute to mitigating and recovering from the outbreak. Groups involved would range from health and human service organizations (i.e., health department, hospitals, American Red Cross) to transportation agencies, law enforcement, and utilities. Decision making in the EOC frequently may need to take place without all of the information needed; a challenge for those in leadership positions. Tabletop exercises and drills are important factors in helping health departments prepare for the crisis management that would be needed as part of a BT response.

11.12 Current and Future Challenges

Public health faces current challenges to meet the mandate in protecting the public from consequences of a BT release. Federal funding has provided critical support in a public health system whose infrastructure has been allowed to decay for many years. This funding must be sustained to provide long-term protection to the public from agents of bioterrorism. Public health must work closely with a wide variety of partners to be able to prepare for and respond to a BT outbreak. The medical, academic, and laboratory communities in particular must work together with public health agencies with each playing a critical role in BT prevention, training, and research and diagnosis. The degree to which the current expertise is woven together at the community level will in large part influence the successful response to a BT attack and will become the legacy of this generation's public health leadership.

References

1. Inglesby, T. V., Grossman, R. and O'Toole, T. A plague on your city: observations from TOPOFF. *Clin. Infect. Dis.* 32, 436–445, 2001.
2. Holtz, T. H., Leighton, J., Balter, S., et al. The public health response to the World Trade Center disaster. In: Terrorism and Public Health. Levy, B. S. and Sidel, V. W. (eds), New York: Oxford University Press, 2003, pp. 19–48.
3. Centers for Disease Control and Prevention. Terrorism preparedness in state health departments – United States, 2001–2003. *Morb. Mortal Wkly. Rep.* 52, 1051–1053, 2003.
4. Thacker, S. B. and Berkelman, R. L. Public health surveillance in the United States. *Epidemiol. Rev.* 10, 164–190, 1988.
5. Birkhead, G. S. and Maylahn, C. M. State and local public health surveillance. In: Principles and Practice of Public Health Surveillance Tevtsch, S. M., and Churchill R. E. (eds), 2nd edn. New York: Oxford University Press, 2000. pp. 253–287.
6. Buehler, J. W., Berkelman, R. L., Hartley, D. M. and Peters, C. J. Syndromic surveillance and bioterrorism-related epidemics. *Emerg. Infect. Dis.* 9, 1197–1204, 2003.

7. Sandman, P. M. and Lanard, J. Risk Communication Recommendations for Infectious Disease Outbreaks. October 2003, pp. 1–8. http://www.psandman.com/articles/who-srac.htm#sect4.
8. Columbia University School of Nursing Center for Health Policy. Bioterrorism & Emergency Readiness. Competencies for all Public Health Workers. pp. 1–23. http://www.cvmc.columbia.edu/dept/nursing/chpnsr/pdf/btcomps.pdf.
9. United States General Accounting Office. Infectious Diseases: Gaps Remain in Surveillance Capabilities of State and Local Agencies. GAO-03-1176T, pp. 1–17. September 24, 2003.
10. Association of Public Health Laboratories. Public Health Laboratory Issues in Brief: Bioterrorism Capacity, October 2002. http://www.aphl.org.
11. Association of Public Health Laboratories. Public Health Laboratory Issues in Brief: Bioterrorism Capacity, August 2003. http://www.aphl.org.
12. Medical Reserve Corps. About the Medical Reserve Corps, June 2008. http://www.medicalreservecorps.gov/about.
13. Emergency Preparedness and Response. Strategic National Stockpile. http://www.bt.cdc.gov/stockpile/index.asp.
14. Blank, S., Moskin, L. C. and Zucker, J. R. An ounce of prevention is a ton of work: mass antibiotic prophylaxis for anthrax, New York City, 2001. *Emerg. Infect. Dis.* 9, 616–622, 2003.

Chapter 12
Public Health Law and Biological Terrorism

Lance Gable and James G. Hodge, Jr.

12.1 Introduction

The recent emergence of new disease threats has acted as a powerful reminder of the dangers that infectious biological agents can pose to the population. Over the past decade, public health and medical communities have been challenged by several novel infectious disease outbreaks. Some of these outbreaks have been naturally occurring, such as the international SARS outbreak in 2003 [1]. Other outbreaks originated from biological agents that were intentionally released into the population, such as the anthrax letters sent to several persons in the United States in the fall of 2001 [2]. These incidents, as well as simulated bioterrorism exercises such as Dark Winter and the TOPOFF drills, have led to increased awareness of potential shortcomings of our public health and health-care systems to respond to emerging disease threats [3–7]. The specter of future outbreaks has prompted Americans to consider a number of legal and ethical issues associated with preparation for and response to biological terrorism.

Bioterrorism involves the intentional use of an infectious agent (e.g., micro-organism, virus, infectious substances, or biological product) to cause death or disease in humans, plants, or other organisms to negatively influence the conduct of government or intimidate a population [8]. Infectious agents provide an attractive tool for potential terrorists. Unlike explosives, bombs and other conventional weapons of terror, the bioterrorist's weapon is often less expensive to obtain, easier to smuggle, easier to spread across a wide segment of the population, and in some cases easier to deploy. Moreover, a highly infectious microorganism can spread rapidly across borders and boundaries, affecting multiple areas. The invisibility of biological weapons further adds to their ability to create fear and havoc. Biological agents may be difficult to detect until after they have exacted serious damage. Most experts agree that there is a plausible risk in the United States of a large-scale bioterrorism attack that could

L. Gable
Assistant Professor of Law, Wayne State University Law School, 471 W. Palmer, Detroit, MI 48202, USA
e-mail: lancegable@wayne.edu

L.I. Lutwick, S.M. Lutwick (eds.), *Beyond Anthrax*,
DOI: 10.1007/978-1-59745-326-4_12, © Springer Science+Business Media, LLC 2008

result in significant illnesses or casualties [9–17]. Consequently, proactive preparations for bioterrorism, even more so than other types of terrorism, involve systematic planning, ongoing training, and redistributions of resources.

The prospect of bioterrorism has galvanized widespread support for improved preparedness within federal, state, and local governments and the health care sector throughout the United States. These efforts have targeted a wide range of relevant and intersecting areas. Strengthening the public health workforce, infrastructure, and capacity available to respond to an outbreak associated with biological terrorism, is critical. Policy-makers have responded by increasing training and funding to these areas [18–20]. Similarly, planners within the public and private sectors have established tactics and procedures to respond to various emergency scenarios. These plans frequently consider methods to improve communications between various emergency responders and others who must have sufficient capability to contact each other in an emergency situation. Preparedness planning efforts targeting bioterrorism have occurred concurrently with initiatives to bolster public health infrastructure for other public health emergencies including natural disasters (e.g., hurricanes) and naturally occurring disease outbreaks (e.g., pandemic influenza). Finally, preparedness planners have considered some of the ethical concerns raised by bioterrorism attacks and their potentially devastating consequences.

A foundational component of these preparedness efforts has been the potential modernization of state and federal public health and emergency response laws. Law is a critical component of a well-developed public health system [21]. Public health law grants public health agencies powers to detect, track, prevent, and contain health threats resulting from bioterrorism and other public health emergencies. However, many existing public health and emergency response laws at the state and federal levels may not be sufficient to address biological terrorism. These laws often do not grant public health authorities the necessary powers to stop an outbreak. Public health laws vary widely across different jurisdictions. As a result, the legal powers ascribed to public health officials may be different in scope and function in different locales. These laws are also commonly targeted to specific diseases or conditions that may not relate to emerging threats [22].

Public health powers typically lie at the state and local levels of government. The federal government plays a more limited role for practical and legal reasons. Public health falls within the state's police powers, an area of state power traditionally reserved to the states under the Tenth Amendment to the United States Constitution [23]. The federal government will normally become involved in localized public health matters only at the request of the state or if the disease has the potential to cross state or international borders, or affect interstate interests. From a practical perspective, this gives state and local officials greater autonomy to enact laws and policies conducive to the needs of their communities, without interference from the federal government.

Responses to bioterrorism, however, will almost certainly involve the federal government, since an infectious disease will rarely be contained within the borders of one state. Indeed, an outbreak may traverse international boundaries as well, which would clearly entail the input of the federal government. Bioterrorism implicates additional concerns beyond public health, including national security and law enforcement considerations. Federal public health and legal authorities may specifically respond to multiple components of a bioterrorism attack, as well as offer guidance and expertise to assist state and local governments in their responses. Thus, responses to bioterrorism require sufficient legal powers at both the federal and state levels, in addition to a well-conceived plan for coordinating these powers to maximize public benefit.

The debate around bioterrorism preparedness has raised salient questions about the role of law in responding to biological threats, highlighted by inherent tensions between protecting the public and upholding individual rights of liberty, privacy, and freedom of association [24]. Balancing these goals requires difficult choices that are further complicated when public health laws are unclear, poorly drafted, or confusing. To assist state and local law- and policy-makers, public health law scholars at the Center for Law and the Public's Health at Georgetown University Law Center and the Johns Hopkins Bloomberg School of Public Health drafted two model state public health acts. The Model State Emergency Health Powers Act (MSEHPA) was drafted quickly after September 11, 2001, with input from the Centers for Disease Control and Prevention (CDC) and multiple national partner organizations [25, 26]. Completed on December 21, 2001, MSEHPA has served as a valuable template for states to modernize their public health laws to address public health emergencies, including emergencies caused by bioterrorism. It provides a modern framework for public health powers, authorizing state and local authorities to engage in a range of activities to address a public health emergency. These measures may restrict temporarily the liberty or property of affected individuals or groups to protect the public's health [27]. To date, 44 states and the District of Columbia have introduced bills based on some or all of the provisions of the MSEHPA, and 38 states and the District of Columbia have passed their respective bills [28].

The Turning Point Model State Public Health Act (Turning Point Act) (completed on September 16, 2003) provides a more comprehensive prototype for state public health law reform [29]. It covers a broad array of topics that extend well beyond emergency situations, including (1) defining and authorizing the performance of essential public health services and functions; (2) improving public health infrastructure; (3) encouraging cooperation between public and private sectors on public health issues; and (4) protecting the privacy of identifiable data acquired, used, or disclosed by public health authorities [29].

A third model law, the Uniform Emergency Volunteer Health Practitioners Act (UEVHPA), as drafted in 2006 by the National Conference of Commissioners on Uniform State Laws, provides a further model for emergency public health governance, organized around the challenge of accommodating health professionals who show up spontaneously at the site of a public health emergency or nearby health facilities in order to provide emergency assistance [30].

The aforementioned Model Acts recognize that an effective public health response to a bioterrorism-related outbreak will demand strong and clear legal powers. In the following sections, we focus predominantly on two specific areas of public health powers authorized under law: (1) restrictions on personal liberty (quarantine, isolation, travel restrictions, privacy) and (2) restrictions on property (decontamination, use of supplies and facilities, disposal of remains). While other areas of law are also relevant to the legal framework needed to address bioterrorism, these two areas feature the most sustained debates and controversies. Each of these powers will be considered in the following sections from a legal and ethical perspective.

12.2 Restrictions on Personal Liberty: Quarantine, Isolation, Travel Restrictions, and Privacy

The release of a highly infectious disease into the population presents government officials with a difficult quandary. Within the climate of fear that may surround such an outbreak, public health authorities must quickly and accurately assess the risk to the population and take measures accordingly to protect the public's health. Under such circumstances, public health authorities may resort to liberty-limiting measures such as quarantine, isolation, travel restrictions, and privacy limitations. Personally restrictive actions are particularly likely when the disease is readily communicable, exceptionally virulent, or is of unknown origin. Restrictions on personal liberty to respond to a public health crisis are constitutionally permissible, but the scope of restrictions and attendant protections against their misuse varies significantly across different jurisdictions.

12.2.1 Quarantine and Isolation

Quarantine and isolation are among the oldest of public health tools. Their use predates modern scientific advances in disease testing and treatment, not to mention modern conceptions of civil liberties. They operate on the most basic principle of infectious disease control—keeping healthy individuals separated from those who have been exposed or infected. In modern times, the mass use of quarantine or isolation has faded as rapid medical tests and effective treatments have become available. When quarantine and isolation have been used, they have been directed predominantly at specific infectious individuals, for example, to control recalcitrant tuberculosis patients [31–34]. Nevertheless, for a disease of unknown etiology or a disease that poses a significant threat to a vulnerable population, quarantine and isolation may still be effective techniques to contain an outbreak. Depending on the scope of the outbreak, large-scale quarantine measures may have to be considered. Modern logistics surrounding enactment of a large-scale quarantine would be complex and possibly unworkable [35].

The terms *quarantine* and *isolation* have engendered a great deal of confusion. The two terms are often used interchangeably, but in actuality represent distinct concepts. The term *quarantine* denotes a compulsory physical separation of an individual or a group of healthy people who have been exposed to a contagious disease to prevent transmission during the incubation period of the disease [21]. Historically, quarantine restrictions were often imposed on travelers to insure that they did not introduce a contagious disease into a country or town. The word itself derives from the Latin term *quadragina* and the Italian term *quarante*, which refer to the 40-day sequestration period enforced on merchant ships during plague outbreaks [21]. The term *isolation*, by contrast, means the separation, for the period of communicability, of known infected persons so as to prevent or limit the transmission of the infectious agent [21]. Precise usage of and differentiation between these terms is vital to insure that those subject to these powers receive appropriate treatment and protection.

The current legal framework authorizing the use of quarantine and isolation in the United States stretches across multiple jurisdictions and levels of government. Quarantine powers were first implemented at the local level, and later the state level, during the colonial period. The federal quarantine statute, first enacted in 1796, authorized the president to assist states in their use of quarantines [36]. The federal government subsequently took control over maritime quarantines [37]. This expanded federal role prompted a debate over whether the federal or state government should administer quarantines—a debate which continues to this day. As discussed below, states claim that their quarantine authority derives from their police power, while the federal government argues that its authority arises from its constitutionally – granted power to regulate interstate commerce.

12.2.1.1 State and Local Quarantine and Isolation Laws

State and local jurisdictions have the primary responsibility for quarantine within their borders. The state quarantine power is derived from the state's inherent police power, reserved to the states under the Tenth Amendment of the United States Constitution. Most public health powers have traditionally been recognized as falling under the jurisdiction of state and local governments. The United States Supreme Court has found that the police powers of the state allow the state to enact regulations to protect the health and safety of its citizens [23]. The use of quarantine and isolation by state and local governments is therefore legally and constitutionally acceptable, provided that these powers are used appropriately to protect public health and safety.

The specific scope of state and local quarantine authority varies considerably between jurisdictions. These differences are evident in the structural distribution of power between the state and local governments and the substantive criteria (or lack thereof) for placing an individual under quarantine. Some states have a centralized public health system that retains most public health powers at the state level, including quarantine and isolation decisions. Other states delegate these decisions to local public health agencies. In these states, quarantine will generally be under the jurisdiction of local public health officials when the disease is confined to a discrete local area. If the outbreak affects more that one community within the state, the state public health authority will usually have the power to implement quarantine or isolation orders. Very few jurisdictions have articulated explicit procedures and policies to determine whether or not an individual should be subject to quarantine. Both the MSEHPA and Turning Point Act propose a systematic process for making this determination that considers the exigencies of the situation. Furthermore, they allow for an appeal of the decision if possible under the circumstances [25, 29].

12.2.1.2 Federal Quarantine and Isolation Law

Federal quarantine powers are much more limited than comparable powers at the state level. The federal government may only apply powers delegated to it under the Constitution. Pursuant to these delegated powers, federal authorities have the ability to prevent the introduction, transmission, and spread of communicable diseases between states and from foreign countries into the United States. The federal quarantine power stipulates that if there is a risk that disease transmission will cross state lines, the federal government has the authority to implement quarantine [38]. The federal government is additionally authorized to cooperate with state and local authorities to enact quarantine to contain an interstate disease outbreak [39]. The federal quarantine response is conducted by the CDC, with assistance from other agencies if necessary, including the Department of Homeland Security (DHS), the Department of Defense (DOD), and the Department of Justice (DOJ).

Federal law establishes a role for a number of federal agencies and departments in the execution of a quarantine order. The Secretary of Health and Human Services (HHS) has statutory responsibility for preventing the introduction, transmission, and spread of communicable diseases from foreign countries into the United States and within the United States and its territories/possessions [40]. Regulations grant the CDC authority to detain, medically examine, or conditionally release individuals reasonably believed to be carrying a communicable disease [41]. The CDC's Division of Global Migration and Quarantine has the specific authority to quarantine individuals seeking to enter the United States. U.S. Customs and Border Protection (CBP) (formerly the U.S. Customs Service) and officers of the U.S. Coast Guard are authorized to assist in the enforcement of federal quarantine orders [42]. Personnel from the U.S. Citizenship and Immigration Services (USCIS) (formerly the Immigration and Naturalization Service [INS]), the CBP, the U.S. Department of Agriculture (USDA), and the U.S. Fish and Wildlife Service (USFW) all assist the CDC in identifying travelers or other persons who may be infected with illnesses that pose a risk to public health [43]. Federal quarantine authority only extends to specific diseases enumerated by executive order [44]. However, this list of diseases can be amended quickly when necessary (e.g., as with SARS in 2003, and pandemic flu in 2005) [45, 46].

The federal quarantine power has rarely been used in modern times. Therefore, it is unclear how widely it could be used to combat a bioterrorism outbreak. Public health law experts have demonstrated concern that the existing legal structures for initiating and managing a large-scale quarantine are inadequate at the federal and state levels [35]. This is problematic because the imposition of a large-scale quarantine will almost certainly involve the use of federal and state powers. Under these circumstances, there is the possibility of confusion and controversy over who is in charge. As past bioterrorism simulations and real emergencies like Hurricane Katrina have demonstrated, if the lines of authority are not clear to officials at all government levels, the public health response can be paralyzed and undermined [3, 4, 47, 48]. Thus, in addition to improving the legal framework within federal and state/local jurisdictions, serious efforts should focus on establishing a coordinated public health response between these jurisdictions.

12.2.1.3 Key Quarantine Considerations

When should public health authorities use quarantine or isolation to restrict individuals during a bioterrorism emergency? The response to this question requires the decision-maker to balance the need for restrictive intervention with the effect it may have on the civil liberties of affected individuals. Modern commentary on the acceptability of quarantine asks whether the risk to the population posed by the disease justifies such a serious loss of liberty [21, 49, 50]. In addition to restrictions on liberty, imposing a quarantine temporarily deprives individuals of their economic livelihood, their right to travel or associate freely with others, and may subject them to stigma and discrimination. In a time of great crisis, public sentiment may strongly support such measures, but public sentiment alone is an insufficient justification to use quarantine powers. These powers may be warranted to prevent the continued transmission of a disease that presents a serious risk to the population. It is important, however, that restrictive powers are not used unnecessarily or as an artifice for discrimination [51]. Past quarantines in the United States have led to violence [52], increased disease transmission among the quarantined population [53], and biased decision making [54]. In one case, a federal court invalidated a quarantine imposed on an area of San Francisco comprised mostly of persons of Chinese descent, finding that the public health officials had used an "evil eye and an unequal hand" in issuing their quarantine order [55].

Restrictive public health powers such as quarantine and isolation should be used as a last resort to halt the spread of an infectious disease. The law can provide a useful normative framework for making quarantine decisions. The MSEHPA, for examples, sets out a list of criteria that should be considered when making a quarantine or isolation decision [25]. In many situations, particularly where the disease is readily diagnosable and treatable, other options may be more defensible from a medical and civil rights perspective. Barbera et al. list three key questions to consider when evaluating a quarantine decision: "(1) do public health and medical analyses warrant the imposition of large-scale quarantine? (2) are the implementation and maintenance of large-scale quarantine feasible? and (3) do the potential benefits outweigh the possible adverse consequences? [35]."

Gostin has outlined several criteria for exercising restrictive public health powers under modern constitutional law [21, 51]:

- *Compelling state interest in confinement.* Public health authorities must only resort to restrictive powers when there is a compelling interest that is substantially furthered by civil confinement. Only truly dangerous individuals (i.e., posing a significant risk of transmission) can be confined. Whenever possible, risks should be assessed through scientific means.
- *Targeted intervention.* Individually restrictive measures should be well targeted to achieving public health objectives. Interventions that deprive individuals of liberty or equal protection without justification may be constitutionally impermissible. For example, placing everyone within a geographic area under quarantine is overinclusive if some members would not transmit infection. Underinclusive interventions that confine some, but not all, potentially contagious persons may be found to be arbitrary or intentionally discriminatory.
- *Least-restrictive alternative.* Public health authorities should not implement extremely restrictive measures such as quarantine and isolation if they can accomplish their objectives through less drastic means (although it is not likely that they would be required to enact extreme or unduly expensive means to avoid confinement).
- *Safe and habitable environment.* Quarantine and isolation are intended to promote well-being rather than to punish. Therefore, individuals being confined should have access to clean living conditions, food, clothing, water, adequate health care, and means to communicate with others outside the quarantine.
- *Procedural due process.* Individuals subject to confinement for public health purposes must be able to access some form of procedural due process depending on the nature and duration of the restraint. Where possible, this process should occur before confinement. If emergency circumstances demand immediate confinement, individuals have the right to request a speedy hearing and counsel to contest their confinement.

12.2.2 Restrictions on Privacy

Public health authorities may also take actions during a public health emergency that limit the right to privacy, including public health surveillance, reporting, and contact tracing. The ability to identify and track the spread of infection is a vital component of the public health response to an infectious disease outbreak. Public health authorities need access to valid and useful information to accomplish these tasks.

In this context, public health surveillance and case reporting are indispensable techniques. Surveillance allows public health authorities to collect, analyze, and interpret health information to search for concentrations of disease [21]. A bioterrorism outbreak could be detected through monitoring large increases in purchases of certain medications from pharmacies, clusters of cases detected by emergency rooms or managed care organizations, or spikes in absenteeism from workplaces and schools. Case reporting is a form of passive surveillance involving the routine submission of data to a public health agency by external sources such as health care professionals and laboratories, often pursuant to mandatory legal requirements [56, 57]. Through disease surveillance and reporting, public health authorities may assess the magnitude of the outbreak and appropriately target resources and tactics [21]. Surveillance and case reporting raise privacy concerns since the reports usually contain identifiable data, which could include a person's name or other identifying characteristics. While using anonymous data instead of identifiable information is preferable to protect privacy, personal identifiers may be necessary to effectively track cases in some circumstances.

Public health authorities responding to bioterrorism may also wish to engage in contact tracing. Contact tracing uses identifiable information to identify and contact persons who have been exposed to potentially infected individuals [21]. Surveillance and contact tracing efforts may be utilized in conjunction with quarantine and isolation measures. This permits public health officials to determine the scope of the outbreak and take necessary measures to reduce the risk of further transmission.

Activities such as public health surveillance, reporting, and contact tracing test the boundaries of the right to privacy. Public health authorities must balance the rights of the individual to control information about their infected status with the rights of the public health authority to collect and use this information to protect others in the community. These tensions may be particularly acute when the biological agent is not well understood. Persons who may have come into contact with the agent may choose to not cooperate with public health officials, fearing that the outcome of their cooperation will be a loss of privacy or liberty. They may also fear the stigma that often accompanies persons or groups subjected to coercive public health powers.

The use of identifiable information in a public health response to bioterrorism is particularly controversial if public health authorities share information with law enforcement agencies. Information sharing between public health and law enforcement agencies may be justified to facilitate a swift response to bioterrorism threats and to apprehend the perpetrators of the outbreak. However, access by law enforcement personnel to identifiable information gathered through public health surveillance further jeopardizes the privacy of these data [58]. Members of the community may be less likely to cooperate with public health officials if they suspect that their data may be revealed to law enforcement officials for purposes unrelated to their health. Furthermore, this type of data sharing may undermine the credibility of the public health system by calling into question its fundamental goals and the justifications for engaging in surveillance activities and data collection in the first place [59].

A bioterrorism outbreak may justify interventions subordinating privacy interests to the common good, but the state must meet several rigorous standards. It must demonstrate that the need for the information is necessary to serve a legitimate public health interest. Also, it must attempt to use the least amount of information necessary to achieve this interest. Finally, it must conduct its activities openly and transparently, and consult with the affected community.

12.3 Restrictions on Property

Law must allow for public health authorities to use coercive powers to manage property under certain circumstances. There are numerous situations that might require management of property in a public health emergency—for example, decontamination of facilities; acquisition of vaccines, medicines, or hospital beds; or use of private facilities for isolation, quarantine, or disposal of human remains. During the anthrax attacks, public health authorities had to close various public and private facilities for decontamination. Consistent with legal fair safeguards, including compensation for takings of private property used for public purposes, clear legal authority is needed to manage property to contain a serious health threat [25].

Once a public health emergency has been declared, the MSEHPA and Turning Point Act allow authorities the power to seize private property for public use that is reasonable and necessary to respond to the public health emergency. This power includes the ability to use and take temporary control of certain private sector businesses and activities that are of critical importance to epidemic control measures. Authorities may take control of landfills and other disposable facilities and services to safely eliminate infectious waste such as bodily fluids, biopsy materials, sharps, and other materials that may contain pathogens that otherwise pose a public health risk. The Model Acts also authorize public health officials to take possession and dispose of all human remains. Health care facilities and supplies may be procured or controlled to treat and care for patients and the general public [25, 29].

Whenever health authorities take private property to use for public health purposes, constitutional law requires that the property owner be provided just compensation. That is, the state must pay private owners for the use of their property [21]. Correspondingly, the Acts require the state to pay just compensation to the owner of any facilities or materials temporarily or permanently procured for public use during an emergency. Where public health authorities, however, must condemn or destroy any private property that poses a danger to the public (e.g., equipment that is contaminated with anthrax spores), no compensation to the property owners is required although states may choose to make compensation if they wish [25, 29]. Under existing legal powers to abate public nuisances, authorities are able to condemn, remove, or destroy any property that may harm the public's health [21].

Other permissible property control measures include restricting certain commercial transactions and practices (e.g., price gouging) to address problems arising from the scarcity of resources that often accompanies public health emergencies. The MSEHPA and Turning Point Acts allow public health officials to regulate the distribution of scarce health care supplies and to control the price of critical items during an emergency. In addition, authorities may seek the assistance of health care providers to perform medical examination and testing services [25, 29]. While the proposed use of these property control measures is not without controversy, they may provide public health authorities with important powers to more rapidly address an ongoing public health emergency.

12.4 Conclusion

The complex and unpredictable threat of bioterrorism demands a serious effort to comprehensively strengthen all areas of public health preparedness. Ongoing changes in public health practice help improve preparedness. Public health authorities at the national, state, and local levels must also be prepared to work together to build a stronger public health infrastructure, ensure adequate training for emergency responders and other necessary personnel, and use new and existing technologies to combat future outbreaks. Moreover, these authorities must understand the role of public health law. Laws are essential to the empowerment, and restriction, of authorities to act in the interests of protecting the public's health prior to, during, and following a bioterrorism event.

Public health law provides the necessary authority for government to engage in public health activities. Likewise, it limits government authority to infringe individual rights related to liberty, privacy, and property. Many existing public health laws do not sufficiently clarify the contours or extent of public health powers. Thus, legal reformation is needed to reflect modern conceptions of public health practice and contemporary constitutional norms.

The MSEHPA and Turning Point Act provide templates for public health law reform. These acts present clear criteria for governmental actions during public health emergencies. They delineate the scope of government public health power, the limits on this power, and the relationships between governments and other actors in emergency response situations. The roles of federal, state, and local governments in utilizing public health powers during public health emergencies must be considered and solidified in advance to avoid confusion or redundancy. Public health authorities need to be able to implement a full range of strategies to combat the spread of infectious diseases through bioterrorism while respecting civil liberties. Revision of state public health laws consistent with this balance will support and strengthen public health responses to future acts of bioterrorism.

References

1. Centers for Disease Control and Prevention. Outbreak of severe acute respiratory syndrome – worldwide. *MMWR Morb. Mortal. Wkly. Rep.* 52, 226–228, 2003.
2. Inglesby, T.V., O'Toole, T., Henderson, D.A., et al. Anthrax as a biological weapon. *J. Amer. Med. Assoc.*, 287, 2236–2252, 2002.
3. O'Toole, T., Mair, M., and Inglesby, T.V. Shining a light on dark winter. *Clin. Infect. Dis.* 34, 972–983, 2002.
4. Inglesby, T.V., Grossman, R., and O'Toole, T. A plague on your city: Observations from TOPOFF. *Clin. Infect. Dis.* 32, 436–445, 2001.
5. Institute of Medicine. *Biological Threats and Terrorism: Assessing the Science and Response Capabilities*: Workshop Summaries. National Academy Press, Washington, D.C., 2002.
6. Trust for America's Health. *Ready or Not: Protecting the Public's Health in the Age of Bioterrorism*, 2007, available at http://healthyamericans.org/reports/bioterror07/.
7. General Accounting Office. *Bioterrorism: Federal Research and Preparedness Activities.* GAO-01-915, 2001.
8. Model State Emergency Health Powers Act 1-104(a) (December 21, 2001), available at http://publichealthlaw.net/MSEHPA/MSEHPA2.pdf.
9. Inglesby, T.V., O'Toole, T., and Henderson, D.A. Preventing the use of biological weapons: Improving response should prevention fail. *Clin. Infect. Dis.* 30, 926–929, 2000.
10. Hughes, J.M. The emerging threat of bioterrorism. *Emerg. Infect. Dis.* 5, 494–495, 1999.
11. Henderson, D.A. The looming threat of bioterrorism. *Science* 283, 1279–1282, 1999.
12. Cole, L.A. The specter of biological weapons. *Sci. Am.* 275, 60–65, 1996.
13. Osterholm, M.T., and Schwartz, J. *What America Needs to Know to Survive the Coming Bioterrorist Catastrophe.* Bantam Dell, New York, NY, 2001.
14. Kellman, B. Biological terrorism: Legal measures for preventing catastrophe. *Harv. J. Law Public. Policy* 24, 417–488, 2001.
15. Kamoie, B. The national response plan: A new framework for homeland security, public health, and bioterrorism response. *J. Health Law* 38, 287–318, 2005.
16. Beinstock, R.E. Anti-bioterrorism research post-9/11 legislation: The USA Patriot Act and beyond. *J. Coll. Univ. Law* 30, 465–492, 2004.
17. Posner, R. A. *Catastrophe: Risk and Response.* Oxford University Press, New York, NY, 2004.
18. Defense Against Weapons of Mass Destruction Act 1996, P.L. 104–201.
19. Public Health Threats and Emergencies Act 2000, P.L. 106–505,.
20. Pandemic and All-Hazards Preparedness Act 2006, P.L. 109–417
21. Gostin, L.O. *Public Health Law: Power, Duty, Restraint.* University of California Press, Berkley, CA, 2000.
22. Gostin, L.O., Burris, S., and Lazzarini, Z. The law and the public's health: A study of infectious disease law in the United States. *Columbia Law Rev.* 99, 59–128, 1999.
23. Gibbons v. Ogden, 22 U.S. 1, 205 (1824).
24. Gostin, L.O. Public health law in an age of terrorism: Rethinking individual rights and common goods. *Health Aff.* 21, 79–93, 2002.
25. Gostin, L.O., Sapsin, J.W., Teret, S.P., et al. The model state emergency health powers act. *J. Amer. Med. Assoc.* 288, 622–628, 2002.

26. The organizations include the National Governors Association (NGA), the National Conference of State Legislatures (NCSL), the Association of State and Territorial Health Officials (ASTHO), the National Association of City and County Health Officers (NACCHO), and the National Association of Attorneys General (NAAG).
27. Hodge Jr., J.G. (2002) Bioterrorism law and policy: Critical choices in public health. *J. Law., Med. Ethics.* 30, 254–261, 2002.
28. MSEHPA State Legislative Activity Table (July 15, 2006) available at http://www.publichealthlaw.net/MSEHPA/MSEHPA%20Leg%20Activity.pdf (viewed February 5, 2008).
29. Tuning Point Model State Public Health Act (September 2003) available at http://www.hss.state.ak.us/dph/improving/turningpoint/PDFs/MSPHAweb.pdf (viewed February 5, 2008).
30. Uniform Emergency Volunteer Health Practitioners Act (October 17, 2006) available at http://www2a.cdc.gov/phlp/docs/UEVHPA.pdf (viewed February 5, 2008).
31. Gostin, L.O. The resurgent tuberculosis epidemic in the era of AIDS: Reflections on public health, law, and society. *Maryland Law Rev*. 54, 1–131, 1995.
32. Jacobs, L.A. Rights and quarantine during the SARS global health crisis: Differentiated legal consciousness in Hong Kong, Shanghai and Toronto, *Law Soc. Rev*. 41, 511–549, 2007.
33. Centers for Disease Control and Prevention. Use of Quarantine to Prevent Transmission of Severe Acute Respiratory Syndrome – Taiwan. *MMWR Morb. Mortal. Wkly. Rep*. 52, 680–683, 2003.
34. Centers for Disease Control and Prevention. Efficiency of Quarantine During an Epidemic of Severe Acute Respiratory Syndrome – Beijing, China. *MMWR Morb. Mortal. Wkly. Rep*. 52, 1037–1040, 2003.
35. Barbera, J., Macintyre, A., Gostin, L.O., et al. Large scale quarantine following biological terrorism in the United States. *J. Amer. Med. Assoc*. 286, 2711–2717, 2001.
36. Act of May 27, 1796, ch. 31, 1 Stat. 474 (repealed 1799).
37. Act of February 25, 1799, ch. 12, 1 Stat. 619.
38. 42 U.S.C. 264, 265, 266-271 (2008).
39. 42 U.S.C. 243 (2008).
40. 42 U.S.C. 264 (2008).
41. 42 CFR 70, 71 (2008).
42. Center for Disease Control and Prevention. Legal Authorities for Isolation and Quarantine, available at http://www.cdc.gov/ncidod/dq/pdf/legal_authorities_isolation_quarantine.pdf (viewed February 5, 2008).
43. Center for Disease Control and Prevention. Division of Global Migration and Quarantine: Field Operations, available at http://www.cdc.gov/ncidod/dq/operations.htm (viewed February 5, 2008).
44. Executive Order 13295.
45. Executive Order 13295 was amended April 4, 2003, to include SARS. (April 9, 2003) *Fed. Regist*. 68, 17255.
46. Executive Order 13375 (amending Executive Order 13295 to include "influenza caused by novel or reemergent influenza viruses that are causing, or have the potential to cause, a pandemic" to the list of quarantinable communicable diseases).
47. Weeks, E.A. Lessons from Katrina: Response, recovery, and the public health infrastructure. *Depaul J. Health Care Law* 10, 251–290, 2007.
48. Greenberger, M. The Alphonse and Gaston of governmental response to National Public Health Emergencies: Lessons learned from Hurricane Katrina for the Federal Government and the States. *Adm. Law Rev*. 58, 611–626, 2006.
49. Gostin, L.O. The future of public health law. *Am. J. Law Med*. 16, 1–32, 1990.
50. Parmet, W. AIDS and quarantine: The revival of an archaic doctrine. *Hofstra Law Rev*. 14, 53–90, 1985.

51. Gostin, L.O., Bayer, R., and Fairchild, A. Ethical and legal challenges posed by severe acute respiratory syndrome: Implications for the control of severe infectious disease threats. *J. Amer. Med. Assoc.* 290, 3229–3237, 2003.
52. Eidson, W. Confusion, controversy, and quarantine: The Muncie smallpox epidemic of 1893. *Indiana Mag. Hist.* 86, 374–398, 1990.
53. Markel, H. “Knocking out the Cholera”: Cholera, class, and quarantines in New York City, 1892. *Bull. Hist. Med.* 69, 420–457, 1995.
54. Risse, G. “A long pull, a strong pull, and all together”: San Francisco and the bubonic plague, 1907–1908. *Bull. Hist. Med.* 66, 260–286, 1992.
55. Jew Ho v. Williamson, 103 F. 1024 (C.C.D. Cal. 1900).
56. Whalen v. Roe, 429 U.S. 589 (1977).
57. Fairchild, A.L., Bayer, R., and Colgrove, J. *Searching Eyes: Privacy, the State, and Disease Surveillance in America*. University of California Press, Berkley, CA, 2007.
58. Gostin, L.O. When terrorism threatens health: How far are limitations on personal and economic liberties justified? *Fla. Law. Rev.* 55, 1105–1170, 2003.
59. Ferguson v. City of Charleston, 532 U.S. 67, 2001.

Chapter 13
Public Health Surveillance for Bioterrorism

Peter N. Wenger, William Halperin, and Edward Ziga

To paraphrase D. A. Henderson, if the public health infrastructure were a living organism, public health surveillance would be its sensory organ system. It receives and processes data from its environment that subsequently impacts on the organism's resulting actions. The appropriateness of those actions is dependent on the "health" of the sensory organs. More formally, public health surveillance is defined as "the ongoing, systematic collection, analysis, and interpretation of health data essential to the planning, implementation, and evaluation of public health practice, closely integrated with the timely dissemination of these data to those who need to know [1]."

Surveillance activities provide evidence-based information vital to subsequent investigative, research, or prevention and control efforts but do not include those efforts [2]. Surveillance is the component of public health practice that provides the information assisting in directing the appropriate response. This applies to any public health surveillance system regardless of its purpose. This chapter will focus the discussion on public health surveillance issues relevant to bioterrorism. For those readers interested in pursuing more information on public health surveillance in general, the authors suggest Teutsch and Churchill's [3] and Halperin and Baker's [4] excellent texts on public health surveillance.

13.1 Consequences of Bioterrorism

Incidents involving bacterial pathogens [5, 6], chemical agents [7], and the September 11, 2001, attack on the World Trade Center in New York City clearly demonstrate the overt vulnerability of civilian populations to terrorist acts. The resulting morbidity and mortality and subsequent psychosocial and

P.N. Wenger
Associate Professor, Departments of Preventive Medicine and Community Health/Pediatrics, University of Medicine and Dentistry of New Jersey/New Jersey Medical School, NJ, USA
e-mail: wengerpn@umdnj.edu

L.I. Lutwick, S.M. Lutwick (eds.), *Beyond Anthrax*,
DOI: 10.1007/978-1-59745-326-4_13, © Springer Science+Business Media, LLC 2008

economic impact on communities can be devastating. Bioterrorism can differ in several significant aspects from other modes of terrorism. Terrorist activities involving chemical agents, small arms, explosive or incendiary devices, or nuclear or radiological weapons are likely to be recognized by first responders such as the police, fire department, emergency medical service (EMS) or Hazardous Material (Hazmat) personnel at the point of attack. The morbidity and mortality caused by these agents are essentially limited to the area in which they are dispersed with secondary effects expected among first responders and in healthcare facilities to which victims are transported.

The covert intentional release of a biological agent, on the other hand, may not have an immediate impact due to the delay between exposure and onset of disease (incubation period). Initial recognition of disease caused by bioterrorist activity will most likely be by medical personnel in emergency departments, clinics, or private practices some days or weeks after release of the agent. Outbreaks of disease caused by bioterrorist activity [8] may initially present similar to many common and naturally occurring outbreaks such as influenza, resulting in further delay in the recognition of the event for what it is. Properties of certain biological agents of terrorism (e.g., smallpox, pneumonic plague, and viral hemorrhagic fevers) include person-to-person transmission. The potential for a sustained outbreak with widespread cases can be great, therefore, unless appropriate interventions that contain the outbreak are implemented. The potential for delayed recognition and response with subsequent dire consequences is substantial. There are many biological agents considered potential bioweapons. The Centers for Disease Control and Prevention (CDC) has developed three categories of biological agents, prioritized as to their potential of bioterrorist use and the severity of disease they may produce (Box 1).

13.2 Surveillance

The response to a bioterrorist incident, including medical, public health, law enforcement, and political interventions are predicated on initial detection of disease associated with the intentional release of the biological agent. Recognition of disease and outbreaks due to either naturally occurring or intentional release of infectious pathogens has depended on astute healthcare providers contacting the appropriate public health agency at the point of initial recognition of cases [1, 2, 9]. For example, if the astute physician in Florida who recognized and reported the initial inhalational anthrax case in the 2001 anthrax outbreak [6] had not either identified or reported the case, it may have delayed recognition of the outbreak for several weeks. This would have delayed implementation of infection control interventions in the affected mail facilities, United States Senate office building, and other contaminated buildings resulting in possible increased morbidity and mortality due to anthrax.

The existence of organized surveillance efforts in a public health agency (e.g., health department) provides the infrastructure for conveying information to facilitate a timely and appropriate response [2]. The threat of bioterrorism has emphasized the need to improve and augment existing surveillance methods and systems to facilitate early detection of disease activity as well as integrate surveillance activity on all levels.

There are over 100 surveillance and public health information systems maintained by different programs at the CDC and hundreds more at the local and state level. Surveillance systems are developed to monitor and disseminate information on many different health-related events involving infectious diseases, chronic diseases, environmental and occupational health, birth defects and injury control. Surveillance for bioterrorist-related disease outbreaks is a component of surveillance for infectious diseases. Fundamental infectious diseases surveillance in the United States has been well established for years, however, surveillance for disease and injury associated with other terrorist-related activity, such as the intentional release of toxic chemical agents and detonation of radiological devices, has not received the same attention. While some disease related to other terrorist activity may be captured in surveillance for bioterrorist activity (e.g., toxic injury due to ricin), systems will have to be designed with these events in mind. Surveillance systems maintained for infectious diseases of public health importance include communicable diseases with epidemic potential, vaccine-preventable diseases, emerging infectious diseases, HIV/AIDS, hospital-acquired infections, tuberculosis, foodborne infectious diseases, antimicrobial-resistant organisms among others. While methods for conducting public health surveillance may differ considerably by program and disease, the general flow of data and information through a surveillance system is schematically represented in Fig. 13.1.

13.2.1 Fundamental Surveillance

The most fundamental surveillance for infectious diseases in the United States is maintained by the National Notifiable Disease Surveillance System (NNDSS). It has been functioning in some form since 1878 [10]. NNDSS seeks reports on diseases caused by many different organisms (Box 2). It is a passive surveillance system in which a healthcare practitioner or a clinical laboratory will report a suspected or confirmed case of a notifiable infectious disease. Reporting is to the local and/or state health department that then passes the information, usually stripped of personal identifiers, on to federal authorities, in this case, the CDC.

Traditionally, data are reviewed on a case-by-case basis at the local level to determine action required on any individual case or local outbreak. A more complete analysis is performed at the state and national levels to detect any unusual patterns that may indicate spread of disease outside the local

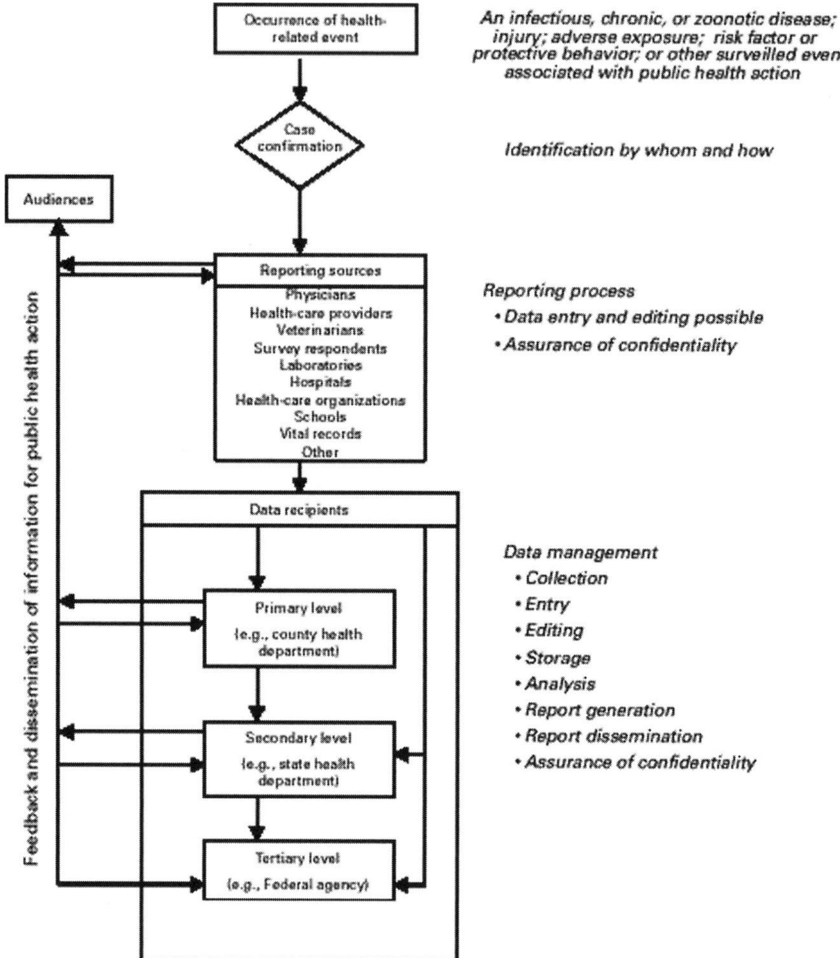

Fig. 13.1 Simplified flow chart for a generic surveillance system
Centers for Disease Control and Prevention. Updated Guidelines for Evaluating Public Health Surveillance Systems: Recommendations from the Guidelines Working Group. MMWR 2001;50(RR-13):8

jurisdiction [11]. The data collected is published as cumulative provisional cases weekly in the *Morbidity and Mortality Weekly Report*(MMWR) and as final corrected data at the end of the year in the annual *Summary of Notifiable Diseases, United States*. Notifiable disease statistics are also available from CDC's National Center for Health statistics in its publication, National Vital Statistics Reports and on the Internet at http://www.cdc.gov/nchswww/.

The Council of State and Territorial Epidemiologists (CSTE), in collaboration with the CDC, recommends the health conditions to be notifiable through the NNDSS. Each state, however, determines whether and how these conditions should be made reportable except for the quarantinable diseases (cholera, diphtheria, infectious tuberculosis, plague, potential pandemic influenza viruses, SARS, smallpox, yellow fever, viral hemorrhagic fevers). Reporting of these infections is required by international regulation [2, 11]. The legal basis requiring reporting of notifiable diseases varies by state, as does the authority for determining which cases are reportable [2, 11]. Depending on the state, reporting of notifiable diseases may be mandated by the legislature, state health officer or epidemiologist, the board of health or some combination thereof [2, 12, 13]. Most states require reporting of all notifiable conditions recommended by CSTE and many have included diseases not included in the NNDSS. For instance, smallpox was removed from the NNDSS list of notifiable diseases in 1988 due to the declared eradication of the disease by the World Health Assembly in 1980; however, most states have reinstituted mandatory reporting of smallpox because of concerns of its use as a bioweapon. The Infectious Disease Committee of the CSTE has since recommended that smallpox be placed under surveillance by all states, territories, and the CDC as part of NNDSS [14]. In addition, many states mandate the reporting of outbreaks due to any pathogen regardless of inclusion in the NNDSS list of notifiable infectious diseases.

13.2.2 Information Technology Impact

Advances in communication and information technology over the past half century have revolutionized the practice of public health surveillance. Notifiable disease reporting was traditionally performing using paper-based data collection forms. In 1984, the CDC in collaboration with the CSTE began testing the Epidemiologic Surveillance Project [15], with a goal to demonstrate the effectiveness of computer transmission of public health surveillance data between state health departments and the CDC. The project developed computer programs using existing disease surveillance systems to transmit data to the CDC on all nationally notifiable diseases. In 1985, the system became a fully interactive computer-based reporting system. By 1989, all 50 states were participating and the project was renamed the National Electronic Telecommunications System for Surveillance (NETSS) [15, 16]. De-identified data is transmitted weekly from all 50 state health departments as well as from New York City, Washington D.C., and five US Territories.

Though the NETSS initiative facilitated disease notification from the state to the federal level, it was clear that the myriad systems that comprise the US public health infrastructure from the local to the federal levels often were not integrated, interfering with the timely flow of information [17]. In 1993, the CDC/Agency for Toxic Substances and Disease Registry (ATSDR) Steering Committee on Public Health Information and Surveillance System convened to implement a major initiative for the creation of integrated public health surveillance and health information systems. Their recommendations are documented in the 1995 report, *Integrating Public Health Information and Surveillance Systems* [18]. Subsequently, the National Electronic Disease Surveillance System (NEDSS) initiative was developed and is currently in the process of being implemented. While NETSS addressed the issue of electronic data transfer from the state level to the CDC, NEDSS has expanded the scope of the initial initiative to include the integration of all related surveillance systems at the local, state and federal level through innovative electronic and information technology. NEDSS "promotes the use of data and information system standards to advance the development of efficient, integrated, and interoperable surveillance systems at federal, state and local levels [19]." The long-term objective of NEDSS [20] is to facilitate development of complementary electronic information systems that automatically gather health data from a variety of sources on a real-time basis as well as facilitate the monitoring of the health of communities. NEDSS will also assist in the ongoing analysis of trends and detection of emerging public health problems and provide information for setting public health policy. The NEDSS architecture will eventually replace the NETSS reporting format. NEDSS currently resides within the Public Health Information Network (PHIN) [21] initiative and serves as its public health surveillance component.

An incarnation of NEDSS, the NEDSS Base System (NBS), is actual surveillance software that may be deployed by state health departments in collaboration with the CDC. As of June 2007 it is deployed to 16 states including Alabama, Arizona, Idaho, Maryland, Maine, Montana, Nebraska, New Mexico, Nevada, Rhode Island, South Carolina, Tennessee, Texas, Virginia, Vermont, and Wyoming [22]. Other states have or are in the process of developing computer-based surveillance data collection and processing systems that are NEDSS-compatible. These systems will eventually be incorporated into a fully integrated surveillance system from the local to national level. The New Jersey Communicable Diseases Reporting and Surveillance System (CDRSS) is an example of a state developed NEDSS-compatible web-based surveillance data collection and processing system that will be discussed subsequently.

13.2.3 Surveillance and the Public Health Infrastructure

A major purpose of surveillance for bioterrorist events is detection at the earliest possible time of infectious diseases occurrences due to the intentional release of bioagents and to disseminate the information promptly to those who will affect appropriate public health, medical, law enforcement, and sociopolitical interventions. Sustainability of a surveillance system wholly dedicated to very rare events such as bioterrorist-related disease outbreaks would be expensive and difficult to maintain. Episodes of naturally occurring infectious diseases of great public health importance are not uncommon and pose many of the same surveillance problems as detecting the intentional release of bioagents.

Severe acute respiratory syndrome (SARS), HIV/AIDS, multidrug-resistant tuberculosis, foodborne disease outbreaks, pandemic influenza, and West Nile virus show the necessity of vigilant and sustained surveillance systems. Surveillance activities require time, money, and most importantly and vastly underappreciated, human resources. Development of new surveillance systems and improvements in existing systems to better detect bioterrorist-related disease activity should include the capacity to monitor for other infectious diseases of public health importance including emerging infectious diseases and vaccine-preventable diseases among others. These systems must have routine surveillance capabilities in order that they survive the extended periods of bioterrorist activity dormancy.

After years of political and financial neglect, our current public health infrastructure is currently under tremendous stress to meet the myriad public health problems posed daily regardless of the demands of bioterrorism security. For example, the authors of this chapter work with the Communicable Diseases Division (CDD) of the Department of Health and Human Services of Newark, New Jersey (NDHHS). Newark is a city of approximately 250,000 residents in a metropolitan area of several million people located about 15 miles from downtown New York City. The residents of Newark are ethnically diverse with a substantial immigrant population. A significant portion of the population exists under the poverty level. All the public health problems found in urban areas are experienced by the city. There are tens of thousands commuters in the city throughout the week including 40,000 students attending the colleges, universities, and graduate schools. In addition, Newark Liberty Airport that services 32 million passengers a year, including 8 million international travelers, and the Port of Newark, one of the largest ports for container ships in the United States, are located within city boundaries. In addition, many vital roadways essential for the nation's commercial transport pass through the city. The potential for bioterrorist activity is great. The CDD of NDHHS manages infectious disease surveillance activities, including surveillance for bioterrorism. Despite funding for biodefense activities, the CDD remains understaffed and financially stressed to meet its' routine, non-terrorist-related public health responsibilities. A case can be made that the advent of substantial funding sources dedicated to bioterrorist-related activity has extended the pre-existing public health resources and divided attention from foundation public health issues. For example, during the smallpox vaccination campaign in early 2003, much of the public health workforce were furloughed from their usual duties to meet the demands required from the campaign leaving their usual responsibilities unfulfilled. The challenge is to develop and maintain surveillance capabilities that meet the daily needs of the community (e.g., vaccine-preventable infectious diseases, foodborne disease outbreaks, etc.) and are flexible enough to detect bioterrorist events. To meet this challenge the CDD/

NDHHS formed an Office of Surveillance and Prevention (OSP) under the direction of the local Health Officer located at the NDHHS. Using state biodefense funding, a fulltime epidemiologist was hired for the OSP and a cooperative consultative arrangement was reached with the Department of Preventive Medicine and Community Health (DPMCH)/University of Medicine and Dentistry of New Jersey (UMDNJ)/New Jersey Medical School (NJMS) and UMDNJ School of Public Health (SPH). This arrangement provides the CDD/NDHSS with additional expertise in surveillance, epidemiology, infectious diseases, and chemical toxins that it was not able to afford to directly employ. Examples of OSP surveillance activities will follow in this chapter.

13.2.4 Indirect Benefits

Most of the discussion of surveillance for bioterrorism involves early detection of disease due to bioterrorist activity; however, surveillance activities can serve other purposes in the face of bioterrorism. Estimating the magnitude of morbidity and mortality in the population due to the bioagent once it has been released and assessing the effectiveness of interventions in limiting the diseases. Surveillance can be used to monitor adverse health events associated with bioterrorism [23] or other major public health events, such as those associated with long-term antimicrobial prophylaxis for specific agents (anthrax) [24] or vaccination campaigns (smallpox [25, 26], influenza [27]). In addition, surveillance information can be used to help focus response assets and assist in efforts to manage community concerns [28].

13.3 Reporting and Collection of Data

13.3.1 Reporting

It is one objective of a public health department to contain an outbreak of infectious disease within a single incubation period of the responsible agent to prevent transmission within the community, limiting unnecessary morbidity and mortality [29]. Early detection of bioterrorist-related activity not only has vital medical and public health implications but also offers the best opportunity for prevention of additional episodes through successful law enforcement intervention. Early detection is crucial in gaining control of any outbreak and early detection is dependent on timely reporting.

Biosensor technology detecting the presence of infectious agents in the environment prior to host infection offers the possibility of very early detection of the intentional release of bioagents. This technology, however, is currently very expensive, uncommon, and not well field tested. At this time, the earliest detection of disease due to infectious diseases, whether naturally occurring or intentionally released, depends on astute frontline healthcare providers and microbiology laboratory personnel.

All US states and territories have laws or regulations mandating the reporting of particular health conditions, including infectious diseases. New Jersey Administrative Code 8:57-1 requires *immediate* telephone reporting by healthcare providers, laboratory directors, and others in positions of authority (e.g., school principals, prison superintendents, etc.) to local public health authorities (if they cannot be located then state authorities) of *suspected* or confirmed cases of 19 different conditions including anthrax, botulism, brucellosis, plague, smallpox, tularemia, viral hemorrhagic fevers, and any outbreak or *suspected* outbreak, including but not limited to, a suspected act of bioterrorism. Recognition of suspected specific diagnosis (e.g., anthrax, plague, or smallpox), however, by frontline providers is difficult due to unfamiliarity with the syndromes associated with these agents or their similarity with the prodromal presentation of other naturally occurring infections. In addition, differential diagnoses are predicated by a physician's index of suspicion, usually determined by commonly occurring diseases and not rare entities.

13.3.2 Confirmation

Definitive diagnoses of infectious diseases require laboratory confirmation, usually by culture or serology, and it is at this point that diagnoses, especially of rare diseases, and reporting commonly takes place by laboratory personnel. Laboratory confirmation of infection involving culture of the agent from affected tissue usually takes several days after obtaining appropriate samples. Serologic evidence is usually not present at initial presentation. Other molecular diagnostic tools, such as polymerase chain reaction (PCR), can significantly shorten the turnaround time in obtaining microbiologic confirmation of a diagnosis. These testing modalities, however, are often not available at a local level, especially for uncommon pathogens and may not be ordered if available due to their expense if a common pathogen is the suspected etiologic agent. The situation is more difficult for laboratory identification of disease due to chemical toxins for which laboratory access is even more difficult and less widely used than for identification of infectious agents. Furthermore, outbreaks are often difficult to appreciate on the provider level and require a greater perspective (e.g., local community, city, regional, state(s), and nation) for recognition. For example, the extent of a recent outbreak of hepatitis A in western Pennsylvania was not recognized until review on a state level [30, 31]. Lack of awareness of reporting responsibilities by those required to report, including the what, when, whom, and how to report, as well as the ease of contact (availability of contact numbers, computer access, or forms) further exacerbate delay in reporting.

13.3.3 Adequacy of Collection

Doyle, et al [32], in an analytical literature review evaluating completeness of notifiable infectious disease reporting in the United States between 1970 and 1999, found that reporting completeness was most strongly associated with the reporter's perception of the seriousness of the disease being reported. This suggests that educational programs for providers and laboratory personnel stressing their public health duties in the effort versus bioterrorism as well as development of diagnostic aids in identifying disease associated with bioterrorist-related agents may be effective in improving conventional provider- and laboratory-based reporting.

13.3.4 Passive versus Active Systems

Reportable disease data is most often collected through a passive reporting system, that is one dependent on the initiative of the reporter and thus prone to under-reporting [1, 32]. Healthcare providers have numerous immediate responsibilities with respect to patient care so it is not surprising that reporting of diseases to public health agencies is often not prioritized. Even though required, the lack or perceived lack of resultant activity by health departments subsequent to case reporting discourages reporter participation. Active surveillance, the collection of data is elicited by the agency operating the surveillance system, is more likely to provide more complete reporting but is much more labor intensive and costlier than its passive cousin. One study [33] evaluated passive versus active surveillance in identifying cases of hepatitis A in Kentucky over a 22-week period. The report demonstrated that nine more cases were identified through the active surveillance system. This resulted in the prevention of an estimated additional seven cases through administration of prophylaxis to the contacts of the nine case-patients. The added benefit of active surveillance does not come without a price. The estimated cost of operating the active surveillance system was approximately six times that of the passive system [33].

While active surveillance may not be sustainable over long periods of time, it can be used over the short term for acute critical issues. This is often referred to as drop-in surveillance. The New York City Department of Health and Mental Hygiene (NYCDOHMH) and CDC performed active syndromic (see below) surveillance in sentinel emergency departments to identify bioterrorist activity in the aftermath of the September 11th terrorist attacks [23]. In Newark, an annual ethnic festival, usually attracting approximately 400,000 people, was scheduled late spring of 2003. Festival organizers expected a sizable contingent from Toronto, at that time experiencing a SARS outbreak. The NDHHS, which maintains passive emergency room surveillance in all five hospitals located in Newark, activated enhanced (collecting data for a specific condition or syndrome, in this case SARS), active surveillance in those same hospitals.

This active enhanced surveillance activity persisted for a period of 3 days prior to the festival (baseline), during the festival, and for 10 days following the festival (one incubation period).

A paper-based data collection tool based on the CDC case definition for SARS at that time was developed by the NDHHS OSP epidemiologist and distributed to appropriate emergency department personnel at each hospital. The form was used for every patient presenting with fever and/or respiratory symptoms during the described period. Health inspectors from the NDHHS visited each emergency department daily and collected the forms and reviewed emergency department logs for any missed possible suspects. The OSP epidemiologist reviewed all data. In addition, EMS personnel assigned to health stations at the festival site received training on evaluating festival attendees for SARS who present with suspicious symptoms. No cases of suspect or probable SARS were identified. At the end of the enhanced active SARS surveillance period, the OSP epidemiologist presented the information obtained to appropriate personnel in participating emergency departments. This surveillance activity not only served its expressed purpose but also fostered increased communication and cooperation between the NDHHS and the area's hospitals.

13.3.5 Personnel and Electronics

It is important for health departments to recognize who is responsible for notifiable disease reporting in their locale and develop close, mutually beneficial relationships with them. In Newark, a significant portion of the community receives initial medical care for acute conditions at local emergency departments. The NDHHS felt, therefore, it would be appropriate to focus initial bioterrorist-related surveillance activities in local emergency departments. The local hospital infection control practitioners (ICPs) are assigned the task of reporting notifiable infectious diseases to the health department in emergency departments and hospitals. One of the NDHHS initiatives was to organize monthly meetings for all the hospitals ICPs, attended by staff from the NDHHS OSP, in which issues of mutual interest are discussed. These meetings have greatly contributed to developing strategies to simplify reporting procedures and increase communication.

Many states have introduced electronic data collection and reporting to increase the completeness and timeliness of reporting. A NNDSS survey conducted by the CSTE in 2001 revealed that 24 of 45 (53.3%) states responding to the survey utilized some form of electronic data transfer in reporting notifiable disease data to state health departments [13]. The number has increased since then. The New Jersey Department of Health and Senior Services (NJDHSS) has developed the CDRSS, a web-based application used to enter, update and track notifiable communicable disease data for the purpose of aggregating and reporting the information to CDRSS system users, as well as the CDC.

CDRSS has been built to conform to NEDSS standards. Users will include ICPs, physicians, laboratories, and local, regional and state public health professionals. CDRSS allows real-time case reporting as well as case retrieval and filtration by various parameters. Summary information is available to all users. An ICP may access summary data on all reportable diseases reported through CDRSS but can retrieve personalized detailed data only on those cases reported from their institution, while a local health officer may retrieve detailed data on all cases reported in their jurisdiction. Data is easily exported to many different programs for the purpose of analysis or presentation. The application has been deployed to the provider level (hospitals [ICPs]) and some microbiology laboratories utilized by New Jersey healthcare providers and is in various stages of deployment to other reporting sources throughout the state. While no formal studies on system effectiveness have been completed at this date, most users have reported a much greater preference for CDRSS over paper-based reporting.

There is great interest in utilizing automated electronic data collection and transmission systems to facilitate early detection of bioterrorist activity. Capturing automated routinely collected data (e.g., billing, electronic medical records or charting, laboratory reports) from emergency departments [34], hospitals, ambulatory-care settings [28, 35, 36], and clinical laboratories for reporting notifiable diseases would complement, not supplant, existing provider- and laboratory-based reporting. In addition, automated electronic data collection would allow sustained data collection from multiple data sources that would ordinarily not be readily available if dependent upon manual data collection. Additional sources to consider include poison control centers, nurse and physician emergency hotlines, over-the-counter pharmacy sales, school and employer absenteeism records, and intensive care unit (ICU) medical records (*see* Table 13.1).

Automated electronic data collection has the potential to augment conventional reporting without additional de novo public health reporting responsibilities to frontline personnel. These systems can be designed to operate in real-time (transfer of data on entering into the system) or batch transfer of data at specified times. Studies of electronic laboratory-based reporting conducted at the University of Pittsburgh Medical Center [37] and the State of Hawaii Department of Health [38] revealed that electronic reports were received, on average, in a more timely manner and were at least as complete as conventional laboratory reporting. A review of five automated electronic laboratory systems, however, revealed problems with data transmission, sensitivity, specificity, and user interpretation [39]. Problems identified included lapses in reporting due to failure or adjustments in data extraction software and lack of uniformity of coding standards between clinical laboratories. Specificity was adversely affected due to automated data extraction errors in extracting culture results if entered in free text, for example, reporting as positive a negative culture result due to the organism's name appearing in free text. In addition, accumulation of duplicate reports, unnecessary reports

Table 13.1 Possible sources of health indicator surveillance data

Data source	Pros	Cons and confounders
Outpatient and emergency department visits	Reflects incidence of disease in the general population	Nonspecific – may be difficult to document definitive information
Intensive care unit diagnoses	Best indicator of rare events like west Nile virus or Hantavirus pulmonary syndrome	Will not capture milder cases
Over-the-counter pharmacy sales	Reflects symptomatology most broadly	Subject to promotions/sales
Clinical lab submissions	Ordered by clinicians	May not be ordered for all (most) patients
Medicare or medicaid claims	Ease of capture data	Problems with timeliness and accuracy
Nursing homes	Reported by medical personnel; immobile population with limited exposure possibilities	Immobility reduces exposure potential; not broadly representative
Systematic testing for specific disease agents in specimens submitted to public health lab	Specificity of diagnoses	Broad screening not likely to capture meaningful data; difficulty getting information on positive samples; not timely
School and work absenteeism	May occur earlier than clinician visits	Nonspecific; delays in obtaining data
Ambulance call chief complaints	Many communities with timely access to data	Nonspecific
Poison information center calls	Ability to access in real-time	Many not be related to infectious diseases
HMO/nurse hotline calls	Occur very early in outbreak	May be difficult to categorize

Reprinted with permission from Biological Threats and Terrorism: Assessing the Science and Response Capabilities: Workshop Summary © 2002 by the National Academy of Sciences, courtesy of the National Academies Press, Washington, D.C.

(e.g., screening rubella serology in pregnant women), and identification of unreportable conditions increased the number of false positives.

The ultimate identification of bioterrorist activity will be realized by investigation of reported diseases through surveillance by local and state health departments. Poor specificity in surveillance reporting will result in unnecessary investigations thus placing undue burden on an already overtaxed public health system. Many local health departments, additionally, do not possess the sophisticated information technology or expertise required to fully participate in automated electronic surveillance. Automated electronic surveillance systems will undoubtedly make important contributions in refining timely surveillance activity, however, there remain many development and implementation issues before its fundamental value will be realized.

13.4 Syndromic Surveillance Methodology

The inherent delays in conventional disease reporting have led to the exploration and development of alternative methods of early detection surveillance systems. Broadly speaking, syndromic surveillance involves monitoring disease or health-related event data that does not require specific medical diagnoses. A syndromic surveillance system collects and interprets data on clinical signs and symptoms that precede formal diagnosis in a way that would identify with sufficient probability an outbreak of public health interest, i.e., bioterrorist event. Data collected for syndromic surveillance could not be used in establishing a specific diagnosis in an individual; however, it may detect patterns of disease in a population that would indicate occurrence of an outbreak earlier than a surveillance system that requires a more definitive diagnosis. Reporting of routinely collected data such as ICD-9-coded chief complaints or initial diagnosis in emergency departments or ambulatory clinic settings may serve as data sources for syndromic surveillance.

13.4.1 Syndrome Classifications

Syndromic surveillance requires the classification of signs and symptoms such as fever, cough or dyspnea or ICD-9 codes into syndromic groups or clusters (detectors) that would be recognized by data extraction programs or personnel. For instance, a syndromic group for lower respiratory tract infections (LRTIs) may include all ICD-9 codes for pneumonia and bronchitis or descriptive terms such as fever, cough, difficulty breathing or combinations of terms such as fever and cough. Since significant variability in assigning diagnostic terms or ICD-9-coding to similar patients exists between providers and clinics, syndromic surveillance can reduce variability in reporting when collecting data from different providers. For instance, one provider may code a patient who initially presents with clinical signs and symptoms of a LRTI with the ICD-9 codes for cough and fever, while another may code it as an unspecified pneumonia and a third may give that patient a more specific diagnosis of viral pneumonia. If all those initial diagnostic ICD-9 codes were included in a syndromic cluster for LRTI that case would be captured while it may have been missed in a surveillance system requiring a more defined diagnosis depending on the patient's provider. In addition, it would allow capture of the suspected diagnosis earlier in the patient encounter.

This methodology, however, would have a corresponding decrease in specificity and thus positive predictive value in identifying an outbreak of LRTI due to any specific pathogen. For example, syndromic surveillance for cutaneous anthrax is more likely to detect cases of cutaneous anthrax in contrast to surveillance for the specific diagnosis. Given the large baseline number of cases of general cutaneous infection that would be identified by syndromic surveillance, however, the number of actual cutaneous anthrax cases that would have to occur for an outbreak to be identified would have to be large. A parallel example would be the detection of bioterrorist-related pulmonary disease during influenza season. The developers and users of any surveillance system will have to decide at what point specificity may be sacrificed to improve timeliness of reporting.

13.4.2 Evaluation of Syndromic Surveillance

It is important to periodically evaluate the sensitivity, specificity, and positive predictive value of these syndromic groups in identifying diseases or outbreaks of public health interest. This can be accomplished by comparison with a "gold standard" such as discharge diagnosis, emergency department or hospital chart review or final microbiology or serology laboratory results. Espino and Wagner at the Center for Biomedical Informatics at the University of Pittsburgh compared two syndromic groups to detect acute respiratory illness [40]. One group was constructed of ICD-9-coded chief complaints and the other of ICD-9-coded diagnoses obtained at a later point in the patient encounter. Performance was measured against review of emergency department records. No difference in sensitivity or specificity was found between the two syndromic groups in identifying actual acute respiratory disease. This suggests that syndromic groups constructed of ICD-9-coded chief complaints, which can be reported early on in the patient encounter, have a role in public health surveillance.

A comparison of syndromic categorization of chief complaint and discharge diagnosis for emergency department visits in US National Capitol Region revealed good overall agreement between the two ($\kappa = 0.639$), however, neurologic ($\kappa = 0.085$) and sepsis ($\kappa = 0.105$) syndrome categories had markedly lower agreement than other syndromes [41].

13.4.3 Electronically-Based Syndromic Surveillance

Data extraction for syndromic surveillance can be done manually as was done by the CDC and NYCDOHMH in the aftermath of September 11th [23]. The procedure, however, is much too labor intensive and expensive to be sustainable over long periods of time. Sustainability of syndromic surveillance depends on the development of automated electronic data transmission systems. An example of a syndromic surveillance system based on real-time automated electronic data collection and transmission is the Real-Time Outbreak and Disease Surveillance (RODS) system developed at the Center for Biomedical Informatics at the University of Pittsburgh [34].

The RODS system adheres to NEDSS specifications and currently operates in multiple cities, states, and countries. It was used during the 2002 Winter Olympics in Utah. In December 2002, RODS software was made available at no cost to health departments and academic institutions; however, it requires the technical resources to maintain real-time electronic disease surveillance systems. The RODS software has been open-sourced since September 2003 and those interested are directed to The RODS Open Source Project website at http://openrods.sourceforge.net/.

13.4.4 Role of Syndromic Surveillance

Syndromic surveillance is not meant to supplant existing provider- and laboratory-based surveillance but to augment these systems. Developing independent but complimentary surveillance systems can serve to confirm and validate information derived from existing systems as well as hopefully improve the sensitivity, specificity, and positive predictive value of overall surveillance in the detection of public health threats. Whether syndromic surveillance is more likely to detect the consequences of bioterrorist activity earlier than astute frontline clinicians or current surveillance systems remains unknown at this time. There is much to be done in exploring this approach to find its ultimate utility in public health surveillance. For those readers interested in pursuing more information concerning syndromic surveillance the authors recommend reviewing the numerous sources found on the CDC website (www.cdc.gov: search under syndromic surveillance).

13.5 Data Analysis and Interpretation

Surveillance system data are observational in nature and distributed over time and space thus allowing public health epidemiologists to describe patterns of disease in the community. It is the analysis and interpretation of the collected surveillance data that enables detection of unusual disease events or trends in the population. Analysis is the application of appropriate methods in aggregating the collected surveillance data and interpretation is the creative assessment of the analysis to detect emerging data patterns [1, 42]. While computer software programs are readily available for automated data analysis choosing the appropriate analytic method as well as the interpretation of analyzed data is wholly dependent on human reasoning. It is vital that epidemiologists involved with the analysis and interpretation of surveillance data understand and be intimately involved with the entire surveillance process. They must know the inherent idiosyncrasies of the data set and its analysis if the interpretation is to be meaningful.

13.5.1 Sentinel Health Events

Analysis and interpretation may be very simple and straightforward. The natural occurrence in the US of most the agents considered most likely to be used in bioterrorism-related activity (Box 1) is so uncommon [43] that one case report is enough to raise a high index of suspicion. These are in essence sentinel health events [44, 45] that signify failure of prevention, in this case, occurrence of a bioterrorist event. The anthrax assault through the US postal system in 2001 is a case in point. Public health authorities recognized quickly after the initial report from Florida that this was not a case of naturally occurring infection and disease.

Even if the agent is not initially recognized, sudden appearance of similar severe disease presentation in unexpected populations should alert authorities to suspicious circumstances and initiate appropriate action. Examples are adult respiratory distress syndrome with fever occurring in healthy young adults or children or in groups of people who work, study, or attended an event in the same location. It cannot, however, be anticipated that bioterrorist-related disease outbreaks will be so obvious. As mentioned earlier, prodromal illness due to many likely bioagents often present like other, naturally occurring pathogens. The episode may, therefore, be difficult to recognize as being a potential bioterrorist-related event, especially if initial numbers are small or occur over a widespread area.

Pathogens commonly causing disease in a community may be used as terrorist episode as was the case in the 1984 outbreak in central Oregon due to intentional contamination of salad bars with *Salmonella typhimurium* [5]. Advances in biotechnology have allowed the genetic manipulation of bacteria and viruses to increase their pathogenicity, virulence, and induce vaccine and antimicrobial resistance. Bioterrorists have the potential to acquire or develop formerly mildly or non-pathogenic microorganisms, which would not be immediately suspected, into bioweapons [46–48]. It is important, therefore, to have surveillance in place with the ability to promptly recognize the early onset of more subtle disease trends that suggest bioterrorist-related activity. In addition, it is essential to have infectious disease and emergency department physicians, ICPs, and clinical toxicologists in place throughout the medical system who are well trained and sensitive to the occurrence of unusual clinical presentations that may indicate terrorist activity or other public health emergencies.

13.5.2 Aberration Detection in Surveillance Data

Detection of bioterrorist-related disease through surveillance activities is often discussed in terms of outbreak or epidemic recognition. Epidemicity is defined as being "relative to the usual frequency of the disease in the same area, among the specified population, at the same season of the year [49]." The terms epidemic and outbreak are often used synonymously although outbreak contains less emotional content to the public.

In syndromic surveillance, an epidemic may be suggested by increases in the number of cases meeting the criteria for a syndromic cluster. This definition of epidemicity demands a comparison between an observed number of cases or health events in a specified population, time and place to what is expected or considered normal. An epidemic may require the presence of an aberration in disease trends. An aberration is defined as the occurrence of health events that are statistically significant when compared to the normal history [42]. Early detection of bioterrorist-related disease through syndromic surveillance requires development of analytic modeling techniques that will reliably detect aberrant signals over time and space using data collected and analyzed in real time or near real time (i.e., data batched and analyzed every 8, 16, or 24 h). The models use historical data over prescribed time intervals in specified populations and locations to predict the expected number of cases or rates of disease that then is compared with the observed number of cases or rates.

There are numerous methodological issues to consider and any method developed or chosen has its own particular advantages and disadvantages. It is vitally important that whatever model is used, it be tested periodically to confirm that it is reliably detecting what it was designed to detect, in this case early evidence of disease trends that may suggest bioterrorist activity. Obviously, this is difficult given the exceedingly low incidence of bioterrorist-related events but it can be accomplished by comparing it versus independent, reliable surveillance systems in early detection of naturally occurring events that may resemble onset of bioterrorist-related disease activity (i.e., historical or real-time seasonal influenza trends) [50].

It is important to remember that while the existence of an aberration may be considered necessary; it is not sufficient for the occurrence of an epidemic [51]. False positive case reports may give rise to aberrant signals in surveillance data. For instance, statistically significant increases in influenza-like illness may not indicate an increase in influenza infection but reflect other non-influenzal respiratory tract viral infections that will be captured as cases of influenza-like illnesses. In this case, laboratory evidence of influenza infection would be required to confirm an influenza epidemic.

While much of the analysis of surveillance data is designed to detect aberrations in disease trends, statistical significance is not a necessary perquisite for detection of bioterrorist activity. The small number of cases (18 definitive cases, 11 of them inhalational, over four states and the District of Columbia over 3 months) associated with the 2001 anthrax attack would not have triggered an alert (statistically significant increase, in this case, in a flu-like prodromal illness) in a local, state, or even national syndromic surveillance system attempting to capture anthrax.

There is no analytic or aberrant detection model that, in and of itself, is capable of identifying an epidemic or bioterrorist-related disease activity. It is the public health personnel responsible for surveillance activities that will ultimately decide on whether or not there is sufficient surveillance evidence suggesting unusual disease activity. One may speculate that improved surveillance may be best accomplished by the proliferation of highly trained, epidemiologically sophisticated infectious disease, toxicology, and other related professionals throughout the medical and public health landscape. This is, in fact, the rationale for the creation of the Epidemic Intelligence Service (EIS) at the CDC. EIS is an on-the-job training program in epidemiology for a cadre of health professionals who then populate medical and public health settings throughout the United States, improving the nations epidemiologic and surveillance capabilities [52].

Advances in molecular biology technology have made important contributions to infectious disease public health surveillance and can assist in rapidly confirming a suspected event. Technologies such as pulsed-field gel electrophoresis (PFGE), restriction fragment length polymorphism analysis, and nucleic acid sequencing have allowed the recognition of related disease outbreaks over widespread geographic, temporal, and convoluted social terrain that would have been difficult to identify on epidemiologic evidence and analysis alone. This has been demonstrated in the recognition of common source multi-state and international foodborne disease outbreaks [53], tuberculosis outbreaks [54, 55], and in the surveillance of nosocomial infections [56, 57].

13.6 Information Dissemination and Communication

13.6.1 Appropriate Reporting of Information

Immediate notification of the proper authorities ("those who need to know") of surveillance information that indicates suspected bioterrorist-related disease is a principal function of the public health surveillance process. Notification and standard operating procedure (SOP) protocols must be clearly established and immediately available to not only those responsible for disseminating surveillance information but to backup personnel in the event regular personnel are unavailable. The protocols should clearly describe who is to be contacted and how for any given situation as well as a hierarchy of contacts if the main contact is inaccessible. Means for emergency and routine communication should be maintained and routinely tested to insure reliability. Recent advancements in communication technology, including the Internet, allow the instantaneous transfer of information, however this technology relies on communication systems that may be vulnerable to interference. Alternative communication channels should be established in lieu of disruption of regular channels during an emergency.

Surveillance information must be presented in a clear, understandable format developed for the recipient of that information. Surveillance information may be distributed to many different recipients with different functions and levels of understanding. Recipients may include physicians, hospital infection control or emergency departments, Office of Emergency Management (OEM) agencies, public health authorities, law enforcement agencies or mass media organizations. The surveillance information should be pertinent to the needs of the recipient so that they may better act on that information without confusion. Distilling data into charts and graphs can simplify and help clarify surveillance information; however, if done improperly the risk of transmission of misinformation is greatly increased. It is recommended that the public health agencies operating surveillance systems work closely with system users to develop methods of information transfer and presentation that are timely, consistent, clear and useful.

13.6.2 Feedback to Surveillance Participants

While prompt dissemination of surveillance information is imperative in any system designed to detect bioterrorist-related disease, the consistent delivery of surveillance information in a context that is useful to the participants and users of the surveillance system(s) is essential for sustainability. Participation in a surveillance system depends on consistent feedback of information to the system's users and the perception that the information is useful. A surveillance system in which data flows in one direction (e.g., little to no feedback to the systems reporters) will undoubtedly experience lack of reporter enthusiasm with resulting reporting delay as well as under-reporting. Timely feedback of information generated by the surveillance system to the reporting entities enhances the chances of reporter participation in the system. In Newark, the OSP epidemiologist in the NDHHS not only forwards the daily emergency department census and admission data to the NJDHSS but distributes the results of the local data analysis to the ICPs at the five participating local hospitals in individual and aggregate format on a weekly basis. The NJDHSS distributes aggregated data on a state and county level collected via the CDRSS through an e-mail list-serve to the state regional epidemiologists who then share the information with interested local parties.

13.6.3 Interorganizational Communications

Close personal communication between representatives of different entities or organizations that are involved in preparedness activities for terrorist events yields great benefits for public health surveillance performance. Within a month of September 11, 2001, the CDD of the NDHHS and the Department of Preventive Medicine and Community Health of the New Jersey Medical School (NJMS) began hosting what initially were Thursday evening sessions of interested public health parties discussing local and regional issues of public health preparedness and response to terrorist activities. Discussions have since included diverse topics of significant public health interest. Participants have included representatives from local hospitals, the New Jersey Medical School and UMDNJ School of Public Health, local Emergency Medical Services (EMS), the New Jersey Poison Information and Education System (NJPIES), healthcare payer organizations, the Port Authority of New Jersey and New York (PANJNY), and the Public Health Service Quarantine Service, among others. Topics have included exercises in specific scenarios (e.g., arrival of a passenger with suspected smallpox infection to Newark Liberty Airport), local public health SARS preparedness, and discussion of specific surveillance issues with respect to agents of bioterrorism, influenza, SARS, and vaccine-preventable diseases. The familiarity engendered during these serial sessions between the representatives of the various agencies has resulted in increased interorganizational cooperation in developing and maintaining improved surveillance communication.

As mentioned earlier, there is currently an effort to integrate the multiple public health data streams on the local, state, and national levels to facilitate early detection of public health issues and emergencies [21]. The Public Health Information Network is the framework in which this initiative is being developed. The alerts and communication component of PHIN is the Health Alert Network (HAN). The purpose of HAN is to ensure that all communities have 24/7 access to timely emergent public health information; the services of highly trained public health professionals; and evidence-based practices and procedures for effective public health preparedness, response, and service [21]. The objective is a seamless rapid alerts and communication system that connects the entire US public health infrastructure; from the local to the national. In New Jersey, HAN is accessed through the New Jersey Local Information and Communications System (NJLINCS) at the password-protected NJ HAN website [58]. Statewide information management resides in the NJDHSS while local management is governed by NJLINCS coordinators located at the county and selected city health departments. Access to the system requires registration through the local NJLINCS coordinators.

13.7 Confidentiality

Surveillance activity, especially on the local and state levels, often requires collection of personal identifying data. Subsequent investigation of infectious disease outbreaks cannot be carried out without person, place, and time data. In the event of bioterrorist activity, information sharing with law enforcement agencies will become necessary. Public health activities, including surveillance, are dependent on the public's acceptance and protecting the confidentiality of personal health information forms the basis of that trust between the public and the public health establishment.

The standard operating procedure (SOP) for surveillance systems must include provisions for maintaining confidentiality of personal health information and consideration of potential uses of data that contain personal identifiers [59], including sharing surveillance data with law enforcement agencies in the event of suspected bioterrorist activities. Protocols must be established restricting access to personal information as well as providing secure storage of data, whether electronic or paper based. Electronic and more traditional data transfer must be made secure and protected from saboteurs and computer hackers. Public health agencies should review the confidentiality and security provisions with all organizations or institutions they may share data with.

The Health Insurance Portability and Accountability Act (HIPAA) of 1996, which took affect April 14, 2003, provides the legal basis addressing the privacy and security of health information. The HIPAA Privacy Rule [60] continues to allow for the existing practice of sharing protected health information (PHI) with public health authorities authorized by law to collect or receive such information to aid them in their activities to protect the public's health. HIPAA requires the development and implementation of policies and procedures to protect the confidentiality and secure the security of personal health information as discussed in the previous paragraph.

13.8 Conclusion

Public health surveillance is an ongoing system of data collection, analysis and interpretation, and then dissemination of that information to those who will act upon it accordingly. It is within this framework, in close harmony with astute healthcare workers in clinical practice and laboratory personnel, that the consequences of an intentional release of a bioweapon will be recognized. This will occur either by direct observation (e.g., a report of a case of anthrax) or through detection of aberrant events (e.g., greater than expected occurrence of severe lower respiratory tract infections). Advances in information technology and the development of innovative surveillance methodology will augment their efforts. It is essential that adequate numbers of people are dedicated to these tasks and they receive the proper training to develop expertise in developing and maintaining surveillance systems with the flexibility to meet the dynamic demands of public health in an ever-changing society. This will only be accomplished through sustained public, political and financial commitment to rebuilding the public health infrastructure.

Information and communication technology has the potential of revolutionizing the practice of public health. They allow the development of novel methods of data reporting and collection, analysis, and dissemination. However the information technology industry has the potential of creating a huge financial drain on public health that may actually impede public health programs. As new methods are developed it is necessary they undergo critical evaluation as to their effectiveness. This can only be accomplished through a public health infrastructure populated with people who understand and are familiar with the intricacies of surveillance. The Institute of Medicine has identified the fragmentation of surveillance systems and lack of integration of public health data and information systems as a critical barrier to the timely flow of information in times of crisis [17]. These technologies provide the tools in which to integrate multiple programmatic public health surveillance and information systems from the local to federal level through the NEDSS initiative. However it is important to remember that those who use them will determine the ultimate value of these tools.

References

1. Thacker, S. B. and Berkelman, R. L. Public health surveillance in the United States. *Epidemiol. Rev.* 10, 164–190, 1988.
2. Thacker, S. B. Historical development. In: Teutsch, S. M. and Churchill, R. E. (eds) Principles and Practices of Public Health Surveillance, 2nd edition. New York: Oxford University Press, 1–18, 2000.
3. Teutsch, S. M. and Churchill, R. E. (eds). Principles and Practices of Public Health Surveillance, 2nd edition. New York: Oxford University Press, 2000.
4. Halperin, H. and Baker Jr., E. L. (eds). Public Health Surveillance. New York: Van Nostrand Reinhold, 1992.
5. Török, T. J., Tauxe, R. V., Wise, R. P., et al. A large community outbreak of salmonellosis caused by intentional contamination of restaurant salad bars. *J. Amer. Med. Assoc.* 278, 389–395, 1997.
6. Brachman, P. S. The public health response to the anthrax epidemic. In: Levy, B. S. and Sidel, V. W. (eds) Terrorism and the Public Health. New York: Oxford University Press, 101–117, 2003.
7. Okumura, T., Suzuki, K., Fukuda, A., et al. Tokyo subway sarin attack; disaster management, part 1: Community emergency response. *Acad. Emerg. Med.* 5, 613–617, 1998.
8. Centers for Disease Control and Prevention. Recognition of illness associated with the intentional release of a biologic agent. *Centers for Disease Control and Prevention*50, 893–897, 2001.
9. Institute of Medicine National Research Council. Intelligence, detection, surveillance, and diagnosis. In: Countering Bioterrorism: The Role of Science and Technology. Washington DC: The National Academies Press, 1–18, 2002.
10. Centers for Disease Control and Prevention. National notifiable disease surveillance system. Available at <http://www.cdc.gov/ncphi/disss/nndss/nndsshis.htm>. Accessed on January 22, 2008.
11. Teutsch, S. M. Considerations in planning a surveillance system. Appendix 2A. In: Teutsch, S. M. and Churchill, R. E. (eds) Principles and Practice of Public Health Surveillance, 2nd edition. New York: Oxford University Press, 27–29, 2000.
12. Chorba, T. L., Berkelman, R., Safford, S. K., et al. Mandatory reporting of infectious diseases by clinicians. *J. Amer. Med. Assoc.* 262, 3018–3026, 1989.
13. Council of State and Territorial Epidemiologists. Nationally notifiable disease surveillance system queriable database: NDSS assessment 2005: State and territorial reporting profiles. Available at <http://www.cste.org>. Accessed on January 22, 2008.
14. Council of State and Territorial Epidemiologists. Position statements 2003: smallpox surveillance (03-ID-03). Available at <http://www.cste.org>. Accessed on January 22, 2008.

15. Centers for Disease Control and Prevention. National electronic telecommunications system for surveillance. Available at <http://www.cdc.gov/ncphi/disss/nndss/netss.htm>. Accessed on January 23, 2008.
16. Centers for Disease Control and Prevention. National electronic telecommunications systems for surveillance-United States, 1990-1991. *MMWR – Morbid. Mortal. Week. Rep.* 40, 502–503, 1991.
17. Committee on Assuring the Health of the Public in the 21st Century. The governmental public health infrastructure. In: Institute of Medicine. The Future of the Public Health in the 21st Century. Washington DC, The National Academies Press, 96–177, 2003.
18. Centers for Disease Control and Prevention. Integrating public health information and surveillance systems. Available at <http://www.cdc.gov/nedss/Archive/katz.htm>. Assessed on January 23, 2008.
19. Centers for Disease Control and Prevention. National electronic disease surveillance system. Available at <http://ww.cdc.gov/nedss/>. Assessed on January 23, 2008.
20. Centers for Disease Control and Prevention. Supporting public health surveillance through the national electronic disease surveillance system. Available at <http://www.cdc.gov/nedss/Archive/Supporting_Public_health_Surv.pdf>. Accessed on January 23, 2008.
21. Centers for Disease Control and Prevention. Public health information network. Available at <http://www.cdc.gov/phin>. Accessed on January 23, 2008.
22. Centers for Disease Control and Prevention. National electronic disease surveillance system base system. Available at <http://www.cdc.gov/phin/activities/applications-services/nedess/nbs.html>. Accessed on January 21, 2008.
23. Centers for Disease Control and Prevention. Syndromic surveillance for bioterrorism following the attacks on the World Trade Center-New York City 2001. *MMWR – Morbid. Mortal. Week. Rep.* 52, 13–15, 2002.
24. Centers for Disease Control and Prevention. Update: Investigation of bioterrorism-related anthrax and adverse affects from antimicrobial prophylaxis. *MMWR – Morbid. Mortal. Week. Rep.* 50, 973–976, 2001.
25. Centers for Disease Control and Prevention. Notice to readers: Smallpox vaccine adverse events monitoring and response system for the first stage of the smallpox vaccination program. *MMWR – Morbid. Mortal. Week. Rep.* 52, 88–89, 99, 2003.
26. Centers for Disease Control and Prevention. Update: Adverse events following civilian smallpox vaccination-United States 2003. *MMWR – Morbid. Mortal. Week. Rep.* 52, 819–820, 2003.
27. Retailliau, H. F., Curtis, A. C., Starr, G., et al. Illness after influenza vaccination reported through a nationwide surveillance system, 1976–1977. *Am. J. Epidemiol.* 111, 270–278, 1980.
28. Pavlin, J. A., Kelley, P., Mostashari, F., et al. Innovative surveillance methods for monitoring dangerous pathogens. In: Knobler, S. L., Mahmoud, A. A. F. and Pray, L. A. (eds) Biological Threats and Terrorism: Assessing the Science and Response Capabilities: Workshop Summary. Washington DC: The National Academies Press, 185–196, 2002.
29. Conrad, J. L. and Pearson, J. L. Improving epidemiology, surveillance, and laboratory capabilities. In: Levy, B. S. and Sidel, V. W. (eds) Terrorism and the Public Health. New York: Oxford University Press, 270–285, 2003.
30. Centers for Disease Control and Prevention. Hepatitis A outbreak associated with green onions at a restaurant – Monaca, Pennsylvania, 2003. *MMWR – Morbid. Mortal. Week. Rep.* 52, 1155–1157, 2003.
31. Walsh, T. Pennsylvania reporting system speeds fight against hepatitis A, November 18, 2003. In: Government Computer News. Available at <http://www.gcn.com/Vol1_no1/daily-updates/24189-1.html>. Accessed on January 23, 2008.

32. Doyle, T. J., Glynn, K. M. and Groseclose, S. L. Completeness of notifiable disease reporting in the United States: An analytical literature review. *Am. J. Epidemiol.* 155, 866–874, 2002.
33. Hinds, M. W., Skaggs, J. W. and Bergeisen, G. H. Benefit-cost analysis of active surveillance of primary care physicians for hepatitis A. *Am. J. Public Health* 75, 176–177, 1985.
34. Tsui, F. -C., Espino, J. U., Dato, V. M., et al. Technical description of RODS: A real-time public health surveillance system. *J. Am. Med. Inform. Assoc.* 10, 399–408, 2003.
35. Lazarus, R., Kleinman, K., Dashevsky, I., et al. Use of automated ambulatory-care encounter records for detection of acute illness clusters, including potential bioterrorism events. *Emerg. Infect. Dis.* 8, 753–760, 2002.
36. US Department of Defense. Annual report, fiscal year 1999, Silver Spring (MD): Walter Reed Army Institute of Research; 1999.
37. Panackal, A. A., M'ikanatha, N. M., Tsui, F. -C., et al. Automatic electronic laboratory-based reporting of notifiable infectious diseases at a large health system. *Emerg. Infect. Dis.* 8, 685–691, 2002.
38. Effler, P., Ching-Lee, M., Bogard, A., et al. Statewide system of electronic notifiable disease reporting from clinical laboratories: comparing automated reporting with conventional methods. *JAMA – J. Amer. Med. Assoc.* 282, 845–850, 1999.
39. M'ikanatha, N. M., Southwell, B. and Lautenbach, E. Automated laboratory reporting of infectious diseases in a climate of bioterrorism. *Emerg. Infect. Dis.* 9, 1053–1057, 2003.
40. Espino, J. U. and Wagner, M. M. Accuracy of ICD-9-coded chief complaints and diagnoses for the detection of acute respiratory disease. *Proc. AMIA Symp.* PMIDI 11833477, 164–168, 2001. www.amia.org/pabs/proceedings/symposia/start.hmtl
41. Begier, E. M., Sockwell, D., Branch, L. M., et al. The national capitol region's emergency department syndromic surveillance system: do chief complaint and discharge diagnosis yield different results? *Emerg. Infect. Dis.* 9, 393–396, 2003.
42. Janes, G. R., Hutwanger, L., Cates Jr., W., et al. Descriptive epidemiology: Analyzing and interpreting surveillance data. In: Teutsch, S. M. and Churchill, R. E. (eds) Principles and Practice of Public Health Surveillance. 2nd edition. New York: Oxford University Press, 112–167, 2000.
43. Chang, M., Glynn, M. K. and Groseclose, S. L. Endemic, notifiable bioterrorism-related diseases, United States, 1992–1999. *Emerg. Infect. Dis.* 9, 556–564, 2001.
44. Rutstein, D. D., Berenberg, W., Chalmers, T. C., et al. Measuring the quality of medical care: A clinical method. *N. Engl. J. Med.* 294, 582–588, 1976.
45. Rutstein, D. D., Mullan, R. J., Frazier, T. M., et al. Sentinel health events (occupational): A basis for physician recognition and public health surveillance. *Am. J. Public Health.* 73, 1054–1062, 1983.
46. Alibek, K. and Handelman, S. Biohazard. New York: Random House, 1999.
47. Garrett, L. Betrayal of Trust: The Collapse of Global Public Health. New York: Hyperion Press, 2000.
48. Miller, J., Engelberg, S. and Broad, W. Germs: Biological Weapons and America's Secret War. New York: Simon and Schuster, 2001.
49. Last, J. M. A Dictionary of Epidemiology. 4th edition. Oxford: Oxford University Press, 2001.
50. Lewis, M. D., Pavlin, J. A., Mansfield, J. L., et al. Disease outbreak detection system using syndromic surveillance data in the greater Washington DC area. *Am. J. Prev. Med.* 23, 180–186, 2002.
51. Stroup, D. F., Wharton, M., Kafadar, K., et al. Evaluation of a method for detecting aberrations in public health surveillance. *Am. J. Epidemiol.* 137, 373–380, 1993.
52. Mullan, F. Plagues and Politics: The Story of the United States Public Health Service. New York: Basic Books, Inc., 1989

53. Mahon, B. E., Pönkä, A., Hall, W. N., et al. An international outbreak of *Salmonella* infections caused by alfalfa sprouts grown from contaminated seeds. *J. Infect. Dis.* 175, 876–882, 1997.
54. Bifani, P. J., Mathema, B., Liu, Z., et al. Identification of a W variant outbreak of *Mycobacterium tuberculosis* via population-based molecular epidemiology. *J. Amer. Med. Assoc.* 282, 2321–2327, 1999.
55. Small, P. M., Hopewell, P. C., Singh, S. P., et al. The epidemiology of tuberculosis in San Francisco – a population-based study using conventional and molecular methods. *N. Engl. J. Med.* 330, 1703–1709, 1994.
56. Roberts, R. B., de Lencastre, A., Eisner, W., et al. Molecular epidemiology of methicillin-resistant *Staphylococcus aureus* in 12 New York hospitals. MRSA Collaborative Study Group. *J. Infect. Dis.* 178, 164–171, 1998.
57. de Lencastre, H., Severina, E. P., Roberts, R. B., et al. Testing the efficacy of a molecular surveillance network: Methicillin-resistant *Staphylococcus aureus*(MRSA) and vancomycin-resistant *Enterococcus faecium* (VREF) genotypes in six hospitals in the metropolitan New York City area. The BARG Initiative Pilot Study Group. Bacterial Antibiotic Resistance Group. *Microb. Drug Resist.* 2, 343–351, 1996.
58. New Jersey Health Alert Network. Available at <http://njlincs.net>. Accessed on January 23, 2008.
59. Snider, D. E. and Stroup, D. Ethical issues. In: Teutsch, S. M. and Churchill, R. E. (eds) Principles and Practices of Public Health Surveillance. 2nd edition. New York: Oxford University Press, 194–214, 2000.
60. Centers for Disease Control and Prevention. HIPAA Privacy Rule and Public Health. *MMWR – Morbid. Mortal. Week. Rep.* 52, 1–12, 2003.

Chapter 14
Psychosocial Management of Bioterrorism Events

David M. Benedek and Thomas A. Grieger

14.1 Introduction

In addition to producing significant toxic and infectious morbidity, a bioterrorist attack will cause widespread social, behavioral, and psychiatric effects. Psychosocial casualties are likely to appear in large numbers in hospital emergency departments or other treatment facilities immediately after learning of an incident creating major challenges for even healthcare facilities with excellent resources [1]. These casualties may continue to present in the months and even years following the event. Beyond those directly exposed to biological agents, emergency responders, other caregivers, relatives and friends of casualties, children and other subpopulations are at substantial risk of developing emotional and behavioral reactions or disorders [2].

Although the healthcare system in the United States is increasingly aware of the potentially devastating effects of bioterrorism, it has not yet had to manage mass casualty situations resulting from biological weapons. The principles of emergency mental health management of bioterrorism events must, therefore, be extrapolated from the available knowledge of the social, neuropsychiatric and behavioral effects of industrial accidents involving toxic exposures, other (non-biological) types of terrorism incidents, natural disasters, and infectious disease outbreaks [3]. Consideration of the experiences of other nations following chemical weapons incidents, knowledge gained during exercises that simulate attacks, and observations of responses to bioterrorism hoaxes can be used to increase understanding and institute preparatory measures.

D.M. Benedek
Associate Professor of Psychiatry, Center for the Study of Traumatic Stress,
Uniformed Services University, Bethesda, MD, USA
e-mail: dbenedek@usuhs.mil

L.I. Lutwick, S.M. Lutwick (eds.), *Beyond Anthrax*,
DOI: 10.1007/978-1-59745-326-4_14, © Springer Science+Business Media, LLC 2008

14.2 Primary and Secondary Prevention

The September 11, 2001 terror attacks on the World Trade Center and the Pentagon dramatically taught Americans painful lessons about the effects of international terrorist activity within their borders. The atrocities considerably reduced the state of denial in most U.S. communities regarding the potential for terrorism and alerted Americans to the specific threat of bioterrorism. Epidemiological studies in the aftermath of these attacks [4] demonstrated increased incidence of mood and anxiety disorders, particularly at the epicenters of the attacks, but also elevated levels of fear, worry, and anger throughout the nation [5, 6].

The emotional consequences of an event are strongly influenced by the manner in which the event is anticipated. While widespread denial has diminished in the aftermath of September 11, bioterrorism remains, to many, incomprehensible. The invisibility of biological agents and the insidious onset of their effects make them especially frightening. Most people, including medical practitioners, would still prefer not to contemplate the nature and extent of destruction that could be caused by a bioterrorism event. The emergency medical personnel and community leaders who will first respond to such an attack will be confronted simultaneously with the consequences of denial, lack of resources, and a profoundly injured sense of fairness and community norms. Without training and preparation, the flexibility, adaptability and decision-making skills critical to effective response may be difficult to mobilize in an atmosphere dominated by feelings of rage, fear, and helplessness.

14.2.1 Primary Prevention

A lack of emotional preparedness would make chaos and disorder more likely after a bioterrorist attack [7]. Primary prevention, therefore, must begin with realistic understanding of the threat, followed by the development of a planned response, the practice (and re-practice) of that response, and the provision of appropriate funding and logistical facilities in support of the plan [8]. These efforts facilitate primary prevention by mitigating a community's sense of helplessness well before an attack ever occurs.

14.2.2 Secondary Prevention

Bioterrorist attacks are likely to create acute, subacute and chronic mental health effects. Most victims will have friends and relatives in the community. An unfortunate outcome for any given patient has consequences for all those with whom the patient is socially joined. When deaths occur, the emotions and psychophysiological changes associated with bereavement may be added to effects elicited by the attack itself even for those who are geographically removed from the event itself [8–10].

Secondary prevention of psychosocial consequences begins at the point of initial triage and treatment. First responders, pre-medical care personnel, and mental health treatment providers must be prepared to provide some level of treatment for individuals with acute (and most often transient) emotional and behavioral disorganization or other symptoms, and monitor members of the population for more protracted symptoms or syndromes. Although emergency medical technicians, paramedics, and police are likely first responders to traditional terrorist attacks (e.g. bombings), emergency room physicians and nurses, epidemiologists, infection control personnel, and infectious disease physicians are likely to be intimately involved with first-response to bioterrorism. For persons developing transient symptoms, these response managers may facilitate recovery by creating a location or locations where symptoms can be observed and monitored sufficiently removed from high tempo triage activity but close enough to permit return for re-evaluation should symptoms worsen. This "holding environment" favors social and psychological recovery.

The purpose of a terrorist attack is to produce terror by creating a sense of chaos. With bioterrorism, this is accomplished through acute disruption of social order and societal expectations regarding accessible and effective medical care. Creating an environment in which emotionally and/or behaviorally disorganized individuals are afforded protection from chaotic conditions created by the attack is one way leaders can contribute to the psychosocial recovery and health of the community as a whole.

Because of the likelihood of numerous acute, subacute, and chronic neuropsychiatric effects, mental health treatment and rehabilitative services (tertiary preventive resources) within the community will ultimately be needed to address psychosocial consequences. These services, including Red Cross disaster assistance, community mental health centers, social workers, home nurses and hospice care providers should be an integral part of bioterrorism response planning and training. The use of these resources can promote adequate care for those suffering psychosocial impacts while emergency and primary care personnel are addressing the life-threatening consequences created by the attack [11]. Combined with the development of an intelligence and information system, a thoroughly rehearsed response plan that provides for effective triage and initial treatment and incorporates community resources beyond the emergency room are measures that decrease community disruption.

14.3 Bioterrorism and Phases of the Traumatic Stress Response

The traumatic stress response has often been divided into four phases. The first phase immediately following (or during) a disaster is characterized by strong emotions including feelings of disbelief, numbness, fear, and confusion associated with high levels of arousal. In the second phase, adaptation to environmental changes as well as intrusive symptoms (unbidden thoughts or recollections of the event accompanied by symptoms of hyperarousal, such as an abnormal startle response) frequently occur. This phase usually last from 1 week to several months. Somatic symptoms such as dizziness, headache, and fatigue, and nausea may also develop here. The third phase is notable primarily for feelings of disappointment and resentment when initial hopes for aid and restoration are not met. The final phase, reconstruction, may last for years. During this phase, survivors rebuild their lives, reestablishing occupational and social identities [3, 12, 13].

Since individuals progress through these phases at variable rates, medical managers must realize that persons can manifest emotional symptoms over different timelines in response to a single event or attack. Moreover, depending upon the severity of trauma, the community's capacity to retain its social organization during response, resources available during the event, and individual coping skills within members of community, varying numbers of the affected population will develop persistent symptoms requiring tertiary treatment.

Microbial and viral agents are invisible and odorless. Exposure, therefore, occurs in the absence of a warning signal. Once suspected, the separation of the infected from the non-infected is likely to require the use of expert evaluation and tests. The uncertainty created by a lack of warning, variability of exposure and incubation period, and the potential use of multiple agents may evoke even a more potent stress response. Terrorists, knowing that these agents are colorless, odorless, and variable in the symptoms they produce, may claim to deploy one agent while in reality deploying a different agent or agents.

Specific agents may also produce pathological consequences or lesions that intensify the stress response. For example, as a viral hemorrhagic fever or a case of smallpox progresses, grotesqueries are produced that generate revulsion and horror. When observed by people naïve to the physical consequences of these illnesses, lasting mental images are created which may be re-experienced in the form of unwelcome intrusive recollections ("flashbacks"). Alternatively, the reaction may be generalized to include fantasies of one's own tortured disfigurement or death [14]. The impact of observing medical grotesqueries has been noted to produce post-traumatic symptoms in children [15], and may generate symptoms in adults. Sick children constitute an especially stressful set of patients. Furthermore, a large influx of very young patients will require mental health staff to have in place specialized treatment and educational materials as well as protocols that are appropriate for assisting children.

14.4 Psychiatric Syndromes and Behavioral Changes in the Aftermath of Bioterrorism

14.4.1 Initial Behavioral Changes

The state of autonomic arousal associated with fear or anxiety precipitates various somatic symptoms. Although signs and symptoms may result from the direct effects of exposure to specific biological agents, it is important to note that very similar symptoms and somatic complaints can occur in individuals neither exposed nor secondarily infected as a consequence of the attack. Some individuals will attribute rapid heart rate, shivering, muscle aches, and shortness of breath (e.g. symptoms of anxiety) to exposure to a toxic agent [16, 17], presenting to care providers for post-exposure treatment upon learning that an attack has occurred.

As stress symptoms can mimic the symptoms of actual exposure to an agent or agents, one challenge for emergency triage workers will be distinguishing between symptoms resulting from direct exposure and those resulting from fear or anxiety. Since both exposed and unexposed persons will seek treatment over time, an understanding of the emotional and behavioral responses (termed the traumatic stress response) to disaster or crisis is as critical to appropriate triage as an understanding of the specific effects of biological agents.

The clinical emotional and behavioral consequences of trauma stem from a combination of social, autonomic and voluntary mechanisms only now being clarified or understood at the molecular level. In the immediate phase, the release of corticotrophin releasing factor (CRF) causing the secretion of adrenocorticotrophin hormone (ACTH), the surge of peripheral catecholamines and activation of brain areas related to perception of threat rapidly follow exposure to extremes of environmental stress. Behavior and cognitive changes correlate with these noradrenergic phenomena [18].

Generally, the immediate impact of acute stress is improved alertness and performance. As preparation and capacity to act in response become inadequate to meet increasing demands, however, the risk of performance and cognitive dysfunction increases. Behavior and thinking may then become overly goal directed, being narrowly focused. Unfortunately, this aroused but focused state results in difficulty shifting goals, scanning alternatives, and changing plans of action [16]. Extreme distress may indeed disrupt cognition to the point of creating chaotic thinking. During these social circumstances the over-focused responses of either flight or immobility may occur. When this response is communicated to others in the immediate social environment, social panic may result [19].

The development of massive group panic is unlikely as pro-social behavior has been the norm after most disasters. In the situation created by bioterrorist attack, however, medical managers must be sensitive to the idea that community leadership will be faced with inadequate resources, inadequate personnel and inadequate experience. These factors, especially when combined, could precipitate maladaptive group panic. Prevention of group or social panic within leaders and medical responders is accomplished by mitigating the impact of these factors. Insuring resource accessibility, planning and over-training with regard to response algorithms are critical to this endeavor. Even without group panic, more common responses of scapegoating or paranoia may still detract from the overall response effort. It is not uncommon for people perceived to have been infected by an invisible agent to be viewed by others with fear or hostility. Stigma and discrimination, for example, have been seen after chemical and radiological incidents and in the aftermath of disease outbreaks [20, 21].

14.4.2 Acute Stress Disease and Posttraumatic Stress Disorder

The immediate alarm response is followed by a cascade of neuronal and intercellular events leading to elevated levels of CRF, increased synthesis of cortisol-related receptors, and activation of protein synthesis in subcortical nuclei of the amygdala responsible for the development of emotionally laden memories (conditioned responses and habits). Hypersecretion of epinephrine also appears to exaggerate and consolidate fear related memories of events. Increased neuronal synthetic activity (neuroplasticity) may play a role in the development of an exaggerated startle response, intrusive thoughts, and low thresholds to autonomic arousal observed in disorders such as Acute Stress Disorder (ASD) and Posttraumatic Stress Disorder (PTSD) [18, 20, 22].

It is less clear how this cascade of neuronal activity relates to social withdrawal also seen individuals with ASD or PTSD. Social withdrawal is a major contributor to the pathological consequences of traumatic experience. One factor that seems to mitigate the psychopathologic effects of these changes is the availability of social supports and a supportive healing environment. The increased neuroplasticity immediately following the recognition of a threat may be indicative of an opportunity for cognitive shift and provide a rationale for rapid psychotherapeutic or pharmacological intervention after a traumatic event. Empirical data to date have not, however, supported the efficacy of such interventions in asymptomatic or pre-symptomatic populations.

The majority of the affected population, whether directly exposed or simply fearing exposure, does not develop either ASD or PTSD. There appear to be early psychological markers for those who may subsequently develop these illnesses. Two studies examined peritraumatic dissociation following terrorist events. These studies have implications for the process of identifying persons at greater risk and for predicting the response of medical personnel in the immediate aftermath of an attack. The first study examined Naval personnel at the Pentagon following the terrorist attack on the Pentagon on September 11, 2001. This population was surveyed 7 months following the event [23]. The second study examined a hospital staff following a 3-week series of random sniper shootings with 10 individuals killed in the Washington, DC area in October 2002 [24]. This population was sampled during the 2-week period that began 5 days after the apprehension of the suspected snipers. The Pentagon staff was assessed with the full version (ten questions) of the Peritraumatic Dissociative Experiences Scale [25] for the period of the attack and an assessment scale for PTSD at the time of the 7-month survey. A high level of peritraumatic dissociation at the time of the event was strongly associated with PTSD 7 months later. An abbreviated scale using the first five items of the 10 item scale was used in the hospital staff sample. A high level of dissociation on this scale was also associated with ASD in this sample (6% of total sample). Higher levels of dissociation were also found in those who reported symptoms consistent with major depression. The association between dissociative phenomena, ASD, and PTSD and the high degree of comorbidity between the disorders suggests a link between difficulty in cognitive processing of the situation at the time of the event and subsequent psychiatric illness.

The hospital staff sample was also assessed with an instrument that measured the degree of perceived safety in routine activities and changes in the number of routine activities altered due to the sniper attacks. Those with ASD reported a nearly two-fold number of reduced activities compared to those who did not meet criteria for ASD [25]. The healthcare workers in this study were not, themselves, directly attacked by the snipers, nor was their actual risk of being shot increased from the relatively low day-to-day risk of meeting with violence in their community. The "exposure" was a consequence of living in the community where attacks occurred and of the media coverage surrounding the event. The emotional and behavioral response to perceived (rather than actual) danger is similar to what may occur in the aftermath of a bioterrorist attack where perceived risk may be considerably greater than actual exposure. Behavioral changes on the part of medical responders in this study, therefore, must be considered in planning for medical response to bioterrorism. During such an event, a proportion of anticipated healthcare responders may substantially modify their behavior patterns (possibly choosing to not come to work) as a result of their perception of risks to themselves or family members as a result of possible exposure in transit to or at work.

14.5 Therapeutic Interventions

14.5.1 Effect of Biological Agents and Therapeutic Responses

Symptoms ranging from lethargy and depression to disorientation, dissociation, depersonalization, hallucinations, paranoia, and cognitive slowing (Table 14.1) have been linked to the direct neurotoxic effects of various biological agents [26, 27]. If available, early medical treatment of those accurately diagnosed as suffering the effects of true exposure or infection should reduce the direct neurotoxic effects of the agent. Those who recover from direct exposure or secondary infection, however, remain at significant risk for the subsequent development of psychological symptoms. Continued surveillance will assist in directing additional psychosocial or psychiatric interventions in this group.

Antipsychotic and anxiolytic medications used in the acute management of delirium due to other etiologies are effective in infectious causes as well. Dose-related side effects of the antipsychotics (such as agitation or somnolence) may be mistaken for primary symptoms of an infectious encephalopathy. Use of the

Table 14.1 Neuropsychiatric syndromes and symptoms with selected biological agents

Biological agent	Syndrome or symptom(s)	Comment
Anthrax	Meningitis, anxiety, confusion	May be rapidly progressive; associated with pulmonary symptoms
Brucellosis	Depression, irritability, headaches	Fatalities associated with CNS involvement
Q fever	Malaise, fatigue, encephalitis, hallucinations	Occurs in 1/3 of patients in advanced cases
Botulinum toxin	Depression, mental status changes, paralysis may be confused with conversion disorder	Associated with lengthy recovery/disability
Viral encephalitides	Depression, cognitive impairment	Other mood changes also reported
All biological agents	Delirium	Acutely impaired attention, memory, and perceptual disturbances

phenothiazines as antiemetic or antipsychotic medications may result in pseudo-parkinsonism or akethisia (fidgeting), or other basal and such disturbances are difficult to interpret and manage in these circumstances. Care must be taken as well to avoid drug/drug interactions between medications that can affect the metabolism and subsequent blood levels of the therapeutic agents. A conservative approach that minimizes the use of psychotropic medications is indicated, therefore, although these medications are helpful in controlling behavior when such control is clinically critical.

14.5.2 Use of Separate Location for Psychiatric Treatment

Within hospitals or other institutions serving as entry points for care, once the need for anti-infectious or other medical treatment measures has been identified and initiated, establishing a location, nearby but separate from the chaos of initial triage and treatment where persons with psychological symptoms can receive respite is appropriate. At this site, clinician or patient-administered screening instruments [28–30] may be utilized to identify persons for whom further follow-up over time may be beneficial. More severe anxiety and mood disorders may not be manifest immediately but may evolve over ensuing weeks. Screening instruments, therefore, if they include patient identification and contact information, may be the most effective tools for tracking this population after discharge from initial care.

Assignment to this location should be accompanied by the reassurance that stress symptoms are normal, predictable and generally transient. Persons here should be informed that such symptoms are not necessarily a harbinger of further somatic symptoms or even a sign of exposure. Many of the initial psychological symptoms associated with trauma will respond to these measures alone. However, symptom based treatment for persistent agitation or insomnia is appropriate [1, 16, 17]. Even though stores of psychotropic medications are less likely to be depleted than those of vaccines or antibiotics, triage, followed by an opportunity for holding and observation will ensure that available pharmacological resources are used only as necessary. This requirement must be balanced against the advantages of rapidly discharging patients from the treatment facility. Caregivers on site, with appropriate guidance from public health and disaster mental health specialists, are best equipped to make decisions about this trade off.

14.5.3 Interventions

Although group debriefing techniques and critical incident debriefings have often been used in the aftermath of natural disasters, school shootings, and terrorist events, there is no convincing evidence that such debriefings reduce the development of psychiatric illness or prevent the development of PTSD [31–33]. Discussions among care providers and emergency responders during the management of an event (situational reports) foster cohesion and group understanding of the unfolding event. These may serve to sustain the performance of persons critical to the management of the event, decrease individual isolation and stigma, and facilitate identification of care team members who may require further mental health attention [16].

Evidence from clinical trials suggests that cognitive behavioral therapy may be valuable. Cognitive behavioral therapy involves education about the nature and universality of symptoms, examination of the precipitants of symptoms (particularly cognitive distortions), and development of reframing and interpretive techniques to minimize further symptoms. Clinical trials for depression, anxiety, ASD and PTSD suggest that even brief therapeutic interventions of this nature may reduce immediate symptoms and diminish the development of long term morbidity [34, 35]. More recent, randomized controlled trials suggest that pharmacotherapy (particularly with selective serotonin re-uptake inhibitors) is effective in reducing posttraumatic symptoms [36, 37]. While much of the initial emotional response may resolve without such intervention, it is important to note that delay in instituting mental health diagnosis and treatment may increase long term morbidity [34–37]. Ensuring availability of individuals trained in assessment and the delivery of treatment for these disorders is therefore critical.

14.6 Appraisal, Attribution, Risk Communication, and the Media

Beyond problems encountered within the emergency room, outreach to the public at large is central to mitigating community attribution and perception of the crisis. A public information plan must include efforts to inform and prepare the public to interpret the nature of the attack and to understand and carry out measures to protect selves, loved ones, and others. Such information campaigns must address the concerns of the public as well as the concerns of caregivers. In mass casualty situations, it is important to remember that loved ones may include pets [38, 39]. It is critical that the information provided be truthful even if it is bad news. If public information programs are discovered to be providing intentionally incorrect information, credibility for the program is lost.

The responsibility for developing public information plans does not rest with emergency and medical care professionals. However, medical and behavioral health personnel should participate in development of these plans since they will have a role in implementation as the message will influence what the community expects from healthcare providers. Robust systems must be in place for dissemination of information during and following the attack. Resilience (and redundancy) of these systems must be tested in advance. Medical personnel should be to deliver consistent and updated information to and through the media. Information from official and unofficial sources prior to, during, and after the terrorist event will shape patients' expectations, behaviors and emotional responses [39]. Rumors may confound information campaigns and lead unexposed persons to seek emergency treatment for various somatic symptoms or for vaccinations or medications. If medical responders accept or perpetuate such rumors, enormous effort and precious resources may be wasted.

It is critical that emergency personnel including physicians acquire access to a secure communication network that connects providers to agencies managing the overall community response, laboratories supporting the medical/epidemiological effort, and the logistical structure that provides personnel, equipment, medications, and vaccines. The delivery of consistent, updated information across multiple channels, via widely recognized and trusted sources will diminish the extent that misinformation shapes public attribution [39, 40]. Clinical personnel should also plan and train for the appearance of media at triage and treatment sites. The media response at these sites may be critical in letting the public know who needs to be examined and which symptoms should prompt urgent attention. Trusted media representatives may serve an important link to the community function by delivering simple, salient, and repeated messages regarding matters of concern if these messages accurately educate the public concerning the nature of the threat, how to act to avoid harm and how to get help. The delivery of practical and reliable information is critical to the development of atmosphere of calmness and hope, and fosters a sense of community and self-efficacy. These elements of calmness, hope, efficacy, along with the establishment of safety (e.g., via prevention, holding environments, and treatment) and the maintenance of social support systems constitute critical elements of immediate and mid-term intervention in the aftermath of incidents of mass violence [41].

14.7 Planning for Mental Health Response

A mass casualty situation occurs when there is a mismatch between demand for and availability of resources. A bioterrorist attack clearly has the potential to create such a situation. Internal debates that develop over allocation of scarce resources once an attack is recognized delay response time and decrease the collaborative response process. This may create demoralization, despair, and reduced confidence in care providers that is subsequently transmitted to the community as a whole. Prevention of demoralization or despair, and lost confidence are most important aspects of the mental health response to terrorism since community disruption and reduced sense of community support are indeed fundamental goals of terrorists.

Realistic plans and exercises must respond to predictable challenges within the parameters afforded by available resources. Medical responders must be practice dealing with many people who seek care although not exposed to the infectious pathogen(s) or toxin(s), and practice assessing and treating such people efficiently and with respect. That unexposed individuals will seek care in great numbers is illustrated by data from the 1995 sarin chemical attack in Tokyo, where the number of individuals presenting to medical authorities with complaints of post-exposure symptoms exceeded the number who required medical treatment due to exposure by a ratio of 4:1 [26].

In the social domain, specific measures to inform individuals about who should seek medical evaluation and care are vital. Successful communication of this message may help reduce the load at the medical triage sites. At emergency triage sites, rapid medical evaluation, treatment, and institution of infection control procedures must be efficiently and effectively implemented. The establishment of holding facilities that provides a recovery environment for those who cannot be immediately sent home is also important. Public health agencies must play an active role in providing community infectious disease control. Such actions will provide a sense of safety and restoration of health to the community as a whole. This sense is critical to the mobilization of any positive psychological and supportive social response within the community.

Of primary importance during initial medical response to a bioterrorist attack is the identification of persons and greatest risk for the development of protracted or more severe psychological symptoms over time. Responders must be aware that, irregardless of population based preventive or psycho-educational efforts, individual factors will determine to a great degree the posttraumatic sequela in any individual. The level of psychological function in the aftermath of trauma is directly related to pre-trauma functioning. Individuals who demonstrate marginal social or occupational performance prior to a disaster are at increased risk, regardless of community preparedness. Persons who have experienced and overcome past traumatic experiences may be more resilient to future traumatic insults. However, if past experiences have resulted in the development of PTSD or other significant symptoms of psychiatric distress, subsequent traumatic exposure may increase the likelihood and severity of future episodes of illness.

Emergency and primary care physicians as well as rescue personnel will be at greater risk as a consequence of biological attack. They will be required to take on the role of first responder both in terms of recognizing the potential problem and responding to the needs of the mass causalities. Even if performing well, they may have to deal with high personal risk and numerous deaths among their patients. This is particularly stressful if these patients are children. It may be difficult for medical professionals who are success-oriented by training to deal with an unavoidable sense of failure in this situation. Provision of psychosocial supports for this group, including appropriate work/rest scheduling, visible and accessible leadership, support groups and early therapeutic intervention, may permit these persons to recognize that their very disturbing emotional responses are normal [42]. Even with such provisions in place, planners must recognize that some charged with the responsibility of managing medical triage and treatment may not respond as rehearsed as a consequence of their own perception of threat.

A final factor distinguishing the overall medical response to a bioterrorist event from either a natural disaster or other even a terrorist bomb detonation may be the need for quarantine or other isolative measures to prevent further infection once the deployment of a biological agent is confirmed. A most recent model for potential impact bioterrorist act is the outbreak of severe acute respiratory syndrome (SARS) in Southeastern Asia and Canada. As would be the case with bioterrorism, the nature of the causative agent, the vector of transmission, and the incubation period were all unknown initially. The only effective preventive measures were quarantine and implementation of hospital precautionary measures. Without a clearer understanding of the illness, it was difficult to determine who should be quarantined and for what period of time. There were no effective antimicrobial treatments and no effective prophylactic treatments for those at risk, including healthcare workers caring for other individuals exposed to the agent. The degree of longstanding impact from this epidemic is difficult to measure, but "secondary" illnesses such as depression relating to the personal and economic impact of the outbreak have already been encountered. Should extensive quarantine be necessary due to bioterrorism, the establishment of a supportive recovery environment will require that reassurance and understandable information about expected symptoms (both physical and emotional), plans for delivery of care and containment approaches are transmitted via a variety of channels to homes, offices, schools, and hospitals wherever triage, treatment, and containment efforts are occurring.

14.8 Summary

Although now more aware of the potential for bioterrorism, the United States has not suffered significant psychosocial or medical consequences from the use of biological weapons within its territories. This has contributed to a "natural" state of denial at the community level. Continued denial will amplify the sense of crisis, anxiety, fear, chaos, and disorder that accompany a bioterrorist event. A key part of primary prevention involves counteracting this possibility before an incident occurs. Doing so will require realistic information regarding the bioterrorism threat followed by the development of a planned response and regular practice of that response.

Unlike natural disasters or other situations resulting in mass casualties, emergency department physicians or nurses and primary care physicians (working in concert with epidemiological agencies), rather than police, firemen, or ambulance personnel, will be most likely to first identify the unfolding disaster associated with a biological attack. This group of medical responders must be aware of its own susceptibility to mental health sequela and performance decrement as the increasing demands of disaster response outpace the availability of necessary resources.

A bioterrorist attack will necessitate treatment of casualties who experience neuropsychiatric symptoms and syndromes. Symptoms may result from exposure to infection with specific biological agents, but similar symptoms may result from the mere perception of exposure or arousal precipitated by fear of infection, disease, suffering and death. Conservative use of psychotropic medications may reduce symptoms in exposed and uninfected individuals, as may cognitive-behavioral interventions. Clear, consistent, accessible, reliable, and redundant information (received from trusted sources) will diminish public uncertainty about the cause of symptoms that might otherwise prompt persons to seek unnecessary treatment. Training and preparation for contingencies experienced in an attack has the potential to enhance delivery of care. Initiating supportive social, psychotherapeutic and psychopharmacological treatments judiciously for symptoms and syndromes known to accompany the traumatic stress response can aid the efficient treatment of some patients and reduce long-term morbidity in affected individuals. Preventive strategies and planning must take into account the idea that specific groups including emergency health care providers and community leaders within the population are at higher risk for psychiatric morbidity. These and other high-risk groups will benefit from the same supportive interventions developed for the community as a whole.

References

1. Hurwitz S, Bergeron N and Benedek DM. Chapter 12: acute psychiatric issues. In McFee RB and Keikin JB, eds. Toxico-Terrorism: Emergency Response and Clinical Approach to Chemical, Biological, and Radiological Agents. New York: McGgraw Hill Medical, 2008, pp 101–108.
2. Becker SM. Are psychosocial aspects of WMD incidents addressed in the federal response plan? *Mil. Med.* 166, 66–68, 2001.
3. Norwood AE, Ursano RJ and Fullerton CS. Disaster psychiatry: principles and practice. *Psychiatr. Quart.* 71, 207–227, 2000.

4. Shuster MA, Stein BD, Jaycox LH, et al. A national survey of stress reactions after the September 11, 2001, terrorist attack. *N. Engl. J. Med.* 345, 1507–1512, 2001.
5. Galea S, Ahern J, Resnick H, et al. Psychological sequelae of the September 11th terrorist attacks in New York City. *NEJM* 346, 982–987, 2002.
6. Schlenger WE, Caddell JM, Ebert L, et al. Psychological retins to terrorist attacks: findings from the national Study of Americans' reactions to September 11. *JAMA,* 288, 581–588, 2002.
7. Lerner M. The Belief in a Just World: A Fundamental Delusion. NY: Plenum Press, 1980.
8. Ursano RJ, Fullerton CS and Norwood AE. Psychiatric dimensions of disaster: patient care, community consultation, and preventive medicine. *Harv. Rev. Psychiatry.* 3, 196–209, 1995.
9. Prigerson HG, Shear MK, Jacobs S, Kasl SV, Maciejewski PK, Silverman GK, Narayan GK, Narayan M and Bremner JD. Grief and its relationship to posttraumatic stress disorder. In Nutt D, Davidson JR and Zohar J, eds. Posttraumatic Stress Disorders: Diagnosis, Management and Treatment. New York, NY: Martin Dunitz Publishers, 2000, pp 163–177.
10. Neria Y, Gross R, Litz B, et al. Prevalence and psychological correlates of complicated grief among bereaved adults after September 11th attacks. *J. Trauma Stress* 20, 251–262, 2007b.
11. Call JA and Pfefferbaum B. Lessons from the first two years of project heartland, Oklahoma's mental health response to the 1995 Bombing. *Psychiatr. Serv.* 50, 953–955, 1999.
12. Lystad M. Perspectives on human response to mass emergencies. In Lystad M, ed. Mental Health Response to Mass Emergencies. New York: Brunner/Mazel, 1998, pp xvii–xviii.
13. Norwood AE and Ursano RJ. Psychiatric intervention in post-disaster recovery. *Dir. Psychiatry* 17, 247–262, 1997.
14. Ursano RJ and McCarroll JE. Exposure to traumatic death: the nature of the stressor, In Ursano RJ, McCaughey BG and Fullerton CS, eds. Individual and Community Response to Trauma and Disaster. New York: Cambridge University Press, 1994, pp 46–71.
15. Shaw JA. Children, adolescents and trauma. *Psychiatr. Quart.* 71, 227–243, 2000.
16. Holloway HC and Benedek DM. The changing face of terrorism and military psychiatry. *Psychiatr. Ann.* 29, 363–374, 1999.
17. Carmeli A, Liberman N and Mevorach L. Anxiety-related somatic reactions during missile attacks. *Isr. J. Med. Sci.* 27, 677–680, 1991.
18. Shalev AY. Biological responses to disasters. *Psychiatr. Quart.* 71, 277–288, 2000.
19. Sime JD. The Concept of Panic. London: David Fulton Publisher, Ltd., 1990.
20. Solomon EP and Heide KM. The Biology trauma: implications for treatment. *J. Interpers. Violence* 20, 51–60, 2005.
21. Becker SM. Meeting the threat of weapons of mass destruction terrorism: toward a broader conception of consequence management. *Mil. Med.* 166, 13–16. 2001.
22. Becker SM. Psychosocial effects of radiation accidents. In Gusev A, Guskova FA and Mettler JR, eds. Medical Management of Radiation Accidents, I. 2nd edition, Boca Raton: CRC Press, 2001, pp 54–69.
23. Grieger TA, Fullerton CS and Ursano RJ. Post-traumatic stress disorder, alcohol use, and safety after the terrorist attack on the Pentagon. *Psychiatr. Serv.* 54, 1380–1383, 2003.
24. Grieger TA, Fullerton CS, Ursano RJ and Reeves JJ. Acute stress disorder, alcohol use, and perception of safety among hospital staff after the sniper attacks, *Psychiatr. Serv.* 54, 1383–1387, 2003.
25. Marmar CR, Weiss DS and Metzer TJ. The peritraumatic dissociative experiences questionnaire. In Wilson JP and Keane TM, eds. Assessing Psychological Trauma and PTSD. New York: Guillford, 1997, pp 67–78.
26. DiGiovanni C Jr. Domestic terrorism with chemical or biological agents: psychiatric aspects. *Am. J. Psychiatry.* 15, 1500–1505, 1999.

27. Franz DR, Jahrling PB, Friedlander AM, et al. Clinical recognition and management of patients exposed to biological warfare agents. *J. Amer. Med. Assoc.* 278, 399–411, 1997.
28. Meltzer-Brody S, Churchill E and Davidson JR. Derivation of the SPAN: a brief diagnostic screening test for post-traumatic stress disorder. *Psychiatr. Res.* 88, 63–70, 1999.
29. Breslau N, Peterson EL, Kessler TC and Schultz LR. Short screening scale for DSM-IV posttraumatic stress disorder. *Am. J. Psychiatry* 156, 908–911, 1999.
30. Brewin CR, Rose S, Andrews B, et al. Brief screening instrument for post-traumatic stress disorder. *Br. J. Psychiatry* 24, 375–380, 2002.
31. Conlon L, Fahy TJ and Conroy R. PTSD in ambulant RTA victims: a randomized controlled trial of debriefing. *J. Psychosom. Res.* 46, 37–44, 1999.
32. Mayou R, Ehlers A and Hobbs M. Psychological debriefing for road traffic accident victims: three year follow-up of a randomized controlled trial. *Br. J. Med.* 176, 589–593, 2000.
33. Rafael B. Debriefing – science, belief and wisdom. In Raphael B and Wilson JP, eds. Psychological Debriefing: Theory, Practice and Evidence. New York: Cambridge University Press, 2000. pp 351–359.
34. Bryant RA, Harvey AG, Dang ST, et al. Treatment of acute stress disorder: a comparison of cognitive-behavioral therapy and supportive counseling. *J. Consult. Clin. Psychol.* 66, 862–866, 1998.
35. Foa EB, Hearst-Ikeda D and Perry KJ. Evaluation of a brief cognitive-behavioral program for the prevention of chronic PTSD in recent assault victims. *J. Consult. Clin. Psychol.* 63, 948–955, 1995.
36. Connor KM and Butterfield MI. Posttraumatic stress disorder. *J. Lifelong Learn. Psychiatry* 1, 247–262, 2003.
37. American Psychiatric Association. Practice Guidelines for the treatment of patients with acute stress disorder and posttraumatic stress disorder. *Am. J. Psychiatry* 161, 1–57, 2004.
38. North CS, Nixon SJ, Shariat S, et al. Psychiatric disorders among survivors of the Oklahoma City bombing. *J. Am. Med. Assoc.* 282, 755–762, 1999.
39. Holloway HC, Norwood AE, Fullerton CS, et al. The threat of biological weapons: prophylaxis and mitigation of psychological and social consequences. *J. Amer. Med. Assoc.* 278, 425–427, 1997.
40. Peters RG, Covello VT and McCallum DB. The determinants of trust and credibility in environmental risk communication: an empirical study. *Risk Anal.* 17, 43–54, 1997.
41. Hobfoll SE, Watson P, Bell CC, Bryant RA, Brymer MJ, Friedman MJ, Friedman M, Gersons BPR, de Jong JTVM, Layne CM, Mague S, Neria Y, Norwood AE, Pynoos RS, Reissman D, Ruzek JI, Shalev AY, Solomon Z, Steinberg AM and Ursano RJ. Five essential elements of immediate and mid-term mass trauma intervention: empirical evidence. *Psychiatry* 70, 283–315, 2007.
42. Raphael B. When Disaster Strikes: How Individuals and Communities Cope with Catastrophe. New York: Basic Books, 1986.

Chapter 15
The Role of the Media in Bioterrorism

David Brown

15.1 Introduction

Journalism in a time of bioterrorism is not essentially different from journalism in any time of crisis. But crisis journalism is different, in degree if not kind, from the reporting of news in ordinary times.

Danger exaggerates tendencies and magnifies traits. Reporting the news in the presence of hazard is harder for its practitioners, and more disruptive to the people who provide the information they seek. Normally difficult aspects of the trade loom larger – the pressure of deadlines, the competition to be first, the need to use human voices to help tell a story. For news sources – which at such moments are likely to include many public officials – the urges to be stingy with information, to be non-committal, and to downplay uncertainty and disagreement are especially strong. The public also is not untouched when life or well-being is at stake. At such times, people pay unusual attention to the news media, which is often a conduit for actual instruction on how to behave.

The problem, however, is not simply that bioterrorism magnifies the timeless difficulty of producing good journalism. There are aspects of bioterrorism that make it particularly vulnerable to bad, misleading or irresponsible journalism. This chapter will describe reasons the subject is perilous, and suggest ways the perils may perhaps be avoided. The practical suggestions are directed primarily to public health officials, scientists, politicians, and their media representatives – and not to journalists – simply because the former groups are the intended audience of the book.

D. Brown
Science Writer, Washington Post, Washington, D. C., USA
e-mail: browndavidm@comcast.net

L.I. Lutwick, S.M. Lutwick (eds.), *Beyond Anthrax*,
DOI: 10.1007/978-1-59745-326-4_15, © Springer Science+Business Media, LLC 2008

15.2 Reporting Science

In many ways, journalism about bioterrorism is little more than a special case of journalism about science. Even when a bioterrorism story involves some broad public policy issue, the subject invariably rests on a substrate of science and technical knowledge. Consequently, understanding policy issues involving bioterrorism – to mention nothing of terrorist events themselves – requires knowledge of biological mechanisms, an appreciation of clinical decision-making in medicine, and a sense of how to conceptualize and evaluate relative risks. Many science reporters are conversant with these subjects, but some aren't. In any case, many stories on bioterrorism are written, produced and edited by journalists unfamiliar, and often uncomfortable, with scientific subjects. Scientists and policy-makers should keep this in mind at all times. Like it or not, they need to realize that to make themselves clear they may have to conduct a running seminar on scientific methods, concepts and reasoning. It goes – almost but not quite without saying – that the sources of information need to be conversant in those areas themselves.

Of all nationally compelling news events, those involving science are the ones in which successful communication most depends on simple command of the facts. Political, constitutional and national security crises may be well-served by the voice of authority, the reassuring (or beguiling) power of rhetoric, and even by the ability to deftly make a weak argument. But scientific crises – which are almost always health crises at some level – require expertise, first and above all. Opinion counts for little when evaluating hazards to life, or devising a response to them. Judgment and authority are useful tools only when wielded by people who know what they are talking about. This is a very hard lesson for policy makers to learn. But it is the first one they must if they want to increase the chance that the news media will do a good job.

What is the importance of the news media doing a good job? Of course, it is impossible to give a good answer to that. But it *is* possible to say how important the public thinks the media is at such times.

Two weeks after the first (and fatal) case of anthrax from a bioterrorism attack using the mail occurred in October, 2001, 78% of Americans sampled in a poll reported they were following the news of it "very closely". This was a level of attention equal to that seen after the events of September 11 that year. Fifty percent said the media was not exaggerating the danger of anthrax; 42% said it was [1]. In the 110 days after the first case, the Office of Communications at the Centers for Disease Control and Prevention (CDC), the government agency coordinating the public health response to the attacks, conducted 23 press briefings and 306 television interviews, wrote 44 press releases, and took 7737 calls from the news media [2]. (Interestingly, 2½ times as many calls came directly from the public – 17,986 in all). The value of a well-informed and well-treated press in such times can scarcely be overstated.

Even when people providing information about bioterrorism are knowledgeable about the scientific issues and experienced in talking to reporters, they would do well to keep two ideas consciously in mind. One a principle and the other an observation, these two ideas are part of the natural mental apparatus of biologists. Their importance in helping guide investigations and solve problems – their heuristic value, in short – is largely unappreciated by non-scientists. A major task of any science communicator is to bring them into public consciousness and keep them there.

15.2.1 The Priniciple of Parsimony

The first is the Principle (or Law) of Parsimony. "One should always choose the simplest explanation of a phenomenon, the one that requires the fewest leaps of logic" and "the principle that entities should not be multiplied needlessly; the simplest of two competing theories is to be preferred" are two definitions of this principle, each converging on the notion that simpler explanations are more likely to be true than complicated ones [3]. When this principle is invoked in scientific argumentation it is often called "Occam's Razor", after William of Occam (1285–1349), a medieval English theologian and logician. Occam (whose name is a Latinized spelling of Ockham, his birth village south of London) criticized what he considered the unwarrantedly complex (and therefore, he thought, likely to be false) writings of his contemporaries. He wrote that when it comes to explaining things, "it is vain to do with more what can be done with less" [4].

Employing Occam's Razor is particularly important (although not infallible) in medical diagnosis, where a physician ideally should account for all the important signs, symptoms and test results presented by the case. The clinician wielding Occam's Razor assumes all newly appearing clinical phenomena are the result of a single disease, not the coincidental occurrence of two or more diseases. Consequently, a single diagnosis that explains all the clinical findings should be exhaustively sought, and abandoned with great reluctance.

Parsimony has two other corollaries besides Occam's Razor. One is that events are likely to unfold in the future as they have in the past – that patterns and mechanisms tend to be stable and relatively unchanging over time. The other is that unusual diseases or presentations of diseases are, by definition, unusual and should not be readily invoked. This idea is captured in two admonitions nearly every physician is told at least once during his training: "common things are still common," and "when you hear hoof beats, don't think of zebras." In sum, the natural impulse of physicians to resist acting on wild or untested ideas runs deep – so deep, in fact, that its power may not be fully appreciated by physicians themselves.

15.2.2 The Bell-Shaped Curve

The second idea that has heuristic value in times of bioterrorism is the bell-shaped curve. It captures the observation that outcomes arising from the same events or conditions are not identical, but differ from one another in ways that can be depicted visually and understood intuitively.

Most outcomes are similar to one another. They inhabit the fat, or humped-up, part of the curve, and define the average. A small number, however, are quite different from the rest, either much less or much more by whatever metric is in use. Those outcomes inhabit the two thin ends, or tails, of the curve. When this pattern is symmetrical on either side of the mean (or average) value it is called a "normal distribution." Normal distributions have specific mathematical properties; for one, the rarity of certain outcomes can be calculated. In that sense, the bell curve can be used to predict the likeliness of future events. Not all biological events have a normal distribution, but many do [5].

15.2.3 Integrating Parsimony and Bell-Shaped Curve

These two ideas – parsimony and the bell curve – are constantly at play in biology and medicine. An intuitive understanding of how the concepts operate in widely divergent biological spheres – and the ability to employ them consciously when facing new or difficult issues – may be the chief benefit for journalists in taking more-than-introductory courses in biology. When it comes to bioterrorism, however, these two concepts are important for opposite reasons.

Bioterrorism dilutes the importance of parsimony. That's because bioterrorism is an unnatural event even if its components – viruses, toxins, organs, medicines – are each natural and at some level behaving in familiar ways. Bioterrorism creates interactions that do not occur on their own. It produces conditions of unpredictable risk; it makes vulnerable people who aren't normally vulnerable; it alters highly evolved mechanisms of transmission, distribution, and protection. The doomsday scenario of a crop-duster laying down a cloud of anthrax spores on Manhattan – an event modeled by inference, if not by name, in a recent journal article – falls entirely outside the natural history of anthrax spores, human beings and Manhattan [6]. It is safe to say that previous experience with anthrax outbreaks is not likely to be very helpful in predicting the outcome of such an event, or in planning for it. Unfortunately, it is hard even to predict *how* unhelpful the past is likely to be.

On the other hand, bioterrorism tends to magnify the importance of the bell curve as an informative idea. Because size of the dose, duration of exposure, mechanism of transmission, and numerous other variables are unknown and unnatural, physicians and public health officials can not easily estimate an individual's risk during a bioterror event. In particular, it is difficult to identify occupants of the left-hand tail of a bell curve that depicts exposure to a pathogen. It's hard to say with confidence who is at very low risk of becoming infected, so that tail tends to be ignored and its occupants mentally swept into the fat part of the curve for safety sake when it comes to decisions about clinical monitoring, prophylactic treatment and other interventions. However, the bell curve that represents the side effects of interventions presents a different story. The existence of the right-hand tail – occupied by the few people who suffer serious side effects of, say, a vaccination – is either tolerable or intolerable, depending on the probability of the threat being guarded against. If the threat is high, then people will tolerate side effects (or at least the risk of them). If the threat is low, they will find side effects burdensome or unacceptable. But if the magnitude of the threat is unknown – is simply "non-zero" – then nobody can gauge whether the side effects experienced are worth the protection gained. This was the central conundrum posed by the federal government's recommendation of smallpox vaccination for certain hospital workers in 2003 [7]. It's useful for people who determine society's response to the threat of bioterrorism (or, needless to say, an actual act of it) to explain how the importance of different regions of the bell curve changes depending on circumstances.

Even if decision-makers do a good job of explaining this, however, they are likely to observe the operation of yet another bell curve – namely, the one that defines what is news and what is not. News is the noteworthy event. On any given day, this is more likely to be the odd and unusual event rather than the common and expected one. If dog-bites-man is the fat and uninteresting part of the human-canine interaction, then the two tails are where the news is: the clichéd man-bites-dog in one tail, and the pack-of-dogs-maul-man in the other tail. In practical terms, this means that even if the balance of events is well explained, the press is always going to devote more attention to the unusual, the dramatic, the damaging. Thoughtful communication with journalists (and, of course, good journalism itself) can keep this natural predilection from obscuring the larger, more subtle truth of events.

So how do these three things – expertise, and the ideas of parsimony and bell-shaped distribution of outcomes – come into play in actual news stories about bioterrorism?

There is only been one bioterrorism event in the United States that is captured national attention in recent times – the anthrax attacks of the autumn of 2001. (The intentional contamination of food with *Salmonella* by the Rajneeshee cultists in Oregon in 1984 was largely a local story [8]). Consequently, the examples in the rest of this chapter are drawn largely from that episode of recent history. The drama was long, with many unexpected turns of event. It captured nearly every important lesson about the media and bioterrorism that is likely to arise in the future.

15.3 US Anthrax Attacks – The Media and HHS

Policy makers and public health officials (and even to some extent, private medical care providers) face a difficult task when biological terrorism threats become real. Without warning they are called upon to describe events, provide advice, anticipate what may happen, and offer reassurance. These jobs are especially difficult when an event has no "natural history" experts can look back to for help. In the early hours and days when even the general trajectory of events is unclear, the tasks can be close to impossible.

It is obvious that under such circumstances, well-meaning and well-informed may give contradictory answers and advice. In order to prevent that, authorities sometimes choose to suppress information, limit access to people who know the most, or simply avoid the press altogether. All three strategies, to varying degrees, were tried during the anthrax attacks.

In terms of public confidence, one of the more damaging incidents occurred the day the outbreak became news, October 4 [9]. Tommy G. Thompson, who at the time was U.S. Secretary of Health and Human Services and the titular leader of most of the federal government's civilian health workers, held a news briefing at the White House after learning of the first case. A 63-year-old man in Florida working as a photo editor at a tabloid newspaper was diagnosed with inhalational anthrax. He was described as an outdoorsman, and Thompson mentioned that "we do know that he drank water out of a stream when he was traveling through North Carolina last week." Several further questions established the man's age, home town, and a few other details. The press conference ended this way:

> Mr. [Ari] Fleischer [White House press secretary]: The final question.
>
> Q: Mr. Secretary, how likely is it that there have been other anthrax cases, in the past year, say, that just simply haven't been diagnosed?
>
> Sec. Thompson: It's entirely possible.
>
> Q: Possible, or—(off mike)?
>
> Mr. Fleischer: Thank you very much.
>
> Sec. Thompson: (To Dr. [Scott] Lillibridge [HHS physician and bioterrorism expert] Would you say it's probable?
>
> Dr. Lillibridge: Possible. As you heighten surveillance, you'll get more.
>
> Q: Can we just ask one other question? When was the last documented case of anthrax in North Carolina?
>
> Sec. Thompson: I don't—
>
> Q: Can you check that?
>
> Sec. Thompson: Well, we certainly will be checking all of that and getting information out as it goes in.

Q: Mr. Secretary, can you explain why he was drinking from a stream: And—(laughter)—should we know that? Why are you giving us that detail?

Sec. Thompson: Just because he was an outdoorsman and there's a possibility that—there's all kinds of possibilities.

Q: Did he contract it that way—Did he contract anthrax by drinking the water?

Sec. Thompson: We don't know. We don't know yet.

Q: Mr. Secretary, have you put—

Mr. Fleischer: Thank you.

Sec. Thompson: Thank you, Ari. [10]

It's little surprise that some listeners left the briefing with the impression there was a reasonably good chance the Florida case was naturally acquired, and that drinking from a stream might have been the route of transmission. It seems quite unlikely that the medical experts believed the former even at this early stage. The latter was virtually impossible given that the patient had inhalational disease and no cases of gastrointestinal anthrax had ever been reported in the United States [11]. However, the reluctance on the part of Lillibridge to provide a fuller explanation that might have appeared to erode Thompson's authority – along with Fleischer's abrupt termination of the briefing – guaranteed that misleading information would be reported, and that it would be attributed to a high administration official.

(Fleischer's unwillingness to extend the press conference may have been something akin to a reflex action. In his role as a political spokesman, leaving facts ambiguous and opinions uncertain is often the explicit goal of an encounter with reporters, and not an unfortunate outcome. However, this should never, ever be the case when the topic is scientific. Science is relatively impervious to spin, and incomplete or misleading answers are easily exposed. Even when there is no intention to deceive – and clearly there was none here – stopping reporters from asking questions about a technical subject when they have many left to ask is done at great peril.)

As it happens, news reports that day and the next generally overlooked Thompson's remark about the stream. In this country, MSNBC, CNN, United Press International, the Washington Times, and the St. Petersburg Times appear to have been the only ones reporting it. Outside the United States, the remark was noted in The Times (London), The Daily Telegraph (London), The Scottish Daily Record, Agence France Presse, and the Spanish-language news service EFE [12]. If people thought there was a good chance the Florida man acquired anthrax by drinking stream water, most were probably foreigners!

This curious result may have occurred because Thompson made his statement at the White House, where foreign news outlets have correspondents but most American newspapers don't. However, it is possible some American reporters didn't mention the remark in their stories simply because they knew it made little sense. The Associated Press, for example, carried a story October 5 in which Jeffrey P. Koplan, director of the CDC, was paraphrased as saying "the patient has no digestive symptoms that would indicate the anthrax came from drinking contaminated water [13]."

Within a week, however, many newspapers – including such influential ones as *The New York Times*, *The Washington Post*, and *USA Today* – had discovered Thompson's statement about the stream. By then nobody found the stream-contagion theory credible, and there was no evidence Thompson's remark had done actual harm. Nevertheless, it was publicized widely. Reporters cited it as evidence in stories whose theme was the federal government's confusing and incompetent performance in communicating with the public [14]. Patricia Thomas, a science journalist commissioned by The Century Foundation to analyze the interaction between government agencies and the press during the outbreak, observed: "As the crisis worsened and spread, Thompson never quite repaired the damage done by his off-the-cuff words about water [9]." Thompson himself was clearly stung by the criticism, telling an audience a year later at the Mayo Clinic's National Conference on Medicine and the Media: "My instincts are to tell you what I know and what is happening. In fact, if you look back at some of the criticism I took last fall, it came about because I was too candid in telling the media what was taking place in our investigation that first day. I was too open with what our scientists were relaying to me and what they were doing. Of course, I never thought I'd have reporters criticizing me for being too open with the facts [15]."

Nevertheless, authority and candor (if that is, indeed, what it was) didn't trump credibility and expertise. While people in the Bush administration apparently believed there was value in having Thompson be the spokesman, he came to the event with little technical grasp of the issues – and demonstrated it immediately. As a main source of information, he was eventually moved aside in favor of various epidemiologists at the CDC, and Anthony S. Fauci, head of the National Institute of Health's National Institute of Allergy and Infectious Diseases. By then, however, considerable damage had been done in terms of public relations. The comment became one of the most memorable anecdotes of the entire outbreak. Worse, it became the pocket-portable symbol of what many people considered – rightly or wrongly – to be the federal government's early mishandling of the crisis. A year later, Thompson's remark was still being cited, albeit indirectly, by a prominent medical journalist, Lawrence K. Altman of The New York Times, in an article criticizing the federal government's press relations on an entirely different matter – smallpox vaccination [16].

If having Thompson be a main source of information early in the outbreak had been the only government miscalculation, then the media's overreaction to his stream comment would be especially objectionable. It was not.

15.4 US Anthrax Attacks – The Media and the CDC

The CDC's press office was barely functional in the first 2 weeks after the initial outbreak. Part of this was simply the result of volume: the office counted 2,229 requests about anthrax and 287 about bioterrorism between October 4 and 18, which is likely to have overwhelmed resources under the best of circumstances [9]. However, there were many other problems, which Thomas describes well in her monograph: "Those who got in touch with a press officer were likely to be referred elsewhere. If they asked about field investigations they were advised to call local officials in Florida, New York, New Jersey, or Washington. (There, press officers in the field sometimes bounced inquiries back to the CDC in Atlanta.) Reporters who asked about the search for the perpetrators were told to contact the FBI, which released prepared statements about the investigation but was otherwise tight lipped. If reporters called to follow up on comments made by Secretary Thompson or to ask about policy issues, they were usually referred to the public affairs office at HHS. And, although they did not realize this was happening, many reporters then had to wait while their requests were vetted by HHS officials in Washington [9]."

The idea that CDC functions as a mere consultant to states and cities in outbreak investigations is little more than a sophistry under normal circumstances. In the anthrax outbreak, it was simply wrong. CDC was at least an equal partner everywhere it sent investigators, from the start. With the outbreak potentially national in scope and with so much attention on the federal government's response to it, for CDC spokespeople to argue that providing information naturally "devolved" to state and local authorities was nothing short of infuriating. (Koplan believes this clarification of federal-versus-state roles in communicating with the media during emergencies is an especially important problem to solve [17]).

Providing reporters efficient access to informed sources is a tall order in a crisis, especially when events are happening in several places and many government agencies are involved. Nevertheless, providing such access is a priority whose importance can scarcely be overstated. Reporters can hardly be expected to abandon a subject simply because they cannot get information on it. Instead, they will turn to experts who are available, but whose knowledge of events is often second-hand or whose opinions may be colored by unstated agendas. Furthermore, policies that produce highly controlled and incomplete delivery of information to reporters lead to hypercritical and retaliatory journalism when things do not go well. Nearly every major news organization produced a story questioning the CDC's credibility and performance in communicating with the public [18]. Regardless of how unfair some of the criticism might have been, this analysis rapidly became part of the accepted history of the event.

Before reflexively limiting information or routing it through a single, scripted source, government authorities should ask: To what end? What is the advantage of such regimentation? What are the hazards of letting epidemiologists, physicians and investigators speak freely and without supervision?

The prime advantage (they are likely to answer) is that when only a few people are allowed to talk to reporters, the chance that contradictory versions of events, or interpretation of them, will emerge is reduced. The press seeks conflict and reports it as news; a difference of opinion is the most rudimentary and common form of conflict. However, forbidding a multitude of informed sources from talking to reporters does not eliminate conflict. It merely transforms the conflict to differences of opinion between taciturn officials and the independent experts, while simultaneously giving the public insufficient information with which to reach its own opinion – not a good combination. An excess of detail and analysis – some of it contradictory – is not likely to produce more public confusion and negative reporting (although, of course, it is impossible to say this with certainty).

The second argument that officials will probably make in defense of controlling the flow of information is that such a policy does not waste the time of people who have other jobs to do. This is undisputedly true. But it is a false economy.

In a true health crisis such as an attack with a biological weapon, an effective public health response and clear communication with citizens are equally important. Any system that puts them in conflict or requires them to compete should be changed. Reassurance, which requires little time or expertise to deliver, is no substitute for information. In fact, unaccompanied by information, or in the presence of events that continue to go badly, reassurance makes people feel isolated and suspicious. The excessive number of calming messages during the anthrax attack drew criticism even from sympathetic quarters. Philip S. Brachman, an epidemiologist and anthrax expert who was retired from CDC after three decades of service, was quoted in one newspaper report: "We have an intelligent public in this country. Don't treat them as children. [Officials] in the beginning got up and said, 'Don't worry.' That's nonsense. What I would do is say, 'We've got a problem, you have every right to be fearful, I'm fearful too, and here's what we're doing' [19]."

Giving the media more information than it asks for or can easily digest is a safer strategy than giving the media the minimum it will tolerate or only what it can understand with no help. Like anyone engaged in acts of construction, reporters are happy to have more building materials than they need. Authorities should not worry that too much information will confuse. In general, reporters will seek and use only the level of detail with which they are comfortable. Bad journalism is almost never the product of too many facts. The prominent science writer Laurie Garrett put it well: "If you build it, we will come. If you have a valid information source that is readily available and easy to get to, with openness and facilitation, it will be used. Most reporters will not search for unreliable facts elsewhere [20]." At the very least, a free flow of information will disarm journalists of their principal complaint in times of crisis – namely, that the people in the know are hiding things.

In a bioterrorism crisis, the CDC should consider designating a high official with scientific expertise – not a member of the communications staff – to function as a kind of *rapporteur* of agency deliberations. Ideally, this person should have some sense of what constitutes news and a fully reported story. He or she would be relieved of regular responsibilities but would otherwise function fully as an insider in agency activities.

Agency officials would continue to brief the press in time-limited sessions. During the anthrax and SARS outbreaks, this was done in daily or near-daily telephone press conferences lasting about an hour. However, there were almost always unanswered questions at the end. The *rapporteur* would remain on the line for an open-ended period to answer them, provide scientific context or background explanations, and generally seek to eliminate ambiguity and misunderstanding. This would enhance clarity and transparency. It would also require planning and institutional courage.

15.5 Getting It Right

The federal government eventually solved the problem of expertise in its communication with the press during the anthrax attacks. But the experts weren't able to end the press's – and the public's – relative lack of understanding about how the outbreak response was being conducted.

Over the course of the 7 weeks between the first diagnosed case (October 4) and the last (November 21), spokesmen for the federal government repeatedly made assessments and predictions that turned out not to be correct. From the press's perspective, this was perhaps the most memorable – the most "thematic" – aspect of the entire event. The illness in the Florida man was initially declared an "isolated case" with "no evidence of bioterrorism [10]." While indisputably true when uttered, these statements on the first day set a pattern of confident assertions overturned by events. In ensuing weeks, pronouncements that a letter containing anthrax spores had to be opened in order to release enough pathogen to cause inhalational anthrax [21]; that postal workers were only at risk for cutaneous anthrax [21]; and that ordinary citizens had nothing to fear from mail all turned out to be wrong [22]. The fact that each successive event inscribed a circle of risk with a wider radius (and with more people in it) did not help the credibility of the speakers or their agencies. A statement by Steven Wiersma, Florida's state epidemiologist, after the first victim died was notably different in tone and content from so much that followed: "I don't want to give anyone the slightest inkling that we know what caused this [23]."

Why did so many assertions turn out to be wrong? There's no certain answer. But my theory is that many smart and experienced people failed to anticipate events such as inhalational anthrax in postal workers and a nearly homebound woman because of an instinctive belief in parsimony. Those things simply seemed so unlikely – without precedent, actually – that planning for them was unnecessary, and perhaps even irresponsible given the likelihood of unintended consequences and morbidities.

The tracks of this thinking are evident in what several high officials said when they were queried by reporters (and others) about why they had not taken steps some believe might have saved lives. Koplan, CDC director, described his and his colleagues' thinking quite clearly several times. In one of the earlier daily teleconferences with reporters, on October 25, he reviewed the entire sequence of events. It was a highly illuminating account of epidemiological thinking.

> Back to this particular outbreak. I think people are somewhat surprised that we're learning things on a day-by-day basis, but that's really no different from any other investigation that we've done this year, 5 years, or over the last 50 years. The way the natural history of these investigations are, you always wish you knew on day 20—on day one what you know on day 20, and it's probably not going to be different here. We learn new things almost daily in this, and try to anticipate, of course, what's coming up the next day or the next week. It's obviously much more difficult when you've got a purposeful intent and someone malicious at the other end engaged in combat on this, and that is different from anything else we have done before.

A little later he describes how the belief emerged that a letter had to be opened to cause inhalational anthrax, and that contact with unopened letters containing powdered bacteria could only cause cutaneous anthrax.

> The letters we had seen or had described to us—we didn't have the letter in hand, but the letters we had had described to us, both the one from The New York Post in New York and then the next set in Washington, D.C., the letter that was in the Hart Office Building that had been addressed to Senator Daschle, were described to us as well-taped, meaning that the seams along that letter were taped in a way that would have minimized, if not eliminated, the ability of a powder to seep out through openings around the letter. You would have to open the letter. And, indeed, we were told that the letter that was sent to Senator Daschle had to be opened by a scissors because of how well it was sealed.
>
> So through this period of time we were still operating on the assumption that in order for a letter to convey this–the anthrax, it had to be either opened by someone who was opening mail, or in some way torn or disrupted in the sorting process, because the concept of a powder in a sealed letter was one that suggested that it would stay in that letter. And that was our epidemiologic experience with the cases we had seen so far. That construct obviously changed markedly with the report of inhalation anthrax in mail workers in the Brentwood facility in Washington where mail was not opened in the places where these individuals were exposed, or seem to have been exposed, and where the disease that they contracted was not cutaneous anthrax, which takes less spores, and is obviously less threatening than inhalational anthrax, and in which the physical characteristics are different. But to get a aerosolization of anthrax requires both air currents flowing around, and some larger quantity of smaller-sized spores to be present, and not easily explained at all by unopened mail. And with that, our current construct on the risk includes, obviously, letters that are unopened as well as letters that are open, that have had, been tampered with or have been maliciously placed in the mail with anthrax spores. [21]

The next day's teleconference featured this exchange about the possible risk from "cross-contaminated" letters – pieces of mail that don't themselves contain anthrax spores but which have come in physical contact with ones that do:

> Reporter: On the cross-contamination possibility... does that mean the public is more at risk, and besides the 200-some different substations, are you looking at expanding the prophylaxis to perhaps whole zip codes?
>
> Dr. Koplan: No, on that latter; just plain no. Let's get back to this issue of cross-contamination versus, you know, prim—whatever we're gonna call them—primary source criminal letters, or mailings. That where you indicated that there is an inhalation case in the State Department that's been reported, I think we all think that that would be highly unlikely to virtually impossible to occur, just by cross-contamination, and as well, without having these letters in hand, but based on what we've seen in other sites, there are probably multiple mailings that have gone out, and, you know, there may be several places in the federal government that have been deemed targets for these letters to go to. So I guess my own personal working hypothesis would be that this is not cross-contamination. It just wouldn't be enough material, infectious material from cross-contamination to do that. [22]

The day after that, Bradley Perkins, the CDC's lead epidemiologist in the Florida anthrax outbreak, was asked about why environmental sampling had not gotten down to the level of the ordinary household.

> Reporter: Can I follow up on the first part of those? What about the idea of homes? Why aren't they being tested and people on Cipro if they also get their mail from the same place?
>
> Dr. Perkins: To date the epidemiology suggests that the cases that have occurred have not occurred as a result of exposure in home settings. And that's why we're not focusing on them at the current time. If the epidemiology changes, we will—we will change along with that epidemiology. [24]

These quotations are a useful peek into the minds of two highly skilled and experienced epidemiologists. They reveal parsimony at work. They also show the unreliability of parsimony in biological terrorism, as the latter two assertions – that cross-contaminated mail, and mail received in the home would not cause inhalational anthrax – would soon prove incorrect. Although the route of exposure of a non-medical hospital employee in New York City was never found, it is likely to have been cross-contaminated mail, as no spores were cultured from her workplace or home. The anthrax source in the case of a nonagenarian woman in Connecticut also remained obscure, but as she rarely left her home and no gross contamination was found in it, the best inference is that she was infected by a cross-contaminated letter carrying a small number of bacterial spores.

A similar failure of intelligent and parsimonious thinking can be expected in any bioterrorism event for the reasons mentioned earlier – they have few or no precedents, and are likely to defy the natural history of the disease in question. Public health officials can count on being wrong much of the time.

The press is likely to focus on the wrongness, and on the "meaning" of the errors. Why? Because the press's only consistent specialty is political analysis, the divination of how events affect power. The journalist James Fallows has described this phenomenon: "No one expects Cokie Roberts or other political correspondents to be experts on controlling terrorism, negotiating with the

Syrians, or other specific measures on which Presidents make stands. But all issues are shoehorned into the area of expertise the most prominent correspondents do have: the struggle for one-upmanship among a handful of political leaders [25]."

This insight is most relevant for the media's handling of matters of foreign or economic policy, but medicine and public health are not immune. The top officials of the New Jersey Department of Health and Senior Services noted this in their detailed account of the state's experience in the anthrax outbreak: "As the situation continued, news reports focused on what decisions were made (e.g., the closing of a facility, use of antimicrobial agents) and how they were made. The media and public were interested in what the response to the event seemed to say about state decision making and readiness to address emergencies in general [26]." If a journalist doesn't really understand the medical, statistical, and biological substance of a disease outbreak, he can at least appear to be knowledgeable about the interaction of individuals and agencies, and how events are believed to be changing their power and image. Much of this coverage is unavoidable. Some of it is even justified and illuminating [27]. In general, though, the public is better served by reporting that tries to reveal the substance of complex events and decisions rather than interpret them. Public health agencies are better served by this approach as well.

There is only one way to keep attention on the substance and that is to reveal the process of decision-making to the press and public as it happens. The best chance of keeping wrong decision and incorrect inferences from becoming the main story is to vicariously allow the non-experts to experience the difficulty and uncertainty of responding to events as they unfold.

This is not necessarily done by opening meetings and conference calls to the press (although letting reporters occasionally witness such events is a good idea). What public health officers and policy-makers need to do is simply describe to journalists how decisions were made. They should not wait until the decisions prove to be right or wrong before they describe the thinking that went into them. They should do it in something close to real time (which regular briefings, such as the CDC's daily teleconferences, offered). Specifically, public health officials should review the choices they considered when facing a set of facts and uncertainties. They should describe what the arguments for each course of action were, directing reporters' attention to the evidence and logic that advocates for each position brought to bear. They should reveal, at least in general terms, the magnitude of disagreement and the steps that led to its resolution – if, in fact, resolution preceded decision. CDC officials did a fairly good job of describing the logic of their thinking and the process by which decisions were reached. It occurred, however, almost entirely after the fact.

The prospect of following these suggestions probably would fill a public health official with horror. But it should not. People appreciate being spoken to candidly. Transparency is increasingly expected in government operations. The public appreciates being treated as intelligent enough to follow a complicated process undertaken on its behalf. The press is less likely to focus on process if it is forced to face the substance in all its difficult and incomplete detail. Observers of all types are less likely to invoke race prejudice, obtuseness, and bad faith – all mentioned at one point or other during the anthrax attacks – if they understand how those in authority made their decisions.

Furthermore, people are more tolerant of uncertainty than decision-makers believe. While officials should be reassuring and do what they can to prevent panic, they should not shield the public from disagreement or discussions of what may happen if things get worse. Disagreement is likely to be uncovered soon enough, and many people's understanding of what constitutes a worst-case scenario is likely to be more frightening than anything the facts support.

15.6 The Potential for Public Panic

On the issue of the threat of public panic, the record of how people behave during mass casualty events may be instructive. The National Science Foundation funded a study in which epidemiologists systematically analyzed the public response to 10 disasters that occurred between 1989 and 1994. These included an underground gas explosion in Guadalajara, Mexico, that killed more than 200 people in 1992; the first bombing of the World Trade Center in New York in 1993; and the Northridge earthquake in California in 1994. The findings were revealing. One of the researchers described a few of the more salient ones:

> Overall, the evidence suggested that victims tend to respond effectively and creatively. What we saw repeatedly in disasters was that victims formed spontaneous groups that have roles, rules, leaders, and a division of labor. This is the phenomenon of emergent collective behavior talked about extensively in the literature on the social science side... The literature and our study show that panic is relatively rare. There's a lot of talk about panic, and there's a general assumption that the public would panic in a bioterrorism event. My question is, where does the data come from to support that? In the events we studied, we were amazed to interview victims and health care workers who commented repeatedly on the absence of panic, complaints, or irrational behavior. Many emergency department workers said, "Gee, I wish things worked this smoothly all the time." Most people talked about an eerie feeling of calm that came over people during life and death moments. Panic happens in disaster movies but typically not in real disasters for reasons that probably are based in evolution. What we witnessed is that ordinary citizens are amazingly capable of avoiding deadly harm. [28]

William Patrick III, a former biological weapons worker quoted in this article also told David Brown of The Washington Post in late October, 2001 that he had not been contacted by government investigators or epidemiologists in the 3 weeks after the first anthrax cases.

Although this evidence is indirect, it suggests that if difficult decisions – and the hazards they create – are explained fully to the press and public, panic and irrational behavior are not likely outcomes. In fact, the usual assurances that things will probably be okay are more likely to seem believable if decision-makers reveal why they feel that way and give at least a hint of how events nevertheless might prove them wrong.

This strategy may improve the image of public health decision-makers during a crisis. But that is not the main reason for it. The chief benefit is that it gives the public a vicarious sense of control. Knowledge tends to allay fears even when uncertainty and danger are part of the knowledge. As evidence of this, public health officials need look no farther than medicine itself. Description and prognostication were what physicians chiefly did before they were able to cure – and people took great solace from that alone.

It is also possible that the act of preparing to describe the logic of a just-made decision to the press may itself be a useful tool in clarifying thinking and bringing unquestioned assumptions into consciousness. One wonders, for example, whether the assumption that mail had to be opened to cause inhalational anthrax – the assumption that may have contributed to the fatal infection of workers at the Brentwood postal facility – would have stood up had there been greater public scrutiny of the assumptions and arguments being made behind closed doors. After all, the first cases of inhalational disease, at the Florida tabloid newspaper office, were not definitively associated with open mail, and in fact no spore-containing letter was ever found there. Similarly, a somewhat more open discussion of the aerosolization potential of finely milled anthrax spores might have directed epidemiologists' attention to the researchers retired from the United States Army's biological weapons program – the only people with first-hand knowledge of the issue – sooner rather than later [29].

But even if the people who deliver information to the press are well-informed and they describe their decisions transparently, that would not guarantee that what appears in the newspaper and on television does not contain misleading information. There are crucial concepts that are second-nature to scientists but which are barely understood by the press and public. It is the job of public health officials to give the press a crash-course in these concepts. The most important one, as earlier suggested, is the usefulness of the bell-shaped curve in understanding the probability of complicated events.

15.7 Is There a Correct Answer?

Reporters and readers like to have concrete answers to questions. One of the more persistent queries, raised after the first case, was: How easy *is* it to contract inhalational anthrax? The answer was frequently given in number of spores, as inferred from experiments on monkeys. The number 8500 was often quoted; so was a range of 2500 to 55,000 spores [30]. Reporters considered this a rather imprecise answer to the question, and at some level it was. As cases of disease occurred without the recovery of infecting letters, the estimates were questioned widely in news stories, and offered as evidence of "how little we know about anthrax." A Knight Ridder story of October 27, 2001 noted that an anthrax expert outside the government "said that officials have overestimated the amount of anthrax necessary – a minimum of 8000 spores – to cause inhalation anthrax [31]." At the CDC teleconference of October 25, a reporter asked: "Are you all doing any work in the labs perhaps with animals to test the assumption that perhaps with this particular form of anthrax it could take less than 8000 spores to cause inhalation disease? [22]"

In fact, the estimates and the events were confusing and contradictory only if one believed there was an absolute threshold for infection. It was clear that most journalists though of infection as analogous to a light switch – a certain number of spores will exert sufficient force to turn the light on, and fewer will not. But this is rarely, if ever, the case with infections, and certainly not with anthrax. The spore numbers are estimates of the number of the dose sufficient to infect 50% of the people exposed – the infectious dose 50%, or ID_{50}. Half the people exposed to it won't become sick and possibly die, so it is far from being the minimum dose necessary to cause infection. Because there is no minimum dose, biologists use this mid-way dose as a measuring stick for the infectiousness of something. While the usefulness of the ID_{50} – and the bell-shaped distribution it implies – is not intuitively obvious at first, once it's grasped many things are easier to understand.

First, it explains why precision isn't possible in describing infectious dose, and thus why imprecision of itself isn't terribly newsworthy. More important, it helps make the two most mysterious cases of the outbreak – the 61-year-old female hospital worker in New York City and the 94-year-old nearly home-bound woman in Connecticut – somewhat less mysterious and frightening. That's because if there is an ID_{50}, there's also an ID_1 – the dose of spores that will infect 1 out of 100 people. For that matter, there's also an $ID_{.1}$ – the dose that will infect 1 in a 1000 – and an $ID_{.01}$ – the dose that will infect 1 in 10,000. So if it turns out that spores can get out of an envelope and stick to other envelopes, and if a fraction of those spores can become airborne again, and if there are a lot of envelopes moving around putting up spores in whatever tiny dose is the $ID_{.01}$ – then it stands to reason that someone among the thousands of postal customers will get infected. In some sense, all those envelopes are out there probing the population for the rare person who's susceptible to such a small dose. The envelopes are looking, so to speak, for the person who occupies the tail of the bell curve – because someone does occupy it. So, it should be no surprise when such a person appears [32].

The New York City patient – a relatively healthy working woman who was not especially old – doesn't present any obvious reasons why she might have been susceptible to a small dose. But the 94-year-old Connecticut woman clearly has the major risk factor of age and its relative immunosuppression. In addition, she had the habit of tearing envelopes in half after opening them, which would have helped reaerosolize spores deposited on the outside through cross-contamination.

Similar confusion surrounded the issue of whether exposed people should undergo a three-dose course of anthrax vaccine after completing a 60 day course of antimicrobials. The large outbreak of inhalational anthrax caused by the accidental airborne release of spores in Sverdlovsk, Soviet Union, in 1979 recorded no infections more than 43 days after exposure [33]. Evidence from monkeys, however, suggests that infection can occur after more than 60 days of latency [34]. Consequently, public health authorities offered vaccine, to be given along with 40 more days of antibiotics, to a large group of people, but did not recommend that they take it. The decision, instead, was left to the exposed people themselves.

This agnostic stance was widely criticized – perhaps with good reason – as being insufficiently clear and authoritative. A *New York Times* editorial called it "an unsatisfactory medical cop-out," and added: "It is disappointing that officials who are in the best position of anyone to make sense of the admittedly sparse data on anthrax are throwing up their hands and leaving the decision to patients and doctors who have far less command of the subject [35]." However, the key piece of data informing any individual's decision was not in the possession of the experts. That piece was the individual's tolerance of risk. What to do depended on whether a person worried about being one of the few people (actually, monkeys) in the tail of the bell curve and wanted to do something about it, or whether he assumed he was in the fat part of the curve where most people reside and was willing to live with the slim chance he was wrong.

It is a subtle point – but one that has the advantage of being a statement of reality. Public health officials could have helped the press and public understand the "unrecommended offer" of vaccine better if they had explained it as yet another decision arising from an understanding of the bell curve – the orderly distribution of events in biological systems in which there are many more average events than exceptional ones.

The suggestion that such a concept could be taught to dozens of reporters on the fly isn't entirely far-fetched. Journalists are used to getting one-on-one telephone tutorials from experts; it's one of the chief privileges of the profession. Daily teleconferences with scientists and public health officials – the only reasonable way to manage news distribution during a bioterrorism event – provide the opportunity. The Internet even makes it possible for someone announcing a decision to help explain it with a diagram or graphic. At the moment, using the Internet to provide journalists with background information during a running news story such as the anthrax outbreak is almost entirely untapped. If there is another event like it, public health officials would be wise to at least post on an easily accessed site a dozen or so scientific papers that form the core evidence base for the disease in question.

Posting the core literature would have many advantages. It would show how information was acquired through observation, experimentation, and extrapolation. It would demonstrate how some interventions (such as the use of anthrax vaccine after human exposure to the bacterium), while "experimental" in a formal sense, is grounded in evidence and not likely to carry much of the uncertainty associated with experimental therapies as commonly understood. It also provides color. The description of the investigation into an anthrax outbreak at a Dickensian goat-hair mill in Manchester, N.H., in the 1950s was both fascinating and informative [36]. The fact that those epidemiologists swabbed anthrax spores off the factory president's desk – which one of the still-living investigators told me – revealed something about the cohabitation of man and spore at all levels of that industry.

The relationship between medicine and the media has never been especially easy or sympathetic [37]. Medicine values privacy and authority. The media seeks to publicize the private and is reflexively suspicious of authority. Medicine values nuance and caveat in communication. The media relishes definitive statements and often cannot tolerate subtlety. Medicine generally attempts to reassure. The media often seeks to present facts in the most arresting and frightening context that can be defended with claims of technical accuracy. The hostility between the two worlds is sometimes profound. The twentieth-century embodiment of medicine's ideals, William Osler, said with more than a little bitterness: "Believe nothing that you see in the newspapers – they have done more to create dissatisfaction than all other agencies. If you see anything in them that you know is true, begin to doubt it at once [38]."

On the other hand, the media does not do a bad job. On ProMED-mail, the main public website for breaking news in infectious disease epidemiology, about 90% of the postings "start with a raw newspaper article." In an analysis of 7 months of activity, 2.6% of outbreak reports from unofficial sources – mostly newspapers – turned out to be wrong. That compared favorably with a 1.7% rate of inaccurate reports from official health agencies [39]. As an independent and occasionally unruly force, the media also has an invaluable role in emergencies, including epidemics. This was noted by numerous observers during the outbreak of severe acute respiratory syndrome (SARS). In China, where control of the disease had consequences for the entire globe, the World Health Organization provided important assistance to local authorities, but "it was the press that kept the focus on and led to the resolute responses that occurred," according to one Western observer [40].

15.8 Lessons

The lessons from the anthrax outbreak were evident soon after it ended. For Sandra Mullin of the New York City Health Department, they were similar to ones another disease had just taught.

> The media blitz surrounding the anthrax situation in New York City and elsewhere has far surpassed the crush of 1999. Nonetheless, West Nile provided a drill of sorts for the challenge public health is now facing. We learned most importantly about the need to address perceptions of risk, to have credible communicators, and to get information out in a timely and consistent way. In the past few weeks, this has meant getting facts out to the public rather than inventing ways to reassure the public. It has also involved acknowledging the seriousness of bioterrorism, but at the same time pointing out that thus far the morbidity and mortality associated with it are far surpassed by preventable illnesses like influenza and human immunodeficiency virus (HIV). Admitting when we do not yet have the answers has also been required. [41]

They're likely to be the lessons learned next time, too.

References

1. The Pew Research Center for the People and the Press, poll released Oct. 22, 2001 at http://people-press.org/reports/display.php3?ReportID = 140, accessed Nov. 3, 2003.
2. Golan, K. S. and Lackey, C. Box 13-1. Communicating about anthrax: some lessons learned at the CDC, in *Terrorism and Public Health* (Levy, B. S. and Sidel, V. W., eds.), Oxford University Press, New York, 2003, pp 253–254.
3. The first definition is from Principia Cybernetica Web at http://pespmc1.vub.ac.be/ASC/PRINCI_SIMPL.html. The second is from HyperDictionary at http://www.hyperdictionary.com/dictionary/principle + of + parsimony, accessed Oct. 27, 2003.
4. Rosoff, L. Roger Bacon, William of Occam and Lord Houghton: guides for the perplexed physician. *Am. J. Surg.* 141, 3–9, 1981. William of Occam also described at http://paedpsych.jk.uni-linz.ac.at/INTERNET/ARBEITSBLAETTERORD/PHILOSOPHIEORD/Occam.html, accessed Oct. 27, 2003.
5. Discussions of the bell-shaped curve and normal distribution can be found at numerous websites, including at the University of the Sciences in Philadelphia at http://www.usip.edu/biology/bs130/normal%20distribution.html; University College London, http://www.ucl.ac.uk/~ucbhtoc/L6%20H'out.html; and the University of Leicester, http://www.le.ac.uk./biology/gat/virtualfc/Stats/normal.htm.
6. Wein, L. M., Craft, D. L. and Kaplan, E. H. Emergency response to an anthrax attack. *Proc. Natl. Acad. Sci. USA*. 100, 4346–4351, 2003.
7. "Donald, A. Henderson, the former head of the global smallpox eradication campaign and now the Bush administration's main adviser on smallpox matters, told the committee [Advisory Committee on Immunization Practices] that the risk of the disease's reappearance is no different now from what it was when the panel last met, in June. 'The risk as appraised is a small one. It is not zero, and that is the worrisome piece,' Henderson said." See Brown, D., "Panel leery of mass smallpox doses; Major risks outweigh benefits of immunizing the general public, experts say", Washington Post, Oct. 18, 2002.
8. Carus, W. S. The Rajneeshees, in *Toxic Terror: Assessing Terrorist use of Chemical and Biological Weapons* (Tucker, J. B., ed.), MIT Press, Cambridge, 2000, pp 115–137.
9. Thomas, P. *The Anthrax Attacks*, The Century Foundation, New York, 2003 This 48-page report available online at http://www.tcf.org/4L/4LMain.asp?SubjectID = 1&TopicID = 0&ArticleID = 221, accessed Nov. 9, 2003.
10. White House Briefing, Oct. 4, 2001, Federal News Service, accessed through LexisNexis.
11. Holmes, R. K. Diphtheria, other Corynebacterial infections, and Anthrax, in *Harrison's Principles of Internal Medicine 15th Edition* (Braunwald, E., Fauci, A. S., Kasper, D. L. *et al.*, eds.), McGraw-Hill, New York, 2001, pp 909–915.
12. Accessed through LexisNexis with search terms: "Thompson" and "anthrax" and "stream" and "North Carolina".
13. Riddle, A. Florida man in critical condition with rare form of anthrax, raising fears about terrorism, Associated Press, BC cycle, Oct. 5, 2001.
14. Stolberg, S. G. Anthrax threat points to limits in health systems, *New York Times*, Oct. 14, 2001; Milbank, D. Government's anthrax muddle: many voices, few facts, *Washington Post*, Oct. 18, 2001; Page, S. White House falters in battle on home front, *USA Today*, Oct. 26, 2003.
15. Thompson, T. G. Bioterrrorism: preparedness and communication, delivered Sept. 20, 2002 at http://www.hhs.gov/news/speech/2002/020920a.html, accessed Nov. 10, 2003.
16. Altman, L. K. At the health department, the messengers still stumble. *New York Times*, Oct. 8, 2002.
17. "State health departments don't like comments on what is happening in their states emanating from Atlanta or Washington. But there probably should be a more obvious federal presence earlier where your suspicion has gone up. If it's anthrax or Q fever or plague, that would be examples. Sure, you could have the state of Florida officials taking

questions, but also make sure that we make some comments from a national perspective." Jeffrey P. Koplan, Telephone interview, Oct. 16, 2003.

18. There are many such articles, including: McClam, E., "CDC criticized for anthrax outbreak", Associated Press, Oct. 23, 2001; Gilbert, C. and Marchione, M., "Terrorism challenges Thompson; Pilloried, praised for crisis handling, he's still determined", Milwaukee Journal Sentinel, Oct. 28, 2001; Mishra, R. and Donnelly, J., "Fighting terror seeking answers/communication confusion/ federal agencies criticized", *Boston Globe*, Nov. 1, 2001.
19. Gilbert, C. and Marchione, M. "Terrorism challenges Thompson; Pilloried, praised for crisis handling, he's still determined", *Milwaukee Journal Sentinel*, Oct. 28, 2001.
20. Garrett, L. Understanding media's response to epidemics, *Pub. Health Rep.* 116 (Supp. 2), 87–91, 2001.
21. CDC teleconference, Oct. 25, 2001 at http://www.cdc.gov/od/oc/media/transcripts/t011025.htm, accessed Nov. 17, 2003.
22. Statements to this effect were made by both Jeffrey Koplan and Julie Louise Gerberding of the CDC in the CDC teleconference, Oct. 25, 2001 at http://www.cdc.gov/od/oc/media/transcripts/t011025.htm, and by Koplan in the CDC teleconference of Oct. 26, 2003 at http://www.cdc.gov/od/oc/media/transcripts/t011026.htm, accessed Nov. 17, 2003.
23. Lebowitz, L., Arthur, L. and Yardley, W. Florida man suffering from anthrax dies, *Miami Herald*, Oct. 6, 2001.
24. CDC teleconference, Oct. 29, 2001 at http://www.cdc.gov/od/oc/media/transcripts/t011029.htm, accessed Nov. 21, 2003.
25. Fallows, J. Why Americans hate the media, *The Atlantic*, February 1996, at http://www.theatlantic.com/issues/96feb/media.htm, accessed Nov. 21, 2003.
26. Bresnitz, E. A. and DiFerdinando Jr., G. T. Lessons from the anthrax attacks of 2001: the New Jersey experience, *Clin. Occup. Environ. Med.* 2, 227–252, 2003.
27. Chen, K., Hitt, G., McGinley, L. and Petersen, A. Ttrial and Error: seven days in October spotlight weakness of bioterror response; health officials were slow to grasp anthrax hazard for D.C. postal workers; Mad dash from Brentwood. *Wall St. J.* Nov. 2, 1, 2001.
28. Glass, T. A. Understanding public response to disasters, *Pub. Health Rep.* 116 (Supp. 2), 69–73, 2001. The word "emergent" in the third sentence is used in its correct sense, meaning "unexpected and suddenly appearing," and not to denote action done quickly and under emergency conditions, which is a common, if regrettable, medical usage.
29. Shane, S. Md. experts' key lessons on anthrax go untapped; Fort Detrick's veteran researchers studied bioweapons for 26 years, Baltimore Sun, Nov. 4, 2001.
30. Defense Intelligence Agency, U.S. Department of Defense, *Soviet Biological Warfare Threat*, Washington, D.C., Publication DST-161OF-057-86.
31. Borenstein, S., Murphy, K. and Goldstein, S. Future cases of anthrax, clues from decontaminated letters will help investigators, Knight Ridder/Tribune News Service, Oct. 27, 2001.
32. Lipton, E. and Johnson, K. The anthrax trail: tracking bioterror's tangled course, *New York Times*, Dec. 26, 2001.
33. Meselson, M., Guillemin, J., Hugh-Jones, M., et al. The Sverdlovsk anthrax outbreak of 1979, *Science* 266, 1202–1208, 1994.
34. Glassman, H. Industrial inhalation anthrax, *Bacteriol. Rev.* 30, 657–659, 1966.
35. Editorial, A muddled message on anthrax vaccine, New York Times, Dec. 20, 2001.
36. Plotkin, S. A., Brachman, P. S., Utell, M., et al. An epidemic of inhalation anthrax, the first of the twentieth century. *Am. J. Med.* 29, 992–1001, 1960.
37. Brown, D. Medicine and the media: a case study. *Pharos*, Summer 1984, 2–7, 1984.
38. Bean, B. B. (ed.) *Sir William Osler: Aphorisms from his Bedside Teachings and Writings*, Charles C. Thomas, Springfield, Ill., p 64, 1951.

39. Hugh-Jones, M. Global awareness of disease outbreaks: the experience of ProMED-mail, *Pub. Health Rep.* 116 (Suppl. 2), 27–31, 2001.
40. Breiman, R. Centre for Health and Population Research, Dhaka, Bangladesh, at "Learning from SARS: Preparing for the Next Disease Outbreak" workshop sponsored by the Institute for Medicine, Oct. 1, 2003.
41. Mullin, S. Public health and the media: the challenge now faced by bioterrorism. *J. Urban Health* 79, 12, 2002.

Chapter 16
Rapid Detection of Bioterrorism Pathogens

David Perlin

16.1 Introduction

Pathogen identification is a crucial first defense against bioterrorism. A major emphasis of our national biodefense strategy is to establish fast, accurate and sensitive assays for diagnosis of infectious disease agents likely to be used in a bioterrorist event. The Centers for Disease Control and Prevention and National Institutes of Health's National Institute of Allergy and Infectious Diseases have identified three priority classes or "select agents" of pathogens and toxins. These are designated A, B, and C, and are likely candidates since they can be easily disseminated, usually in aerosol form, require small numbers of organisms or molecules to cause disease, and result in rapid morbidity and mortality.

The challenge for most infectious diseases specialists is that these agents are rarely encountered in normal practice, many are seen in remote outbreaks in distant countries, and one (smallpox) has been eradicated with the last case observed several decades ago. As our first line of defense, the vast majority of physicians may not be able to distinguish the early events of a bioterrorist event from other atypical pneumonias or cutaneous infections. The challenge of rapid pathogen or toxin recognition is to aid physicians in the diagnostic process and to help identify at an early stage a potential deliberate outbreak [1]. Such assays will ensure early and appropriate treatment of infected patients, and will alert public health authorities and law enforcement to help contain an outbreak.

A major lesson of the October 2001 anthrax outbreak was that aggressive therapeutic intervention saves lives, since highly virulent organisms like anthrax can respond well to antimicrobial therapy when diagnosed in the early stages [2, 3]. Unfortunately, the early signs and symptoms of many of these diseases are nonspecific so it is critical that highly sensitive and reliable tools are available to identify infected individuals. The first step toward effective patient and

D. Perlin
Public Health Research Institute, UMDNJ-New Jersey Medical School, 225 Warren Street, Newark, New Jersey, USA
e-mail: perlinds@umdnj.edu

L.I. Lutwick, S.M. Lutwick (eds.), *Beyond Anthrax*,
DOI: 10.1007/978-1-59745-326-4_16,

public health control is to identify rapidly the infecting pathogen and its source. Some of these select agents are highly transmissible in the early stages of disease and it is critical to identify infected patients to limit the risk to the remainder of the population. In some cases, such as hemorrhagic fever with Ebola virus, it is hypothesized that patients become infected through contact with an infected animal. Yet, the natural reservoir of the virus is unknown, as is the manner in which the virus first appears in a human at the start of an outbreak [4]. Whether the initial source can be elucidated or not, rapid diagnostic procedures are critical to support infection control measures that monitor and limit the spread of infectious diseases agents [5, 6]. Finally, accurately defining the scope and progression of an infectious disease outbreak helps mobilize resources more efficiently and eases public anxiety that can lead to panic [7].

16.2 Limitation of Conventional Diagnostics

Rapid clinical diagnosis and aggressive preemptive therapy can limit the fatalities associated with a biological agent of mass destruction [8, 9]. Most clinical laboratories, however, still rely upon culture-based technology with phenotypic endpoints, approved by FDA and/or CDC. These assays can take several days for definitive results. In addition to time delays, these techniques often lack adequate sensitivity and specificity and some organisms are difficult to isolate in culture. Delays often translate into the initiation of empiric therapy in the absence of positive pathogen identification. The problem is not limited to a bioterrorism outbreak as hospital and public health laboratories, confounded by inadequate and slow methodology for pathogen detection, often have difficulty identifying pathogens. When occurring with very ill and/or immunocompromised patients, these delays can increase morbidity and mortality.

In a bioterrorist event, like many naturally occurring disease outbreaks, there is a need to obtain rapid pathogen identification from clinical specimens but also from environmental specimens to minimize fomite-based transmission. Time delays measured in days can prevent adequate public health measures from being instituted to contain an outbreak. Such delays also subject exposed individuals to needless stress and anxiety. The inadequacy of phenotypic-based diagnostic assays is illustrated graphically by the "gold standard" public health laboratory-testing algorithm that was in place for positive identification of *Bacillus anthracis* from environmental samples during the October 2001 anthrax outbreak (Fig. 16.1a). A complicated matrix of phenotypic and biochemical assays required 3–5 days for a positive endpoint. What was needed was a streamlined approach that could progress from primary specimen to a positive or negative outcome in a matter of hours or less (Fig. 16.1b). Rapid diagnostics have finally come of age and offer exceptional promise in this regard for accurate pathogen identification.

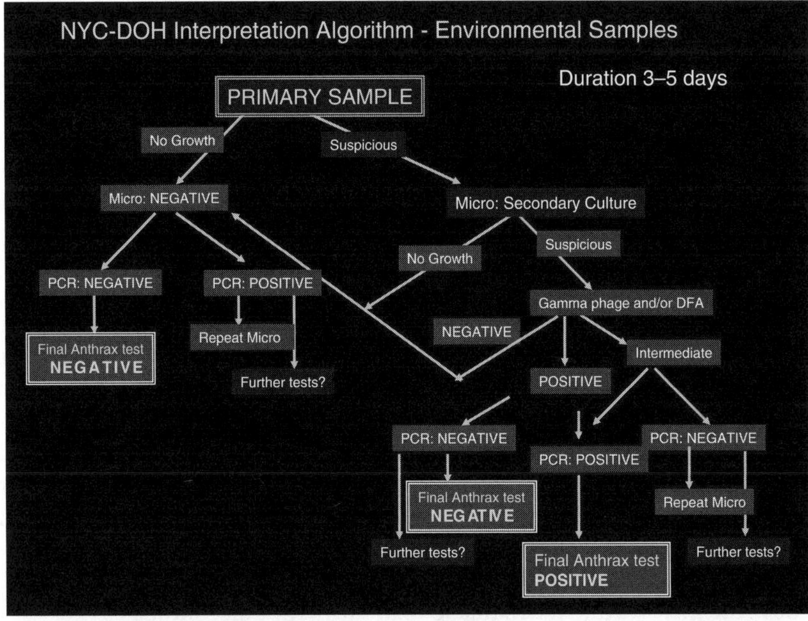

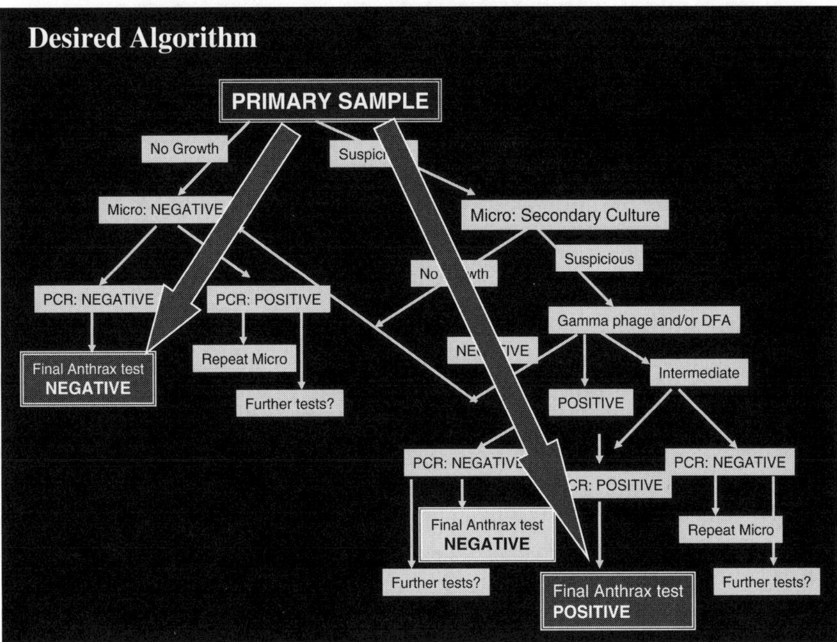

Fig. 16.1 (**a**) Schemes for identification of *Bacillus anthracis*. New York City Department of Health interpretation algorithm for identification of *Bacillus anthracis* from environmental samples based on CDC guidelines. (**b**) Desired pathway for identification of *Bacillus anthracis*

16.3 Rapid Identification Methods

Rapid identification assays can be loosely divided into tests that either utilize antigen-antibody or other antibody-specific binding to identify a specific pathogen or genetic tests that identify pathogen-specific DNA or RNA sequences.

16.3.1 Serologies: Antigen–Antibody Interactions

Serological techniques have been invaluable for detecting active infections with organisms that are difficult to culture and for documenting previous infection/immunity. While conventional serodiagnosis has a limited ability to detect acute infections with select agents, it is invaluable for monitoring disease kinetics and dispersion of these agents within exposed or high-risk populations, especially where asymptomatic infections are frequent. Such information is crucial to therapeutic intervention and prophylaxis, as well as to isolation protocols in the context of a biological attack. Serodiagnosis is particularly useful for mass screening of infectious diseases because such techniques are generally simple to perform, inexpensive and amenable to high throughput technologies. The assay takes advantage of the exquisite sensitivity and specificity of antigen-antibody interactions. Antigen capture assays represent a somewhat more recent addition to serological techniques. These methods have been useful for rapidly diagnosing acute infections where antigen levels are relatively high, especially in the urine where they may be concentrated.

The Enzyme Linked Immunosorbent Assay (ELISA) has become the workhorse of most clinical laboratories. It relies on specific antigen-antibody interactions to identify a pathogen [10]. Typically, a preliminary test can be performed quickly, usually within 3–4 h. A positive ELISA test can be confirmed by performing a Western Blot with target-specific antibodies or by an immunofluorescent antibody (IFA). Unfortunately, pathogen antigen production or a host antibody response is not always robust enough to permit reliable testing, especially in the early stages of an infection. In addition, a false positive result with an ELISA test can occur due to interference from other antibodies. Although the ELISA test is highly specific, an antibody response may not be detected in either the early or late stages of a disease. Improved sensitivity may be obtained by expanding the class of antibodies detected to IgG, IgA and/or IgM classes of antibodies [11].

ELISA platforms are especially well suited for toxin detection and, when combined with procedures such as time-resolved fluorometry, sensitivities of 4–20 pg/mL can be obtained in a typical 2 h assay for molecules such as botulinum type A or B neurotoxin and *Staphylococcus aureus* enterotoxin B [12]. A newer format for antigen-antibody detection where the detector antibody is labeled by chemiluminescence facilitates an even greater sensitivity [13]. In one approach, target antigen is first complexed to paramagnetic beads coated with capture antibody and then identified using a detector antibody. An electrochemical flow cell with photon detector is used to detect the target-antibody interactions with detection limits approaching 200 fmol/L and dynamic ranges of six orders of magnitude [10]. More recently, a novel type of biosensor for rapid pathogen identification has been described using B cells as sensing elements. This system know as CANARY (cellular analysis and notification of antigen risks and yields) utilizes B lymphocytes genetically engineered to express both cytosolic aquorin, a calcium-sensitive bioluminescent protein, and membrane bound antibodies specific for a given pathogen or toxin [14]. Interactions of antigen with antibody elevate intracellular calcium levels resulting in light emission by the cytosolic aquorin molecules. The system responds in a fashion that is more rapid, sensitive, and specific than most antigen detection systems, and has been shown to detect *Yersinia pestis* in less than 3 min at levels of 50 colony forming units [14].

16.3.2 Antigen–Non-Antibody Target Interactions

In recent years, the recognition that pathogens can evoke specific T-cell responses has been used to develop assays such those used in the enzyme-linked immunospot assay (ELISPOT) T-SPOT TB® and Quantiferon-TB for the diagnosis of latent tuberculosis infection. The exquisite sensitivity of these assays in which signature TB peptides elicit specific interferon gamma release makes them applicable to immunosuppressed individuals, while the specificity of the assay overcomes problems such as prior vaccination with Bacille Calmette-Guérin (BCG). These assays cannot distinguish between drug sensitive and resistant forms of TB, but are particularly valuable in following diseases transmission in settings where multidrug resistant (MDR) or extremely drug resistant (XDR) strains are prevalent.

Enzymatic activity has been used for some time in the detection of microorganisms. For example, the presence of significant levels of *Helicobacter pylori* in gastric secretions has been made using the detection of urease activity of the bacillus. Although bacterial urease production is not unique to *H. pylori*, the other urea producers are not found in the human stomach, the site of replication of *H. pylori*.

An example of a bioterrorism antigen detection system utilizing a specific enzymatic interaction with a substrate rather than binding to an antibody is the micromechanosensor reported by Liu, et al. [15]. The functional nature of a toxin is detected utilizing microfabricated cantilevers [16]. In this proof of concept model, botulinum neurotoxin B is detected by its activity as a endopeptidase, cleaving its neurotarget synaptobrevin 2 (also referred to as VAMP 2). The reporting system detects the large change in resonance frequency of the vibrations of the cantilever following release of the agarose bead, which is bound to the cantilever by synaptobrevin. The cantalever system is most sensitive in gaseous or vacuum milieus and the fluid medium damps the vibration to some degree. It can detect botulinum toxin at 8 nM concentration within 15 min and is applicable to on-chip electronic technology that greatly increases sensitivity.

16.3.3 Genetics: Exploiting Genomic Differences

Genomic differences between microbes offer an alternative to culturing for detection and identification of pathogens by providing species-specific DNA targets that can be accurately resolved by molecular methodology. Nucleic acid-based molecular approaches for pathogen identification overcome many of the deficiencies associated with conventional methods by exploiting both large- and small-scale genomic differences between organisms. Polymerase chain reaction (PCR)-based amplification of highly conserved ribosomal RNA (rRNA) genes, intergenic sequences, and specific toxin genes is currently the most reliable approach for identification of bacterial, fungal and many viral pathogenic agents. When combined with microarray or fluorescence-based oligonucleotide detection systems, these molecular approaches provide quantitative, high fidelity analysis [8, 17, 18]. Most importantly, these genetic probing systems offer rapid turn around time (1–6 h) and are suitable for high throughput, automated multiplex operations critical for use in clinical diagnostic laboratories.

The need for rapid diagnostics was never more apparent than during the severe acute respiratory syndrome (SARS) epidemic of the spring of 2003. In the early stages of the epidemic, physicians and public health officials were relatively helpless to contain a fast moving, globally spreading epidemic of severe atypical pneumonia caused by an unknown respiratory agent. Once the viral agent was identified, genomic sequences of the SARS coronavirus (CoV) were used to develop a diagnostic assay within days that rapidly (within 1–2 h) and reliably identified the SARS CoV in a range of clinical and environmental specimens [19]. Armed with molecular tools, physicians and public health officials in China and Canada, hit hardest by the disease, could confirm the cause of rapidly spreading atypical pneumonias, monitor virus levels in patients and explore potential sources for the outbreak [20–23]. This single event highlighted the importance of rapid molecular diagnostics in outbreak control and disease management, signaling the arrival of a new era in diagnostics.

16.3.3.1 Attributes of a Comprehensive Diagnostic Test

An effective diagnostic assay must be rapid, sensitive and specific as well as being simple and robust to facilitate use in clinical and public health laboratories. Assays should detect a wide variety of pathogens and, where possible, have capacity to detect "designer" organisms (heterologously expressed toxin or virulence genes) created through recombinant technologies. Genetic-based molecular assays are currently in development that not only include all category A through C pathogen and toxin genes but also include a wide range of common bacteria, viruses and fungi. With this approach, it is possible to recognize in clinical (respiratory secretions, blood, urine, tissue), environmental (including letters, nasal swabs and hair) and food or water samples the presence of a pathogenic organism that is present as a homogeneous population or is cloaked by dispersion within a large population of nonpathogenic organisms. It is also possible to detect unnatural events such as the expression of a lethal toxin gene (such as a botulinum toxin genes) in a recipient nonpathogenic organism such as *Escherichia coli* or *Bacillus subtilis*. Similarly, a mixed powder containing anthrax-laden spores in a background of 99.9% *B. subtilis* spores would be perceived as harmless, until the 0.1% *B. anthracis* component began to cause disease. Such complex mixtures can be easily resolved by molecular diagnostics.

Specificity and sensitivity are also key elements of the diagnostic assay. When specific probes are used, they must be shown to interact only with their designated targets to avoid false positive responses. The advent of real-time self-reporting probes capable of allele-specific sequence discrimination at the level of a single nucleotide allows these probes to react with exceptional fidelity [24, 25]. Sensitivity is a major requirement especially because in early stages of a disease few pathogens may be present for detection. Some pathogens like *Francisella tularensis*, the etiological agent of tularemia, need only a few organisms to cause lethal disease [26].

16.3.3.2 DNA Microarrays

Microarrays of nucleic acids were developed to utilize the enormous amount of information provided by genome projects but have clear potential in mass screening and diagnostics [27, 28]. A microarray allows thousands of targets to be analyzed simultaneously, being particularly useful for novel virus identification and characterization. Microarrays consist of gene and genome-specific nucleic acid fragments, either cloned gene segments or long (70–80 mers) oligonucleotides, which are fixed to a glass slide or other solid matrix such as those used for computer chips [29]. One such product is the GeneChip®, a high density, oligonucleotide-based DNA array developed at Affymetrix. Target DNA or RNA is labeled and hybridized to complementary DNA sequences on the microarray. Scanning lasers are used to detect high affinity interactions and each addressable position corresponds to a known target.

The application of this maturing technology may be best illustrated during the outbreak of SARS during early 2003. To assist in trying to identity the pathogen, the CDC referred specimens containing the unknown agent to many laboratories, including that of Dr. Joseph DeRisi. DeRisi had developed a microarray chip called Virochip containing nucleic acids specific for numerous viruses known to cause human disease. Hybridization of the unknown virus genome segments to the chip revealed the presence of a previously uncharacterized coronavirus. Subsequent molecular characterization and phylogenetic sequence comparisons confirmed that the virus was a new member of this family [30, 31].

Microarray technology is powerful but also expensive, technically demanding and labor intensive. Amplifying the sample above background is critical to achieve dependable results. A highly purified nucleic acid sample is best for the assay as interfering substances may limit hybridization. False positive interactions can usually be minimized through careful microarray development with suitable redundancy of targets. It is best, however, to verify independently "positive hits" with a different technique. Like any hybridization-based assay, target specificity is critical, although absolute fidelity can be fine tuned. Allele-specificity at the level of single nucleotide changes can be desirable for subtyping of species [32]. The ability to detect imperfect matches within a family is equally desirable for the discovery of new disease agents and variants of old ones (SARS CoV). Of course, genetic microarrays like other genetic approaches can detect the presence of toxin genes, but they cannot be used to directly detect toxins.

A trend toward fully automated microfluidic applications involving chip-based capillary electrophoresis that can perform in-line reagent dispensing, hybridization, and detection significantly reduces sample sizes and improves accuracy [33]. The combination of array hybridization followed by direct viral sequence recovery provides a general strategy for the rapid identification and characterization of novel viruses and emerging infectious diseases. The ability of DNA microarrays to identify either multiple gene targets from single or multiple pathogens in a single sample has the capacity to transform detection of emerging pathogens. It is particularly useful to evaluate rapidly changing disease agents such as influenza [34]. New platforms such as the GreeneChipPm, which is a panmicrobial microarray comprising 29,455 sixty-mer oligonucleotides, is suitable for comprehensive detection of a wide range of vertebrate viruses, bacteria, fungi, and parasites [35]. This technology has the potential to transform blood testing by providing an integrated platform for comprehensive testing that replaces multiple individual assays [35, 36].

16.3.3.3 Real-Time Probes

The simplest PCR form involves the use of specific primers to amplify a known target fragment of DNA or RNA and detection the product with an intercalating dye. This approach relies upon the specificity of linear DNA-DNA or DNA-RNA hybridization probes in the amplification process. Probe-target hybridization is highly temperature dependent, however, and, depending on the nucleotide composition of the probe, random annealing can pose a problem. Sequences with high G + C contents are especially vulnerable since the temperature profile for annealing is shifted and false priming may occur.

In general, standard PCR-based amplification is insufficient for identification purposes due to relatively high levels of false positive results. A solution to this problem is the use of fluorescent probes such as the 5′ endonuclease, adjacent linear and hairpin oligoprobes and the self-fluorescing amplicons that require high fidelity binding to target sequences for detection [18, 37–39]. Such high fidelity probes, especially self-reporting probes, have additional advantages in that both PCR amplification and detection can be done in a sealed tube, greatly reducing the possibility of contamination. They can also be used in real-time assays in which product formation is continuously monitored and validated. This is an important consideration for a clinical microbiology lab because PCR amplification has the potential to amplify small amounts of target DNA from contaminating organisms or even human DNA. Real-time PCR does not require post-PCR sample handling, preventing potential PCR product carry-over contamination and facilitating high throughput assays. Real-time PCR assays using high fidelity probes are also rapid (0.5–2 h), quantitative and have a large dynamic range exceeding 1 million-fold of starting target.

Probing systems including LightCycler™ [40, 41], TaqMan™ [42] and Molecular Beacons [24, 43] are widely used to identify pathogens in real-time assays. The LightCycler system measures the fluorescence resonance energy transfer (FRET) between two linear oligonucleotide probes labeled with different fluorophores in a glass capillary tube format. The probes are hybridized to the target in a head-to-tail motif during the annealing stage of the PCR which bring the fluorophores in a close proximity, causing a transfer of energy resulting in an emission of a detectable fluorescent light. TaqMan probes are linear oligonucleotides that contain a 5′ reporter dye and 3′ acceptor with overlapping emission-absorption spectra. The reporter dye remains quenched by the 3′ acceptor, while hybridized to its target. Cleavage of the 5′ reporter by 5′ nuclease activity of Taq DNA polymerase results in strong fluorescence signals. TaqMan can be utilized in a 96 well format, amenable to high throughput screening. One limitation of FRET-based systems is that multiplexing is more limited since several quenchers in the same reaction are required and spectral overlap can be a problem. Molecular Beacons are small, single stranded nucleic acid hairpin probes that brightly fluoresce when bound to their targets [43]. The probes possess a stem and loop structure in which the loop contains a complementary target sequence. The stem forms by the annealing of short complementary nucleotide sequence arms adjacent to the target sequence. A fluorophore is covalently linked to one end of the stem sequence with a quencher covalently linked to the other end. In free solution, Molecular Beacons do not fluoresce because the stem structure keeps the fluorophore close to the quencher and fluorescence energy is absorbed and released as heat. In the presence of target DNA, however, the loop sequence anneals to the target and a probe-target hybrid is formed forcing the stems containing the fluorophore and quencher apart, and fluorescence occurs. Molecular Beacons are better suited than most linear probes to monitor authentic amplicons in PCR reactions because a single nucleotide mismatch can prevent a Molecular Beacon from binding to its target and lighting up [24]. Both TaqMan and Molecular Beacons can detect single nucleotide changes and are highly suitable for allelic discrimination [24, 44].

16.3.3.4 Multiplex Assays

A single multiplex reaction assay that combines numerous probes and is capable of identifying multiple pathogens is a more efficient and cost-effective approach for a clinical microbiology lab, greatly expanding the capacity of pathogens being surveyed. Multiplex assays require that probes representing different targets can be reliably resolved in the same reaction tube or well. Typically, different probes are labeled with a range of fluorophores that have unique emission spectra that can be discerned with discrete optics or dispersed onto an array for detection. When dealing with fluorophores, the spectral properties of the probe-target hybrid must be significantly different from the unbound probes to permit unambiguous probe identification. LightCycler™, TaqMan™ and Molecular Beacon probes are all suitable for multiplex assays. The ability to multiplex PCR by probe color and melting temperature (T(m)) greatly expands the power of real-time analysis. Novel labeling techniques are evolving quickly that will allow more than 50 targets to be simultaneously evaluated in a single reaction. For example, MassTag PCR, which has been used detect viral hemorrhagic fever, is a multiplex assay in which microbial gene targets are coded by a library of 64 distinct mass tags. Nucleic acids are amplified by multiplex PCR using up to 64 primers, each labeled by a photo-cleavable link with a different molecular weight tag. After separation of the amplification products from unincorporated primers and release of the mass tags from the amplicons by UV irradiation, tag identity is analyzed by mass spectrometry [45].

16.3.3.5 Target Selection

A number of target sequences have been proposed for the identification of pathogens likely to be used in a bioterrorist event. Some targets are specific to a single species, subspecies, toxin or virulence factor (Table 16.1). Other targets can be used more generally such as ribosomal RNA (rRNA) genes or heat shock genes. These genes contain highly conserved DNA sequences (usually required for function) interspaced with variable regions that have been widely utilized in species-specific genetic assays. Ribosomal genes in fungi and bacteria have conserved sequences that are ideal for universal primer targeting, contain variable sequence regions that are species-specific, and are present in high copy-number tandem repeats [46]. The gene for the small-subunit ribosomal RNA (16 S-like) has been especially useful in evolutionary studies of distant phylogenetic relationships, remaining quite stable during evolution of all organisms [47]. The 16 S-like ribosomal genes can be amplified from total DNA isolated from essentially any organism using a single set of primers recognizing the conserved regions of the gene.

DNA or RNA from a wide variety of organisms can be amplified using a single set of "universal" PCR primers that bind to conserved regions of these genes. Species determination may then be performed by analyzing the

Table 16.1 Targets for real-time detection of toxins and secretion systems

Name	Organism	Gene(s)
Ricin	*R. communis*	*RTA & RTB*
Staphylococcus Enterotoxin B	*S. aureus*	*entB*
Botulinum A	*C. botulism*	*BoNT/A*
Botulinum B	*C. botulism*	*BoNT/B*
Botulinum C	*C. botulism*	*BN/C1*
Botulinum D	*C. botulism*	*BoNT/D*
Botulinum E	*C. botulism*	*BotE*
Botulinum F	*C. botulism*	*BotF*
Botulinum G	*C. botulism*	*BoNT/G*
Difficile A	*C. difficile*	*ToxA*
Difficile B	*C. difficile*	*ToxB*
Perfrigens Type A	*C. perfrigens*	*cpE*
Epsilon toxin	*C. perfrigens*	*extD*
Shiga toxin 1 & 2	*E. coli*	*STX1 & 2*
Listeriolysin	*L. monocytogenes*	*hly1*
Diptheria	*C. diphtheriae*	*Tox*
Yersinia translocon proteins	*Yersinia spp.*	*YorB, YorD, LcrV*
Pseudomonas translocon proteins	*P. aeruginosa*	*PopB, PopD, PcrV*
Shigella translocon proteins	*S. flexneri*	*IpaB, IpaC*
EPEC translocon proteins	*E. coli*	*EspB, EspD*
Salmonella translocon proteins	*Salmonella spp.*	*AF056246*
Xanthamonas translocon protein	*X. campestris*	*HrpF*

species-specific sequences contained in regions within the resulting amplicons [48]. There are advantages to both types of targets. Specific targets can be detected in samples that are heavily contaminated with nonpathogenic bacteria. They also make it possible to detect virulence factors inserted into normally innocuous bacteria. "Universal" target amplification approaches have the advantage that they can be more easily multiplexed. A single set of primers serves to amplify multiple species, permitting the development of more general diagnostic assays. The same two approaches can be used to develop targets for viral detection assays, although "universal primers" are generally more restricted to bacteria, fungi and specific families of viruses.

16.3.3.6 Sample Processing

Sample processing development is an integral component of a successful diagnostic program. During a bioterrorist event, depending on its size and duration, a public health lab may need to process tens of thousands of specimens. Rapid nucleic acid extraction from clinical and environmental samples will be critical for downstream molecular evaluation. Extraction of genetic materials must be automated, ultrasensitive and have high throughput capability to process and organize large sample populations. The detection of nucleic acids from infecting microorganisms or viruses in whole blood, tissues, respiratory secretions, urine, and other body fluids can be influenced by numerous factors. Sample preparation depends on the type of biological material that vary in consistency and viscosity. Highly viscous samples (such as mucous) can be difficult to handle and process. Bacterial and fungal spores are encased in a heat and largely chemical resistant shell, making the isolation of nucleic acids troublesome. New cell and spore disruption techniques involving mechanical, chemical, enzymatic and thermal treatments have improved extraction efficiencies markedly [48–51].

All of these procedures are suitable for robotic high throughput processing. When possible, liquid biological samples should be centrifuged to concentrate bacteria, spores and fungi prior to nucleic acid extraction, increasing purity and efficiency. Anticoagulants such as EDTA, heparin or citrate can limit product formation by interfering with the PCR as can large excesses of free genomic DNA. Differential surface-based binding procedures have been developed to purify and concentrate target DNA away from genomic DNA and host-associated inhibitors, improving sensitivity. Magnetic bead technology is an ideal choice for nucleic acid isolation and purification because of its greater affinity for nucleic acids than other conventional methods. It reduces the risk of sample cross contamination found in other extraction methods by eliminating centrifugation and other manual steps during the extraction and purification process. Magnetic bead based nucleic acid extraction can be performed from micro ($<100\,\mu$L) volume samples, is completely automated for high throughput and can rapidly isolate purified nucleic acid in about 1 h. Commercial systems such as MagNA Pure LC™, KingFisher™ and NucliSens easyMAG™ are readily available in clinical laboratories for extraction of both DNA and RNA from a wide range of pathogenic bacteria, viruses and fungi present in clinical samples. These standardized products allow for highly efficient target capture and are scalable over a wide range of nucleic acid levels. The GeneXpert® System is a bench-top sized fully self-contained microfluidic system for sample extraction and nucleic acid detection.

The Cepheid MIDAS II (microfluidic DNA analysis system) provides rapid, on-site testing for bioterror pathogens from environmental samples. It automatically processes biological samples, extracts the nucleic acid, and prepares it for testing. The system then transfers the extracted nucleic acid and PCR reagents to a real-time thermal cycler with eight independently programmable reaction sites. All of the critical processes of the analysis are performed in a closed microfluidic system, including post-analysis clean-up and decontamination. This technique allows for continuous, automated operation over an extended time with an assay time is less than 30 min for pathogen detection.

16.3.4 Validation of Diagnostic Assays

One of the primary outcomes of rapid diagnostics development is to facilitate therapeutic intervention by detecting infectious agents early in infection. This goal requires that a new molecular detection technique be optimized for both sensitivity and specificity, and be validated. An important consideration is to be able to quantitatively compare culture and antigen-based detection in individuals with molecular probes. Once molecular diagnostic approaches are validated, the new diagnostic tools can be refined and used to assess earlier predictors of disease such as elevated temperature or measurable immunological responses. Ideally, validation of a new diagnostic should occur by statistically demonstrating its equivalence or superiority to conventional detection methodology on clinical samples.

Typically, such validations are best determined from clinical specimens obtained from patients in endemic areas of disease. For most select agents, human infections are rare and occur in remote regions outside the USA, making validation on human populations impractical. A partial solution is to use well-developed animal infection models to both optimize and provide initial validation for new diagnostic tools. The primary advantage of an animal infection model is that infection and progression of disease can be more precisely defined. The goal of optimization studies in animals is to achieve the highest possible level of detection while maintaining fidelity of identification in the absence of false positives.

16.4 In Place and on the Horizon

Rapid advances in the genomic sequencing of bacteria and viruses over the past few years have made it possible to consider sequencing the genomes of all pathogens affecting humans as well as the crops and livestock upon which our lives depend. The Chem-Bio Non-Proliferation program of the US Department of Energy began a large-scale effort of pathogen detection in early 2000 in an effort to provide biosecurity at the 2002 Winter Olympic Games in Salt Lake City, Utah [52, 53]. Molecular assays were developed at the Lawrence Livermore National Lab for likely bioterrorist agents by utilizing whole genome comparison methods to recognize unique regions of pathogen genomes suitable for identification. Genetic-based rapid assays were developed for all major threat list agents for which adequate genomic sequence is available, as well as for other pathogens requested by various government agencies. The assays were validated by CDC and were used at the 2002 Winter Olympics [52, 53]. The program continues to add new pathogens to expand the diversity of the detection platform.

The Olympic air monitoring utilized 15–20 monitor stations over an area centered on Salt Lake City. Filters were removed on a 4 h basis and tested for genome fragments of bioterrorism pathogens. During the screening period, a sample collected at the city airport was positive by initial screening. The airport was alerted regarding the potential for evacuation, but confirmatory tests were negative [53]; the cause of the false positive test result was not specified.

In 2003, the US Department of Homeland Security expanded this program into BioWatch, a multicity (initially 20) program. From this "early warning" system, there has been one report of a positive assay. The incident originated in Houston, Texas where air filters detected genomic evidence of *F. tularensis*, the cause of tularemia, on air monitoring filters between October 4 and 6, 2003 [54]; subsequent assays were negative. The source of the positive test was not clear but tularemia is endemic in the state. The $60 million/year system was expanded to 31 cities in late 2003. Yet, it has been criticized for being unable to detect small releases of pathogens [55].

In July 2003, the United States Postal Service employed at mail processing centers a high throughput Bio-agent Detection System (BDS) developed by Northrop Grumman Company. The automated system samples air from critical points around the mail sorting machines. The air is drawn through a spinning membrane of chemically enhanced water that removes contaminants. DNA is then sampled by PCR probing methodology developed by Cepheid, Inc. The system is fully automated with run completion in 30 min. If a biological agent is detected, a system alert is generated that that shuts down operations. BDS was developed initially for anthrax, but it is being expanded to include other pathogens and will be adapted for toxins, as well.

The Science Applications International Corporation is developing a biosensor that combines advanced genomic and signal processing techniques to identify all known, newly emergent, and bioengineered pathogens (including all viruses, bacteria, fungi and protozoa). Known as TIGER (triangulation identification for genetic evaluation of risks), the biosensor uses mass spectrometry to determine the mass of core genetic material selectively extracted from a pathogen. TIGER uses specialized algorithms to read a pathogen's genetic signature. The sensor then checks the pathogen's mass against the masses of known pathogens in its database. This system differs from most antibody-based biosensors that cannot detect unknown or bioengineered pathogens.

An antibody-based microarray, which can be fabricated with a wide range of pathogen or toxin-specific antibodies, is a rapidly emerging approach that hold great promise for disease detection proteomics [56]. Similarly, mass spectrometry-based proteomics is emerging as an important tool, which can be used to study protein-protein interactions on a small and proteome-wide scale and generate quantitative protein profiles from diverse species [57, 58]. The ability of mass spectrometry to identify accurately thousands of proteins from complex samples will continue to improve and impact biology and medicine [57].

Direct nucleic acid detection methods may not be sufficiently sensitive to detect pathogens that are either present at low levels in body fluids or tissues. A promising approach to assess host-pathogen interactions at a very early stage of infection is to develop a signature for the host's immunological response. Both PCR and antigen capture assays require the presence of the causative agent. A number of recent studies suggest that there is a pathogen-specific difference in the innate host immune response and that these differences are detectible by transcriptional profiling with DNA microarrays [59]. In this approach, a molecular immunological signature or bar code-like response would be generated that corresponds to a given pathogen.

In conclusion, rapid advances in diagnostic technology have facilitated real-time multiplex detection of a wide range of human pathogens. A range of platforms are now available in clinical and public health laboratories with the most advanced chip-based detection systems largely confined to academia. Finally, as miniaturization of technology is a rising trend, it is likely that many of the diagnostic platforms will also emerge in deployment of handheld point-of-care devices suitable for rapid detection of agents of bioterrorism or naturally occurring epidemic diseases.

References

1. Perdue, M.L. Molecular diagnostics in an insecure world. *Avian Dis.* 47(Suppl. 3), 1063–1068, 2003.
2. Brookmeyer, R. and Blades, N. Prevention of inhalational anthrax in the U.S. outbreak. *Science* 295, 1861, 2002.
3. Luper, D.C. Anthrax 2001 – lessons learned: clinical laboratory and beyond. *Clin. Lab. Sci.* 15, 180–182, 2002.
4. Nyamathi, A.M., Fahey, J.L., Sands, H. and Casillos, A.M. Ebola virus: immune mechanisms of protection and vaccine development. *Biol. Res. Nurs.* 4, 276–281, 2003.
5. Mothershead, J.L., Tonat, K. and Koenig, K.L. Bioterrorism preparedness. III: state and federal programs and response. *Emerg. Med. Clin. North Am.* 20, 477–500, 2002.
6. Franz, D.R. and Zajtchuk, R. Biological terrorism: understanding the threat, preparation, and medical response. *Dis. Mon.* 48, 493–564, 2002.
7. Blendon, R.J., Benson, J.M., DesRoches, C.M., et al. The impact of anthrax attacks on the American public. Medscape General Medicine 4, 2002. Available at http://www.medscape.com/viewarticle/430197.
8. Firmani, M.A. and Broussard, L.A. Molecular diagnostic techniques for use in response to bioterrorism. *Expert Rev. Mol. Diagn.* 3, 605–616, 2003.
9. Broussard, L.A. Biological agents: weapons of warfare and bioterrorism. *Mol. Diagn.* 6, 323–333, 2001.
10. Andreotti, P.E., Ludwig, G.V., Peruski, A.H., et al. Immunoassay of infectious agents. *Biotechniques.* 35, 850–859, 2003.
11. Raja, A., Uma Devi, K.R., Ramalingam, B. and Brennan, P.J. Immunoglobulin G, A, and M responses in serum and circulating immune complexes elicited by the 16-kilodalton antigen of *Mycobacterium tuberculosis. Clin. Diagn. Lab. Immunol.* 9, 308–312, 2002.
12. Peruski, A.H., Johnson 3rd, L.H. and Peruski, L.F. Rapid and sensitive detection of biological warfare agents using time-resolved fluorescence assays. *J. Immunol. Methods* 263, 35–41, 2002.
13. Yang, H., Leland, J.K., Yost, D. and Massey, R.J. Electrochemiluminescence: a new diagnostic and research tool. ECL detection technology promises scientists new "yard-sticks" for quantification. *Biotechnology* 12, 193–194, 1994.
14. Rider, T.H., Petrovick, M.S., Nargi, F.E., et al., A B cell-based sensor for rapid identification of pathogens. *Science* 301, 213–215, 2003.
15. Liu, W., Montana, V., Chapman, E.R., et al. Botulinum toxin type B micromechanosensor. *Proc. Natl. Acad. Sci. U.S.A.* 100, 13621–13625, 2003.
16. Fritz, J., Baller, M.K., Lang, H.P., et al. Translating biomolecular recognition into nanomechanics. *Science* 288, 316–318, 2000.

17. Peruski Jr., L.F. and Peruski, A.H. Rapid diagnostic assays in the genomic biology era: detection and identification of infectious disease and biological weapon agents. *Biotechniques* 35, 840–846, 2003.
18. Abravaya, K., Huff, J., Marshall, R., et al. Molecular beacons as diagnostic tools: technology and applications. *Clin. Chem. Lab. Med.* 41, 468–474, 2003.
19. Zhang, J., Meng, B., Liao, D., et al. De novo synthesis of PCR templates for the development of SARS diagnostic assay. *Mol. Biotechnol.* 25, 107–112, 2003.
20. Chowell, G., Fenimore, D.W., Castillo-Garson, M.A. and Castillo-Chavez, C. SARS outbreaks in Ontario, Hong Kong and Singapore: the role of diagnosis and isolation as a control mechanism. *J. Theor. Biol.* 224, 1–8, 2003.
21. McIntosh, K. The SARS coronavirus: rapid diagnostics in the limelight. *Clin. Chem.* 49, 845–846, 2003.
22. Zhai, J., Briese, T., Dai, E., Wang, X., Pang, X., Du, Z., Liu, H., Wang, J., Wang, H., Guo, Z., Chen, Z., Jiang, L., Zhou, D., Han, Y., Jabado, O., Palacios, G., Lipkin, W.I. and Tang, R. Real-time polymerase chain reaction for detecting SARS coronavirus, Beijing, 2003. *Emerg. Infect. Dis.* 10, 300–303, 2004.
23. Abdullah, A.S.M., Tomlinson, B., Cockram, C.S. and Thomas, G.N. Lessons from the severe acute respiratory syndrome outbreak in Hong Kong. *Emerg. Infect. Dis.* 9, 1042–1045, 2003.
24. Mhlanga, M.M. and Malmberg, L. Using molecular beacons to detect single-nucleotide polymorphisms with real-time PCR. *Methods* 25, 463–471, 2001.
25. Tyagi, S., Bratu, D.P. and Kramer, F.R. Multicolor molecular beacons for allele discrimination. *Nat. Biotechnol.* 16, 49–53, 1998.
26. Conlan, J.W., Chen, W., Shen, H., et al. Experimental tularemia in mice challenged by aerosol or intradermally with virulent strains of *Francisella tularensis*: bacteriologic and histopathologic studies. *Microb. Pathog.* 34, 239–248, 2003.
27. Anthony, R.M., Brown, T.J. and French, G.L. DNA array technology and diagnostic microbiology. *Expert Rev. Mol. Diagn.* 1, 30–38, 2001.
28. Zammatteo, N., Hamels, S., De Lougueville, F., et al. New chips for molecular biology and diagnostics. *Biotechnol. Annu. Rev.* 8, 85–101, 2002.
29. Ekins, R. and Chu, F.W. Microarrays: their origins and applications. *Trends Biotechnol.* 17, 217–218, 1999.
30. Rota, P.A., Oberste, M.S., Monroe, S.S., et al. Characterization of a novel coronavirus associated with severe acute respiratory syndrome. *Science* 300, 1394–1399, 2003.
31. Ksiazek, T.G., Erdman, D., Goldsmith, C.S., et al. A novel coronavirus associated with severe acute respiratory syndrome. *N. Engl. J. Med.* 348, 1953–1966, 2003.
32. Ferrari, M., Sterirri, S., Bonini, P. and Crenonesi, L. Molecular diagnostics by microelectronic microchips. *Clin. Chem. Lab. Med.* 41, 462–467, 2003.
33. Ivnitski, D., O'Neil, D.J., Gattuso, A., et al. Nucleic acid approaches for detection and identification of biological warfare and infectious disease agents. *Biotechniques* 35, 862–869, 2003.
34. Quan, P.L., Palacios, G., Jabado, O.J., Conlan, S., Hirschberg, D.L., Pozo, F., Jack, P.J., Cisterna, D., Renwick, N., Hui, J., Drysdale, A., Amos-Ritchie, R., Baumeister, E., Savy, V., Lager, K.M., Richt, J.A., Boyle, D.B., García-Sastre, A., Casas, I., Perez-Breña, P., Briese, T. and Lipkin, W.I. Detection of respiratory viruses and subtype identification of influenza A viruses by GreeneChipResp oligonucleotide microarray. *J. Clin. Microbiol.* 45, 2359–2364, 2007.
35. Palacios, G., Quan, P.L., Jabado, O.J., Conlan, S., Hirschberg, D.L., Liu, Y., Zhai, J., Renwick, N., Hui, J., Hegyi, H., Grolla, A., Strong, J.E., Towner, J.S., Geisbert, T.W., Jahrling, P.B., Büchen-Osmond, C., Ellerbrok, H., Sanchez-Seco, M.P., Lussier, Y., Formenty, P., Nichol, M.S., Feldmann, H., Briese, T. and Lipkin, W.I. Panmicrobial oligonucleotide array for diagnosis of infectious diseases. *Emerg. Infect. Dis.* 13, 73–81, 2007.

36. Petrik, J. Microarray technology: the future of blood testing? *Vox Sang*. 80, 1–11, 2001.
37. Wilhelm, J. and Pingoud, A. Real-time polymerase chain reaction. *Chembiochem* 4, 1120–1128, 2003.
38. Mackay, I.M., Arden, K.E. and Nitsche, A. Real-time PCR in virology. *Nucleic Acids Res*. 30, 1292–1305, 2002.
39. Cockerill 3rd, F.R. Application of rapid-cycle real-time polymerase chain reaction for diagnostic testing in the clinical microbiology laboratory. *Arch. Pathol. Lab. Med.* 127, 1112–1120, 2003.
40. Loeffler, J., Haymeyer, L., Hebart, H., et al. Rapid detection of point mutations by fluorescence resonance energy transfer and probe melting curves in *Candida species*. *Clin. Chem*. 46, 631–635, 2000.
41. Bell, C.A., Uhl, J.R., Hadfield, T.L., et al. Detection of *Bacillus anthracis* DNA by LightCycler PCR. *J. Clin. Microbiol.* 40, 2897–2902, 2002.
42. Brandt, M.E., Padhye, A.A., Mayer, L.W. and Holloway, B.P. Utility of random amplified polymorphic DNA PCR and TaqMan automated detection in molecular identification of *Aspergillus fumigatus*. *J. Clin. Microbiol.* 36, 2057–2062, 1998.
43. Tyagi, S. and Kramer, F.R. Molecular beacons: probes that fluoresce upon hybridization. *Nat. Biotechnol.* 14, 303–330, 1996.
44. Tapp, I., Malmberg, L., Rennel, E., et al. Homogeneous scoring of single-nucleotide polymorphisms: comparison of the 5′-nuclease TaqMan assay and molecular beacon probes. *Biotechniques* 28, 732–738, 2000.
45. Palacios, G., Briese, T., Kapoor, V., Jabado, O., Liu, Z., Venter, M., Zhai, J., Renwick, N., Grolla, A., Geisbert, T.W., Drosten, C., Towner, J., Ju, J., Paweska, J., Nichol, S.T., Swanepoel, R., Feldmann, H., Jahrling, P.B. and Lipkin, W.I. MassTag polymerase chain reaction for differential diagnosis of viral hemorrhagic fever. *Emerg. Infect. Dis.* 12, 692–695, 2006.
45. Anthony, R.M., Brown, T.J. and French, G.L. Rapid diagnosis of bacteremia by universal amplification of 23S ribosomal DNA followed by hybridization to an oligonucleotide array. *J. Clin. Microbiol.* 38, 781–788, 2000.
46. Wagar, E.A. Defining the unknown: molecular methods for finding new microbes. *J. Clin. Lab. Anal.* 10, 331–334, 1996.
47. Greisen, K., Loeffelholz, M., Purohit, A. and Leong, D. PCR primers and probes for the 16S rRNA gene of most species of pathogenic bacteria, including bacteria found in cerebrospinal fluid. *J. Clin. Microbiol.* 32, 335–351, 1994.
48. Bauer, M. and Patzelt, D. A method for simultaneous RNA and DNA isolation from dried blood and semen stains. *Forensic Sci. Int.* 136, 76–78, 2003.
49. Grant, P.R., Sims, C.M., Krieg-Schneider, F., et al. Automated screening of blood donations for hepatitis C virus RNA using the Qiagen BioRobot 9604 and the Roche COBAS HCV Amplicor assay. *Vox Sang*. 82, 169–176, 2002.
50. Loeffler, J., Schidt, K., Hebart, H., et al. Automated extraction of genomic DNA from medically important yeast species and filamentous fungi by using the MagNA Pure LC system. *J. Clin. Microbiol.* 40, 2240–2243, 2002.
51. Read, S.J. Recovery efficiences on nucleic acid extraction kits as measured by quantitative LightCycler PCR. *Mol. Pathol.* 54, 86–90, 2001.
52. Slezak, T., Kuczmarski, J., Ott, L., et al. Comparative genomics tools applied to bioterrorism defence. *Brief. Bioinform.* 4, 133–149, 2003.
53. Center for Infectious Disease Research and Policy. BioWatch program aims for nationwide detection of airborne pathogens. Available at http://www.cidrap.umn.edu/cidrap/content/bt/bioprep/news/biowatch.html. Accessed February 6, 2004
54. ProMED-mail. Tularemia, air sensor detection – USA (Texas). ProMED-mail 2003; 23 October: 20031023.2657. October 23, 2003. Available at http://www.promedmail.org. Accessed February 6, 2004.

55. CNN News. U. S. unveils bioterror sensor network. Available at http://www.cnn.com/2003/US/11/14/bioterror.sensores.ap/. Accessed February 6, 2004.
56. Borrebaeck, C.A. and Wingren, C. 2007. High-throughput proteomics using antibody microarrays: an update. *Expert Rev Mol Diagn*. 7, 673–686, 2007.
57. Aebersold, R. and Mann, M. Mass spectrometry-based proteomics. *Nature* 422, 198–207, 2003.
58. Gavin, I.M., Kukhtin, A., Glesne, D., Schabacker, D., Chandler, D.P. 2005. Analysis of protein interaction and function with a 3-dimensional MALDI-MS protein array. *Biotechniques* 39, 99–107, 2005.
59. Simmons, C.P., Popper, S., Dolocek, C., Chau, T.N., Griffiths, M., Dung, N.T., Long, T.H., Hoang, D.M., Chau, N.V., Thao le, T.T., Hien, T.T., Relman, D.A. and Farrar, J. Patterns of host genome-wide gene transcript abundance in the peripheral blood of patients with acute dengue hemorrhagic fever. *J. Infect. Dis.* 195, 1097–1107, 2007.

Chapter 17
Plant Pathogens as Biological Weapons Against Agriculture

Forrest W. Nutter and Lawrence V. Madden

17.1 Introduction

17.1.1 Background

U.S. agriculture is vulnerable to attacks by terrorists [1, 2]. Biological warfare involving the use of plant pathogens as weapons has the potential to have severe negative impacts on public health, as well as the political, social, and economic sectors of our agricultural economy [3–8]. While it is a given that human populations can be the targets of bioterrorism (e.g., the *Bacillus anthracis* events in 2001), it is not widely appreciated that livestock and agricultural crops are also at risk from attack by bioterrorists via the deliberate introduction of plant pathogens harmful to U.S. crops while the crop is still developing in the field [4, 9–14].

Numerous events throughout history have dramatically affected global food safety and security due to the accidental or natural introduction of threatening pathogens. The events leading up to the *Escherichia coli* 0157 outbreaks in U.S. spinach and lettuce in 2006, and the similar outbreaks in apple cider in the early 1990s are but three examples of outbreak due to a series of so-called "natural events" that led to these outbreaks [15, 16]. Another "natural" event was the introduction of the fungal pathogen that causes Asian soybean rust into the U.S. in 2004 via hurricane Ivan [17].

Agricultural bioterrorism can be defined as the intentional use of a biological organism as a weapon to strike (with terror) against a target human population by adversely impacting a nations agricultural biosecurity. If agricultural bioterrorism is part of an enemy's offensive strategy, then agricultural biosecurity must be a critical part of the defensive strategy. This will require a sound infrastructure and a coordinated effort among highly trained personnel to protect U.S. agriculture from attack by biological organisms (deliberately introduced or otherwise) [13, 14, 18]. The United States National Research

F.W. Nutter
Department of Plant Pathology, Iowa State University, Ames, Iowa, USA
e-mail: Fwn@iastate.edu

L.I. Lutwick, S.M. Lutwick (eds.), *Beyond Anthrax*,
DOI: 10.1007/978-1-59745-326-4_17, © Springer Science+Business Media, LLC 2008

Council (NRC) concluded in a 2002 report that U.S. agriculture is vulnerable to bioterrorism directed against U.S. agriculture and that the nation has inadequate biosecurity plans to deal with agricultural bioterrorism [18, 19]. Moreover, the 2002 NRC Report "*Countering Agricultural Bioterrorism*" concluded that "As of spring 2002, no publicly available, in-depth interagency or interdepartmental plans have been formulated for defense against the deliberate introduction of biological agents directed at U.S. agriculture". This stark realization was reiterated in 2004 by then U.S. Health Secretary Dr. Tommy Thompson. Upon his departure from his Cabinet Post, he gave this somber warning: "I for the life of me cannot understand why the terrorists have not attacked our food supply, because it is so easy".

17.1.2 Needs Assessment

The potential for (and consequences of) deliberate bioterrorism attacks directed at U.S. agriculture needs to be recognized as a serious potential threat to the U.S. and its agricultural economy [1, 6–9, 19, 20]. Such attacks could come from foreign or domestic terrorists [7, 10, 11, 18–23]. Although efforts to deter and prevent the introduction of new and emerging agricultural pathogens and pests at our borders have been significantly increased since September 11, the potential for bioterrorists attacks remains an Achilles heel that greatly threatens U.S. agricultural biosecurity. We as a nation cannot afford to be overconfident. Efforts to prevent or deter acts of agricultural bioterrorism, by themselves, cannot ensure the biosecurity of U.S. agriculture [8, 18, 20, 24–26].

On a positive note, several key efforts have been undertaken by USDA National Program Leaders to correct these vulnerabilities. With regards to plant pathogens, two anti-bioterrorism programs have been established. First, The National Plant Diagnostic Network (NPDN) was established in June 2002 (http://npdn.ppath.cornell.edu/Mission.htm) to link all plant disease diagnostic laboratories throughout the U.S. to better communicate (in real time) the presence of agricultural threats found in the U.S. The NPDN provides the infrastructure to: (i) facilitate intra- and inter-regional diagnostic collaboration, (ii) make accurate and rapid diagnoses/identifications, and (iii) gather temporally and geospatially-referenced diagnostic data. The mission of NPDN is to enhance national agricultural biosecurity by quickly detecting new and emerging pathogens and pests that threaten U.S. agriculture. The NPDN has tremendous potential to facilitate the rapid exchange of critical diagnostic information within and among the five Regional Diagnostic Centers. During crises, the exchange of real-time information concerning the rapid detection of emerging diseases and pests, the documented (real-time) geographical distribution (i.e., GIS disease/pest prevalence maps), and the predicted distribution and establishment of new and emerging (and endemic) diseases and pests, will be paramount to effectively mitigate potential impacts. This newly created federal agency has significantly increased and improved coordinated efforts that have greatly increased U.S. preparedness within and among key federal and state Department's of Agriculture, and U.S. Land Grant Institutions. As a result, the NPDN system now provides the critical infrastructure needed to communicate the early detection and reporting of plant pathogens that potentially threaten U.S. crop biosecurity. Early detection is a critical first step that underpins decisions concerning mitigation response and recovery plans [27].

The second key USDA initiative also commenced in June 2002 when President Bush signed into law, The Public Health Security and Bioterrorism Preparedness and Response Act of 2002. This legislation established much-needed regulations governing the possession, use, and transfer of biological agents and toxins that have been determined to have the potential to pose a severe threat to public health and safety, including threats to plant (crop) health. Moreover, this Act established the authority of the Secretary of Agriculture to establish a "select" list of biological agents that the Secretary has determined can pose a real threat to plant health (Table 17.1). The Act further requires that all persons in possession of any listed biological agent must notify the Secretary of such possession within 60 days of the publication of that

Table 17.1 The select agent plant pathogen list, as determined by interim and final rules in 2002, 2005, and 2008

2002	2005	2008
Liberobacter africanus (Citrus greening diseases)	*Candidatus Liberobacter africanus*	*Candidatus Liberobacter africanus*
N/A	N/A	*Candidatus Liberobacter americanus*
Liberobacter asiaticus	*Candidatus Liberobacter asiaticus*	Removed from list
Peronosclerospora philippinensis (Philippine downy Mildew of corn)	*Peronosclerospora philippinensis*	*Peronosclerospora philippensis* (and its *synonym P. sacchari)*
Phakopsora pachyrhizi (Asian soybean rust)	Removed from list	N/A
Plum pox potyvirus	Removed from list	N/A
Ralstonia solanacearum, race 3, biovar 2 (Potato brown rot)	*Ralstonia solanacearum,* race 3, biovar 2	*Ralstonia solanacearum,* race 3, biovar 2
Sclerophthora rayssiae var. zeae (Corn brown stripe downy mildew)	*Sclerophthora rayssiae* var. zeae	*Sclerophthora rayssiae* var. zeae
Synchytrium endobioticum (Potato wart disease)	*Synchytrium endobioticum*	*Synchytrium endobioticum*
Xanthomonas oryzae pv. oryzicola (Rice bacterial leaf blight)	*Xanthomonas oryzae pv. oryzicola*	*Xanthomonas oryzae* (all pathovars including *pv. oryzirola, and pv. oryzae)*

Table 17.1 (continued)

2002	2005	2008
Xylella fastidiosa (citrus variegated chlorosis strain)	*Xylella fastidiosa* (citrus variegated chlorosis strain)	*Xylella fastidiosa* (citrus variegated chlorosis strain)
N/A	N/A	*Phoma glycinicola* (Red leaf blotch of soybean)
N/A	N/A	*Phytophthora kernoviae* (Tree bleeding stem disease)
N/A	N/A	*Rathayibacter toxicus* (Gumming disease of grasses)

N/A = not applicable (not on the select agent list) at that time.

regulation. Section 212 of the Act also established the manner in which persons who require the possession of a select agent for purposes of research can safely acquire, use, transfer (transport), handle, and dispose of select agents. Thus, the Secretary of Agriculture was given oversight to ensure the availability and biosecurity of biological agents for research, education, and other legitimate purposes. Still, challenges remain concerning the development of suitable threat surveillance systems, new pathogen detection tools, the capability for real-time disease monitoring (mapping), as well as the establishment of coordinated information delivery systems to meet future challenges in crop biosecurity.

17.2 Weaponization of Plant Pathogens

The term “weaponization” cannot be found in today’s dictionaries, however in the context of plant pathogens, the “weaponization of plant pathogens” can be simply defined as “the use of a plant pathogen as a weapon to threaten the ability to produce a safe and affordable food supply”. Unlike the situation with many human pathogens, there are few obstacles to the weaponization of plant pathogens [17, 19]. First, many of the estimated 50,000 plant pathogens that occur in nature are already highly infectious and aggressive. Second, plant pathogens are rarely harmful to the human perpetrators, and therefore, plant pathogens can be easily acquired, transported, and handled, without fear of harm to the handler. Because plant diseases have rarely been successfully eradicated, it is relatively easy to obtain pathogen isolates from diseased plants known to occur in other areas of the world, and through modern transportation systems, plant pathogen isolates can be brought into the U.S. and introduced into a farmer’s field within 24–48 h after pathogen isolates (inoculum) was collected [17]. It is also very easy to culture and increase pathogen inoculum in a laboratory [28]. Third, once an agricultural pathogen is introduced to a new area, attribution can be extremely difficult because of the potentially long time it may take to detect and correctly identify the presence of the introduced threatening pathogen or pest. The database of genetic fingerprints for plant pathogens is much less extensive than that for human pathogens [29], so determining the origin of an introduced pathogen would be a slow process at best. Alone or collectively, each of these factors make U.S. crops highly vulnerable to deliberate attack [12, 17, 18].

Because nature has developed an arsenal of highly infectious plant pathogens that are already extremely fit (epidemiologically) to cause high levels of disease (injury) that will translate into direct and/or indirect crop loss (damage), we do not feel it is necessary that the definition for "weaponization of plant pathogens" requires the inclusion of any process or attempts to modify pathogen genetics to create more devastating pathogens. It should be noted, however, that although bioterrorists groups will likely lack the knowledge base and biological facilities to attempt to improve upon what nature has already provided (as far as creating more devastating plant pathogenic weapons), it is possible that state-sponsored biological warfare programs could attempt to genetically alter a plant pathogen in terms of:

- *Expanding the host range for pathogenicity* – i.e., the ability to cause disease in specific host species has been expanded to include new plant host species (species-level).
- *Increasing pathogen virulence* – i.e., enabling the pathogen to cause disease in host cultivars (varieties) that were previously resistant to the pathogen (cultivar/variety-level).
- *Increasing pathogen aggressiveness* – i.e., creating a pathogen that has an increased capacity to cause more disease (injury) with respect to time, resulting in greater damage (crop loss). The components of pathogen aggressiveness that might be altered through selection and/or genetic modification include: (i) an increase in infection efficiency (i.e., a higher percentage of pathogen dispersal units that successfully complete in infection process, (ii) a shorter incubation period, (iii) a faster rate of lesion expansion/larger lesions, (iv) a shorter latent period, which is the time from infection to the time new dispersal units are formed, and (v) a higher sporulation capacity, which in medical terms is a higher R_0 (More Secondary Cases).
- *A new ability* for a pathogen to be acquired and transmitted by insects (vectors) and/or expanding the number of insect species that can successfully acquire and transmit the pathogen.
- *A new or increased ability* to produce toxins and/or other harmful byproducts that adversely affect human and animal health.

To date, there are a number of infectious clones of plant pathogenic viruses that could be genetically manipulated (in theory) to alter the pathogenicity, virulence, aggressiveness, toxin-producing ability, or insect acquisition/transmission capabilities of a plant pathogen [30, 31]. Whereas the acquisition and movement (transport) of plant pathogens is regulated by The Public Health Security and Bioterrorism Preparedness and Response Act of 2002, this Act does not regulate the acquisition of purified proteins and commercially available DNA components (subclones) that could be reassembled to produce infectious virus.

For example, the in vitro assembly of double-stranded DNA viruses such as those of the poxvirus, herpesviruses and many bacteriophages [30], plus the chemical synthesis of poliovirus using purified cDNA [31] components, has already been accomplished. Thus, legally acquiring or developing the purified components of regulated (select agent) plant pathogens remains a potential threat to agricultural biosecurity. The ability to build a plant virus from scratch with added or enhanced capabilities to cause greater disease damage (crop loss), and/or express proteins/plant products that are injurious to humans or livestock is a scary scenario indeed! It is important to keep in mind that if contaminated dog food can lead to a nationwide scare and loss of animal pets (dogs), as a result of accidental and/or negligent actions (as occurred in 2006), then it is indeed just as plausible, (or even more so) for disease outbreaks in crops to be the result of deliberate attacks. The vulnerability of U.S. crops to such attacks must be taken seriously. The key point here is that any "accidental" or "natural" series of historical events that have lead to accidental or natural disease outbreaks of a new agricultural threat can just as easily be set into motion by deliberately initiating a set of events that will also lead to similar (or even more) devastating consequences than previous accidental or naturally-occurring outbreaks.

17.2.1 Food Supply as a Target for Biological Weapons

The use of biological weapons agents to reduce or eliminate an enemy's food supply is not a new concept [5–8, 17]. Plant pathogens and insects have been the subject of substantial investments in offensive biological (i.e., anticrop) weapons research, especially between WWI and the signing of the Biological Weapons Convention in 1972. nations that signed this document have pledged "not to develop, produce, stockpile, or otherwise acquire or use biological agents for military purposes" [1]. Still, because of the potential negative impacts of plant pathogens on crops yields, foreign and domestic markets, and the potential to sustainability increase the costs of production (due to the need for new or more expensive plant management practices), several countries in the twentieth century have continued to explore the use of plant pathogens as potential weapons when waging war [17]. For example, even after 1972, Iraq and the former Soviet Union continued to develop biological weapons for use against an enemy's food supply [1–3]. Moreover, dissident radical groups have threatened to use pathogens, "agents", or "compounds" against crops for a range of purposes. Realistically, however, even a massive outbreak of a plant or animal disease in the United States would not cause mass famine; the U.S agricultural sector is too diverse, too resilient, too productive, and too closely regulated for this to be a realistic possibility [7–14, 18–20]. Still, the deliberate introduction of any one of a number of plant pathogens can wreak havoc on the U.S. agriculture economy (see next Sect. 17.2.2), and reduce consumer confidence in our nation's ability to produce a safe and affordable food supply (see Sect. 17.2.3 and 17.2.4).

17.2.2 The U.S. Agricultural Economy as a Target for Biological Weapons

It has been estimated that the accidental or intentional introductions of harmful biological agents continues to cost the U.S. economy, public health, and the environment more than 100 billion dollars annually [32]. Rational decision-making demands a detailed cost-benefit analysis of mitigation-response, and crop protection tactics [33]. When an introduced pathogen is first discovered, infected and possibly exposed plants are culled ("rogued"), and fungicides can be used to treat plants in neighboring areas (even for low-value-per-acre plants) to prevent infection. This method is expensive and more often than not, it fails to prevent future infections, especially for pathogens in which pathogen inoculum is wind-dispersed and can be disseminated long distances before initial sources (epicenters) are detected. Moreover, agrichemicals applied as even a short-term response measure can have negative environmental consequences. As emphasized earlier, damages incurred as the result of accidental or natural events can also be incurred if threatening plant pathogens and/or pests are deliberately introduced. The use of biological weapons to attack livestock, crops, or ecosystems offers an adversary the means to wage a subtle, yet potentially devastating form of biological warfare [11, 21, 34].

A successful bioterrorist attack on U.S. agriculture could have severe economic consequences [6–8, 13, 17]. The most damaging impact would be the loss of international markets for U.S. crop commodities and other plant-based materials. Member nations of the World Trade Organization retain the right to ban imports of plant materials that may introduce plant pathogens not presently found within their borders [27]. Thus, importing countries that are themselves free of a specific, highly contagious plant pathogen will routinely impose phytosanitary trade restrictions on countries where these specific, "high risk" pathogens are known to occur (or were recently detected). This can result in billions of dollars in lost trade and mitigation costs, as illustrated by the following recent U.S. examples:

17.2.2.1 Karnal Bunt of Wheat

Karnal bunt, caused by the fungus *Tilletia indica*, resulted in severe economic consequences to U.S agriculture. About 80 countries have banned wheat imports from regions reported to have karnal bunt, even though this disease does not have a large direct effect on wheat yield [35]. When the disease was first discovered in Arizona and surrounding areas in 1996 (probably from an accidental introduction from Mexico), there was an immediate threat to the $5.9 billion per year U.S. wheat industry, since about 50% of wheat produced in the U.S is exported. Because of this threat, the regulatory branch of USDA, the Animal and Plant Health Inspection Service (APHIS), immediately directed efforts to contain (quarantine) the outbreak within the original small, infested farm area and begin efforts to eradicate the pathogen. Over $60 million was spent between 1996 and 1998 by APHIS on this quarantine and eradication effort. It is estimated that growers in the affected area lost well over $100 million from lost sales and increased production costs [35]. In this case, the localized nature of the outbreak and rather slow infection rate of the fungus allowed the United States to convince its trading partners that none of the contaminated wheat was entering the global market, and wheat exports from areas in the U.S. free of karnal bunt continued largely unaffected as before. Unfortunately, karnal bunt was discovered again, this time in Texas, and a new round of costly quarantine and eradication efforts was initiated.

17.2.2.2 Citrus Canker

In addition to the costs that result from reduced international and domestic demand, the costs of containment can also be quite substantial. The introduction of exotic plant pathogens may elicit rapid and aggressive attempts to contain and eradicate the new threat. Unfortunately, quarantine and/or eradication measures can potentially cause more economic damage in the short term than the disease itself. Even for agricultural commodities that are not exported in large volumes?, an outbreak of a phytosanitary-listed disease can invoke vigorous eradication efforts that can have tremendous negative economic effects. However, despite these costs, such interventions are often justified, because, if highly infectious exotic pathogen becomes endemic, the long-term mitigation costs are often much greater than the costs of containment. If containment efforts fail (as most do), however, then mitigation efforts may become a necessity. For example, efforts to eradicate citrus canker in Florida (caused by the bacterium *Xanthomonas axonopodis* pv. *citri*) have cost federal state, and the citrus industry, approximately 100 million dollars per year since containment and eradication efforts were first initiated in 1994. By the time the citrus canker eradication program was halted in 2006, the total cost was approaching one billion dollars for a citrus crop with an annual crop value of 8 to 9 billion per year in Florida alone (Tim Gottwald, USDA-ARS scientist, personal communication). As of 2008, the citrus canker eradication program was the largest eradication program for a plant pathogen in U.S. history.

17.2.2.3 Potato Cyst Nematode

The potato cyst nematode (PCN) was first detected in the U.S. on April 13, 2006, in a soil sample collected from a potato grading station in Blackfoot, Idaho. The early detection of this pest is credited to the Idaho Department of Agriculture's participation in the USDA Cooperative Agricultural Pest Survey (CAPS) surveillance program that is jointly managed by USDA's Animal and Plant Health Inspection Service (USDA – APHIS) and participating state departments of agriculture. Through extensive sampling, the extent of the infestation in Idaho was traced back to seven potato fields in Idaho. Potatoes and tomatoes are the crops principally affected by this soil-borne pathogen. At high population densities, this organism can cause poor potato growth, resulting in a substantial reduction in tuber size, as well as up to 80% reductions in yield.

In August 2006, state and federal officials announced the establishment of a regulatory area that was approximately 10,000 acres near Shelley, ID. Potato growers within this regulated production area were advised to have their fields sampled and tested for potato cyst nematode (before harvest) in an effort to speed the delivery (legal transport) of their potatoes to market. Because pathogen "cysts" that contain eggs of the nematode reside in the soil, an Emergency Action Notice was issued by USDA - APHIS that restricted the movement of soil and potatoes from specific Idaho facilities, including the potato processing facility where PCN cysts were first detected. The movement of cyst-infested soil particles adhering to field equipment has been also shown to be a primary means of dispersing this nematode species (including PCN) to other fields and regions. Thus, growers located within the regulated area were required to have all field equipment cleaned and sanitized before field equipment was allowed to leave a potato field.

To date, there is an ongoing statewide survey to determine the extent of the PCN infestation in Idaho, and to ensure that potato production in Idaho is PCN-free to maintain foreign markets. To achieve this goal, an integrated disease management program is recommended that includes: the ongoing testing of potato fields for PCN (more than 50,000 soil samples from approximately 355 fields and facilities to date), the purchase and use of nematicides to eradicate PCN populations within PCN-infested potato fields, the recommendation that potatoes not be grown in PCN-infested fields for seven years (7-year crop rotation), and the recommendation that only a PCN-resistant potato cultivars should be grown after the 7-year potato-free period has ended. These practices have, and will continue to be followed by potato growers at a substantial cost. The USDA-APHIS-Plant Protection and Quarantine (PPQ) Director of Invasive Species and Pest Management, Dr. Osama El-Lissy, has estimated that approximately $30 million dollars will be spend on eradication and other survey (testing) activities by the end of crop year 2008 (personal communication). Moreover, the estimated cost to achieve the eradication of PCN is estimated to be approximately $50 million over a 6–7 year post-detection time span.

17.2.2.4 Citrus Greening

In September 2005, Citrus Greening Disease (also known as Huanglongbing, or yellow dragon disease) was first diagnosed in the U.S. on a pomelo tree located near Homestead, Florida. Immediately, the state's $9 billion citrus industry was alerted to the potential of incurring devastating losses from this plant disease [36]. Why is this plant disease so catastrophic?

- Infected citrus tree cannot be cured
- Post-infection survival of citrus trees is 3–5 years
- Mature trees will produce significantly less fruit until tree death

- Infected developing trees will not reach maturity (fruit production), thereby causing a tremendous loss on orchard investments
- Eradication efforts for this pathogen in the past have all failed due to delayed detection that allowed for secondary spread to occur beyond initial disease outbreak
- The insect vector for this pathogen (the Asian citrus psyllid, *Diaphorina citri*) serves as the primary mechanism for pathogen dissemination and is an efficient insect vector.

This bacterial disease, caused by *Candidatus Liberobacter asiaticus* (Asian strain), is thought to have originated in China in the early 1900s [37]. The bacterium itself is not harmful to humans, but severe losses in citrus trees have occurred due to epidemics in Asia, Africa, the Arabian Peninsula, and Brazil (see http://ipmworld.umn.edu/chapters/tsaigreening.htm). There are three strains of this pathogen: an Asian strain (*Canditatus Liberobacter asiaticus*), an African strain (*Canditatus Liberobacter africanicus*) and a recently described American strain (*Canditatus Liberobacter americanus*). Because the Asian strain is now present in the U.S. (as of September 2005), the Asian strain has been dropped from the USDA Select Agent List, but the African and American strains have been added (Table 17.1). The African strain remains on this list and the American strain that causes citrus greening was added to the Select Agent List in 2008.

The three pathogen strains that cause citrus greening are primarily disseminated (acquired and transmitted) by two species of psyllid insects, one of which (Asian citrus psyllid), has been present in Florida since 1998. Thus, an insect vector required for pathogen spread was already present and well established (geographically) in citrus production areas before the pathogen was introduced into the U.S.

17.2.3 Loss of Consumer Confidence in a Safe and Affordable Food Supply

Many of the animal diseases that are potential bioterrorist threats are caused by viruses, for which there is no practical therapy once the animal is infected. Therefore, transmission cannot be interrupted by treatment, but only by culling diseased and exposed animals or by vaccination (when that is an option – see below). In contrast to animals, about 75% of plant diseases are caused by fungi, and these can be controlled, to varying degrees of effectiveness by eradication [38]. However, if eradication efforts fail (which they often do), then integrated disease management tactics, such as the application of fungicides and/or the use of resistant cultivars may be needed in subsequent growing season to mitigate disease risk (and yield loss) [38–42]. For many high-value-per-acre crops (e.g., fruit and vegetables, ornamentals, etc.), fungicides are used routinely to control endemic diseases. Some fungicides can move systemically within plants and can arrest the infection process during the early phases of infection. More commonly, however, fungicides are applied to the surfaces of plants and are used prophylactically to provide short-term protection from fungal infection [38]. The use of fungicides and other integrated management tactics will negatively impact production costs, which can severely reduce U.S. competitiveness in global markets [17, 33, 38], as well as raising the price of food (plant and animal) that U.S. consumers will pay at the grocery store.

The remaining 25% of pathogens known to cause disease in plants are bacteria, phytoplasmas, nematodes, and viruses. Many of these organisms cannot be cost-effectively controlled by agrochemicals and/or the use of eradication tactics [38–42]. Such pathosystems create unique challenges when first introduced to a new geographic area, and can be a drain on the U.S. economy.

17.2.4 The Use of Plant and Human Pathogens as Biological Weapons to Adversely Affect Human/Animal Health

One of the worst-case scenarios would be for bioterrorists to use plant pathogens that can produce toxic agents (toxins, alkaloids, carcinogens, mutagens, etc.) as weapons to affect human health. Fungi that produce mycotoxins harmful to humans and animals, such as aflaxtoxin (produced by *Aspergillis flavus)*, fumonicins (produced from *Fusarium spp*.), and ergosterol (an alkaloid from the fungus *Claviceps purpurea*), have all been shown (via natural events) to be responsible for human suffering. This is especially true for *Claviceps purpurea*, which causes a disease in humans called Ergotism or Saint Anthony's Fire. This name originates from the pain and suffering experienced by victims caused by the constriction of capillaries in extremities (fingers, toes, nose). Ergot poisoning occurs when humans accidently ingest bread made from contaminated flour that is ground from seed obtained from rye plants infected with this fungus. In this pathosystem, fungal infections occur while the crop is still developing in the field [41, 43].

17.2.5 The Use of Plant Pathogens as Weapons to Instill Fear and Mistrust of the U.S. Food Supply

Crops that are harvested and sold on the fresh market, such as small and large fruit crops and fresh vegetables, could potentially be used as a delivery system for human pathogens. For example, strawberry production intended for the U.S. market is highly concentrated in two valleys in California. Human pathogens introduced into an agricultural crop while the crop is still in the field, especially if introduced just before crop maturity, (Point C, Fig. 17.1) are more likely to survive in or on the crop until they are purchased on the fresh market and ingested. Plant and/or human pathogens could also be deliberately introduced just prior to harvest (Point D), during storage on the farm (Point E), or

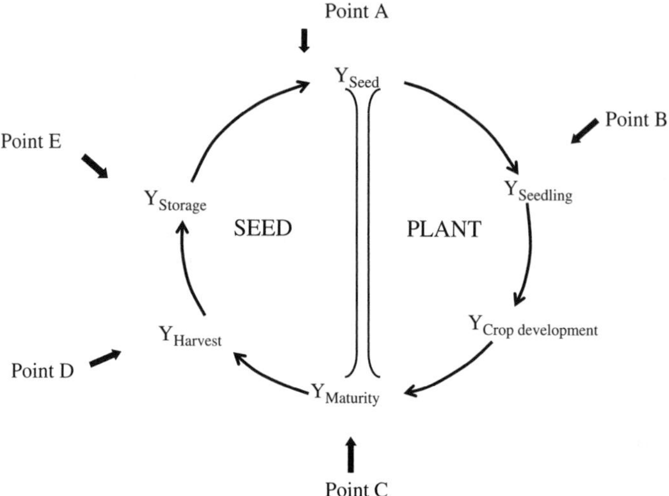

Fig. 17.1 Typical crop production cycle in which plant pathogens (inoculum), could be introduced at a number of vulnerable points during crop development. Y_{Seed} indicates the percentage of seeds infected or infested with a plant pathogen and introduced into a crop at planting, $Y_{Seedling}$ indicates the percentage of seedlings infected at that growth stage, and so on. Human pathogens could also be introduced during any stage of crop development

during transit once the crop leaves the farm. Moreover, conditions during transport, storage, and retail marketing of produce are likely to be favorable for pathogen survival in order to maintain high produce quality [17]. Similarly, lettuce used for nearly all fast food restaurants (as well as in grocery stores) is also produced in rather small, concentrated cropping areas and could be used by bioterrorists as an effective delivery system for human pathogens. In a book chapter published in 2005 by Nutter and Madden, they predicted nearly a year in advance, the scenario regarding the *Escherichia coli* 0157:H7 in spinach outbreak in 2006 that resulted in 205 confirmed illnesses and three deaths. Imagine the fear, panic, and economic harm that would occur if such scenarios were to occur on a regular basis in the US.

17.3 Use of Plant Pathogens as Biological Weapons in the War on Drugs

The deliberate introduction of plant pathogens has found a niche in the war on drugs as a means to destroy narcotic "crops" before they can be harvested [44–46]. There is also a sizable market for the use of plant pathogens as "bioherbicides" to eradicate weed plants (biological control) in commercial crops. This technology has resulted in the development of many bioherbicide products that are used with the intention of replacing chemical herbicides. Such products are now commercially available in many countries. Most of these biocontrol products are highly specific and do not affect non-target plants or other non-target organisms.

In an attempt to control the source of illegal drugs, the U.S. has sponsored research to develop and use plant pathogens as biological herbicides to eradicate narcotic crops. In some cases, plant pathogens have been altered to increase the pathogenicity, virulence, and/or the pathogen aggressiveness of bioherbicide products to cause greater levels of plant injury to targeted weed or plant populations over a shorter period of time [45]. Transferring virulence genes into endemic microorganisms could potentially tip the host-parasite evolutionary balance in the favor of the pathogen, resulting in severe plant disease epidemics in targeted weed and narcotic plant populations [44]. One example of creating and enhancing bioherbicides to destroy fields of narcotic plants is the Nep1 gene from the wilt pathogen, *Fusarium oxysporum*. This gene has been used to enhance the bioherbicidal effects of the biocontrol agent, *Pleosporum papaveracea*, to eradicate opium poppy [45]. In another example, the inherent virulence of *Colletotrichum coccodes* was increased ninefold. Moreover, injury to target weed populations (*Albutilon theophrasti,* northern joint retch) occurred over a shorter period of time (increase aggressiveness). This plant is a serious weed threat in cotton because this weed species has developed resistance to chemical herbicides. Introducing the Nep1 gene, which encodes a phytotoxic protein into *C. coccodes* [44], resulted in faster plant death than using *C. coccodes* without the Nep1 gene.

The pathogen delivery system, i.e., how the pathogen is brought into contact with the target host population (deposition), is also a critical component of a biological control-based weed/narcotic plant control program [34]. The delivery system for a threatening plant pathogen would also be of tremendous interest to the bioterrorist. For example, a stable granular formulation of the plant pathogen *Fusarium oxysporum* has been developed for the eradication of opium poppy (*Papaver somniferum*) [34]. This pathogen delivery system utilizes a wheat flour-kaolin (clay-based) granular formulation. This formulation was found to have a significantly longer shelf life than similar bioherbicide products used to infect this narcotic plant species. Thus, the concept of developing improved pathogen delivery systems to lengthen the time period of pathogen survival, coupled with the development of more virulent and aggressive pathogen isolates to develop bioherbicides, can also be used as a template to develop and deliver biological weapons that more effectively destroy crop plants [45, 46].

The term "biological warfare agents" (biological weapons) was defined in 1969 by the UN Secretary General as being "living organisms, whatever their nature, or infective material derived from them, which are intended to cause disease or death in man, animals, and plants, and which depend for their effects on the ability to multiply in the person, animal, or plant attacked" [19, 47]. This definition is rather imprecise in that it leads the reader to think in terms of biological weapon (BW) agents can potentially affect just a few individuals (man, animals, plants), rather than large populations of humans, animals (livestock and pets), and plants (crops). The UN Secretary General's definition of BW agents is somewhat limited in scope in that the pathogenic effects of many plant pathogens do not require that the BW agents possess the capability to multiply within the host (plant). Indeed, a number of biological weed control agents (mostly fungi) have been developed and used in an inundative strategy to infect and destroy their targeted weed (or illegal drug) hosts [19, 44]. The inundative strategy does not rely on the capability of biological control agents to reproduce and disseminate. Furthermore, some plant pathogens produce byproducts (toxins, alkaloids, mutagens, carcinogens, etc.) that are harmful to both animal and human populations. Again, plant pathogens by themselves cannot infect and cause disease in human and animal populations (which is a clear safety advantage for perpetrators handling plant pathogens as opposed to human pathogens). Most plant pathogenic agents previously considered for use as biological weapons, however, possess extremely fast reproductive rates, and can cause severe crop destruction in a short period of time [5–9, 19]. Asian soybean rust, for example, caused by the fungus *Phakopsora pachyrhizi*, can double in disease intensity (severity) every 2–8 days, depending upon environmental conditions (Nutter, unpublished) (Table 17.3).

17.4 Generating Disease Epidemics

The agricultural biosecurity of U.S. crops can be thought of as a system of linked subsystems, namely: crop production, storage (on farm), transportation, processing, storage (processed product), product transportation, and marketing. In this chapter, we address the vulnerability of U.S crops during the crop production process, i.e., while the crop is still in the field.

A typical crop production cycle beginning with seeding (Point A) is shown in Fig. 17.1. The "Y" indicates the proportion of the seed (or plants) that are infested or infected with a plant pathogen. Although (i) seed certification programs, (ii) phytosanitary restrictions (e.g., quarantines) prohibiting the importation of seed from countries that are known to have specific threatening pathogens, and/or (iii) the use of chemical or biological seed treatments can all act to reduce the probability that an accidental introduction via infested or diseased seed (Y_{Seed}) will occur, there is still a risk that seed could be used as a vehicle to deliberately introduce new, threatening agricultural pathogens. This is because a substantial amount of the seed planted in the U.S. is actually produced in other countries where there may be relatively little oversight with regards to the biosecurity of seed production enterprises. Thus, there is a potential scenario for a bioterrorist group to introduce an exotic seed-born plant pathogen into the U.S. via seed [9]. For seed born pathogens, the spatial pattern of diseased seedlings would initially be random in the developing crop (Point B in Fig 17.1, $Y_{Seedlings}$). Nutter et al. [48] used this "infected seed" delivery approach to generate epidemics of varying intensity in barley, caused by Barley stripe mosaic virus using BSMV-infected barley seed. An initial seed lot of barley that was found to have 64% BSMV seed-infection was blended with healthy seed to establish seed lots with known levels of BSMV-infected seed (0%, 0.1%, 1%, 5%, 15%, 45%, and 60%). The seeds were planted in replicated plots, and disease incidence (percentage of infected plants) was determined. Since the rate of plant-to-plant spread (r) was constant across all seed infection levels, the different levels of Y_0 (seed infection levels), resulted in a range of BSMV-infected plants by harvest time. The approach used to generate virus epidemics of different intensities also facilitated the development of stimulus (BSMV incidence): yield response models [48, 49]. The relationship between the initial level of seed infection (x) and barley yield (y) was then determined using least square regression. Barley yield was reduced by approximately 9.37 kg/acre for each one percent increase in BSMV seed infection ($R^2 = 72\%$) in year 1 of the study, and by 6.97 kg/acre ($R^2 = 68\%$) in year 2 of the study.

While it might seem that little biological knowledge is needed to deliberately initiate plant disease epidemics, a little biological knowledge coupled with the use of epidemiological principles and models can greatly increase the probability of a successful biological attack when using plant pathogens as weapons [28, 50–55]. For example, if seed infection (Y_{Seed}) is zero in a plant pathosystem, then a plant pathogen could be deliberately introduced into the crop anytime between the seedling stage ($Y_{Seedling}$, Point B) and crop maturity ($Y_{Maturity}$, Point C). Questions that would arise for the bioterrorist would be when to introduce pathogen inoculum, the type of dispersal unit (spores, sclerotia infected plant parts, infested crop debris), how much inoculum ($Y_{Introduced\ source}$) is needed per unit crop area, how to best deliver pathogen inoculum to the intended target crop, and finally what environmental conditions (e.g., temperature, relative humidity, leaf wetness duration) are needed to optimize infection efficiency (i.e., optimize the number of successful infections divided by the number of pathogen dispersal units (such as spores or sclerotia). In general, the earlier a pathogen is introduced into a crop, the more time there is for pathogen and host populations to interact, results in higher end-of-season disease intensity levels and greater yield loss [39, 49]. Thus, epidemiological theory can be used to generate more severe plant disease epidemics (see Sect. 17.4.1) to determine how much inoculum is needed. Section 17.4.5 addresses how to determine where and when environmental conditions are most suitable to optimize infection efficiency. While not likely, plant pathogens that infect seeds could be introduced into the field after the crop has matured, but before it is harvested ($Y_{harvest}$). It is also possible that pathogens causing storage rots could be introduced while being temporally stored on the farm.

17.4.1 Model Selection

In order to optimize the probability that an epidemic will be successfully generated, the biology of the pathogen must be considered and coupled with a pathogen growth model that best describes disease increase for a given pathosystem [56–59]. The dynamics of pathogen growth may vary considerately, but two general models proposed by Van der Plank [56] can serve as a recipe to identify the most efficient strategy to use in generating plant disease epidemics. These are the monomolecular and the logistic growth models [56–58]. In the first model (the monomolecular model), the amount of disease in a crop at the end of the growing season is related to the amount of inoculum present at the start of the season. This model has been termed the monomolecular model, because of the analogy to monomolecular chemical reactions of the first order. It is also referred to as the simple interest model, because disease increases in a fashion similar to money invested at a simple interest rate of return. Because the rate of plant-to-plant spread is slow in such pathosystems, the addition of more inoculum (such as spores or sclerotia) to the cropping system will result in higher levels of disease intensity at the end of the growing season [48, 51]. The model can be written as:

$$dy/dt = IR(1 - y)$$

The absolute rate of increase in disease (y) with time (t) in a crop is proportional to the amount of inoculum present in the crop (or the amount of inoculum deliberately introduced into the crop) (I), the efficacy of the inoculum in causing disease (R) as affected by the environment and/or plant host resistance, and the proportion of diseased tissue or plants (y) in the crop subtracted from the total amount of plants or plant tissue available (1.0). Thus, it is possible to influence dy/dt, and thus the amount of disease present at the end of the season, by manipulating I and/or R. Post-detection sanitation practices, chemicals, or biocontrol agents could be used to affect I and/or R in an attempt to mitigate the impacts of introduced pathogens. This is because, in plant pathosystems in which the rate of plant-to-plant spread is low or close to zero, disease management strategies that reduce initial inoculum (Y) will be the most effective in reducing disease risk [38, 42, 56].

In the second model, the logistic model, the absolute rate of disease increase (dy/dt) is related to the current level of disease (y), the apparent rate of increase during the season (r), and the proportion of healthy tissue or plant units not yet infected (1–y) [56, 57, 59]. Because two or more pathogen disease cycles occur within the same season (polycylic), Van de Plank [56] referred to this situation form of disease increase as being analogous to money that earns compound interest. This model is written as:

$$dy/dt = ry(1 - y)$$

Moreover, because the objective of a bioterrorist might be to achieve high levels of disease intensity at one or more points during the growing season (t), this model can be used most effectively if we have estimates of r and y. For example, if the plant pathogen has a high apparent infection rate (r), as with late leaf spot of peanut (*Cercosporidium personatum*), then according to Table 17.2, a high disease intensity can best be generated by using this pathogen in production areas that have both a susceptible target host (peanut) and a favorable environment that would optimize the apparent rate of infection (r). Thus, in pathosystems that best fit the logistic model, optimizing factors that increase r

Table 17.2 Theoretical effect of changes in initial level of disease (y) or rate of infection (r) on the absolute rate of infection (dy/dt)

	Effect of
When r is	Change in y on dy/dt
High	Small
Low	Large

have a greater effect on optimizing the overall rate of epidemic development, as opposed to increasing the amount of introduced inoculum (y) deliberately introduced into a crop. Conversely, for pathogens with a low apparent infection rate, it is more efficient to use tactics that affect y (i.e., add more inoculum) to generate high levels of disease intensity. Thus, the use of epidemiological principles can greatly improve the probability of a crop bioterrorist generating plant disease epidemics to attach a nation's agricultural economy [57, 58].

At the higher end of the technology that could be used to initiate a plant disease epidemic, Nutter and Gottwald (unpublished) used a remotely piloted aircraft to inoculate a field of wheat in Byron, Georgia with the fungal pathogen that causes leaf rust (*Puccinia recondita* f. sp. *tritici*). Leaf rust of wheat is a "high r" pathogen, so just a few grams of spores goes a long way in terms of generating severe epidemics. The experiment was conducted in order to study the spatial spread and disease development of a plant disease epidemic originating from a line source of infected wheat plants. Urediniospores of the wheat rust fungus were "harvested" by gently tapping infected wheat seedlings with a sterile implement to dislodge rust urediniospores onto a sheet of aluminum foil. The urediniospores were then funneled into a sterile vial and transported to Byron, Georgia. Within three hours of harvesting the urediniospores, the spores were mixed with a special petroleum-based oil, and applied as an aerosol to wheat plants from a height just a few centimeters above the wheat canopy using a remotely-piloted (drone) aircraft equipped with a sprayer. Ten days later,

Table 17.3 Effect of year and season on the rate (slope) of soybean rust disease development with respect to time and doubling time (days), y-intercept, R^2, and root mean square error

Variety	Year	Season	Intercept	Slope	R-square	RMSE	Doubling time (days)
G8587	1981	Summer	–6.16	0.080	0.91	0.625	8.7
TK5	1981	Summer	–6.30	0.120	0.93	0.583	5.8
G8587	1980	Spring	–11.16	0.155	0.94	0.831	4.5
TK5	1980	Spring	–9.27	0.157	0.95	0.649	4.4
G8587	1980	Fall	–9.96	0.159	0.95	0.705	4.4
TK5	1981	Spring	–10.46	0.163	0.98	0.363	4.3
G8587	1980	Summer	–17.98	0.164	0.64	2.293	4.2
G8587	1981	Fall	–8.12	0.168	0.87	1.232	4.1
G8587	1981	Spring	–10.78	0.177	0.85	1.188	3.9
TK5	1981	Fall	–8.23	0.220	0.81	1.821	3.2
TK5	1980	Fall	–13.76	0.262	0.96	0.900	2.6
TK5	1980	Summer	–26.23	0.331	0.76	2.431	2.1

there was a line source of leaf rust pustules in a wheat field that was 100 miles from where the fungal spores were actually produced. From a research perspective, the experiment was a success in that a range of wheat rust disease intensities with respect to distance from the line source was generated (i.e., disease gradients were created perpendicular to the line source of infected wheat plants). Although a few cars drove by during the field inoculation experiment, no suspicions were apparently aroused. From a forensics point of view, however, such nonrandom spatial patterns of disease intensity in a field may, in some cases, be evidence of a deliberate attack. However, a "line" source of disease in a field might not always be the result of a deliberate event. For example, in crops that are sprayed with fungicide, a plugged spray nozzle could also result in a line source of disease in a field. Additionally, a spatial pattern of point sources (foci) along fence lines close to access roads might also be evidence that a pathogen was deliberately introduced. Moreover, the presence of disease gradients within crops (i.e., disease intensity decreases with respect to distance from a line or point source) could definitely indicate where law enforcement personnel and scientists should first look for evidence of a deliberative introduction. This is because the presence of a disease gradient points to part of the gradient or "epicenter" (highest disease intensity) where evidence of a deliberate introduction would most likely be found. Pathogen-specific sampling protocols and chain of custody protocols are needed before pathogen isolates are obtained for identification, sequencing, and characterization, etc. To date, such protocols are sorely lacking. However, with appropriate sampling and timely disease/pest assessment/detection protocols, a determination can be made as to whether the introduction of a plant pathogen was by a natural, accidental, or deliberate (bioterrorism) event (Fig. 17.2).

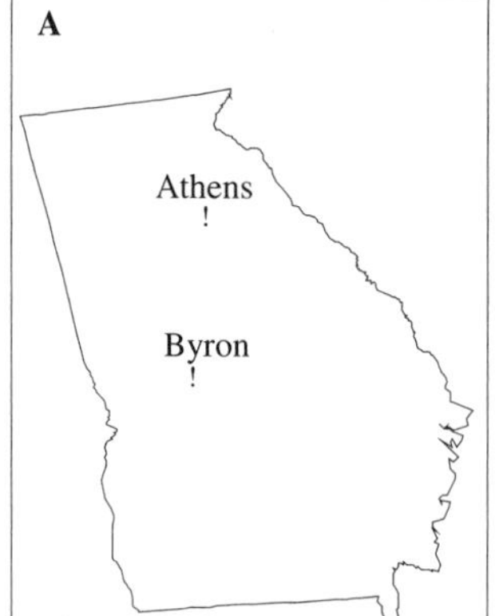

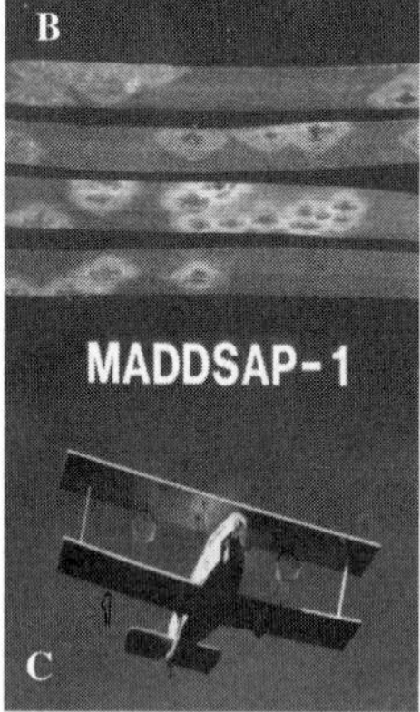

Fig. 17.2 An epidemic of wheat leaf rust (*Puccinia recondita* f. sp. *tritici*) was generated in a wheat field in Byron, Georgia, U.S. (**a**) by harvesting urediniospores of leaf rust from infected wheat seedlings produced in a greenhouse in Athens, Georgia (**b**). A Microbial Agent Dispensing (remotely-controlled) Drone (MADDSAP-1) was used to spray a suspension of wheat rust spores onto a susceptible wheat crop

17.4.2 Varying the Effectiveness of Initial Inoculum

If the bioterrorist wants a specific pathogen to be found and recognized as an attack on the agricultural economy to invoke expensive quarantine and eradication efforts, detectable a pathogen population (inoculum) level can be deliberately established to obtain a desired threshold of disease intensity, (i.e, above a disease detection threshold). If a bioterrorist does not want the pathogen to be found until well after a point in time that eradication would still be possible, then multiple, small, discrete, and well-dispersed introductions within and among crop fields may be established. Nutter et al. [51] used this technique to establish specific disease levels of spot blotch *Cochliobolus sativus* in barley. This was accomplished by inoculating field plots of barley with different numbers of *C. sativus* spores per 150 m^2 of plot area. A fourfold increase from one inoculum density to the next resulted in a linear increase in disease intensity (severity) on the susceptible cultivar Larker. Disease also increased linearly on the resistant cultivar Dickson, but the increase in disease inoculum levels severity in response to increasing was much smaller compared to the susceptible cultivar, indicating that more spores per plot were needed in Dickson barley plots than on Larker to obtain similar disease levels [51].

One major consideration for the use of plant pathogens as weapons is the viability (infection efficiency) of inoculum that was produced at one geographical location for future use at another geographic location. Some plant pathogens can remain viable for a long period of time (Curve A, Fig. 17.3). Such pathogens have an advantage in that inoculum can remain highly infectious (i.e., can cause in many infections) well after the inoculum has been collected (whether in the laboratory or in the field). Pathogens that are more sensitive to the environment after collection may have survival curves similar to Curve B in Fig. 17.3. If pathogen survival is just a matter of hours or even a few days, this would indicate that a bioterrorist must first reproduce (increase) pathogen inoculum locally in a clandestine laboratory or greenhouse. Conversely, if a pathogen has a survival curve similar to Curve A, pathogen inoculum could be produced a long distance from the target crops. For example, Patil et al. [60] reported that the survival curves for soybean rust under laboratory and field

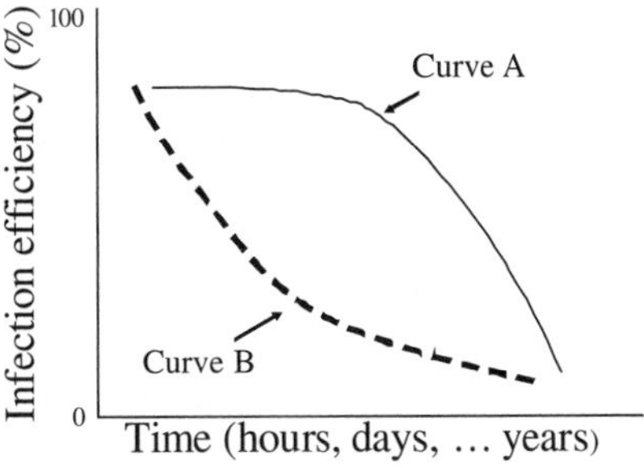

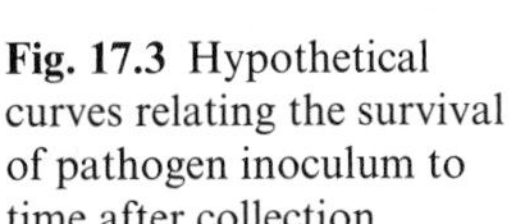
Fig. 17.3 Hypothetical curves relating the survival of pathogen inoculum to time after collection

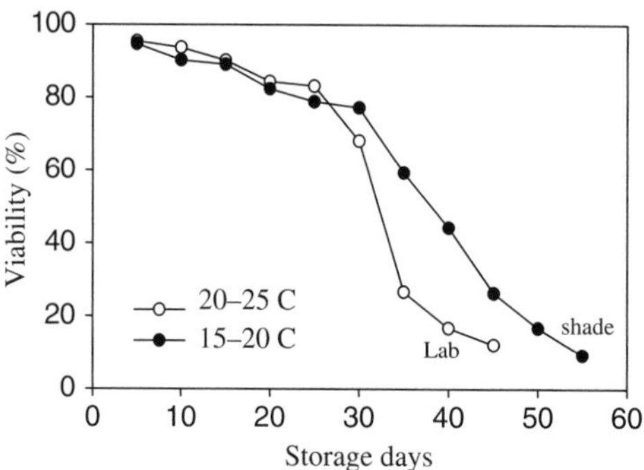

Fig. 17.4 Relationship between storage time and viability of soybean rust spores based on numerical data from Patil et al. [60]

conditions (shade) maintained 80% viability for approximately 30 days after spores were collected from infected plants (Fig. 17.4).

Methods to introduce a pathogen will likely have one major drawback for bioterrorists – that is, the pattern in which inoculum is introduced may not be typical of a natural occurrence [61–64]. Spraying spores onto plots may result in a pathogen population being distributed in a non-random pattern (e.g., the occurrence of "patterns" of disease foci along a fence row or a line source of disease across a field via the use of a hand-based ground sprayer or using a drone aircraft as we did with wheat rust of wheat. A random pattern of diseased plants resulting from pathogen inoculum released from higher altitudes may result in a random pattern of disease foci, however, some yield compensation by neighboring healthy plants can occur in many pathosystems, which would result in less yield loss per unit inoculum that was introduced into a crop. On the other hand, aggregations of diseased plants or pathogen populations may not allow for yield compensation and more yield loss would occur per unit of inoculum if inoculum was introduced in aggregated patches [39, 86]. However, the deliberate distribution of small disease patches overa large geographic area may decrease the probability that every single deliberate introduction performed by a terrorist group will be detected early enough for eradication to still be achievable.

17.4.3 Time of Inoculation

The stage of crop development at which a pathogen population is introduced may greatly affect overall yield loss as well as one or more yield components. For example, inoculating barley with *Cochliobolus sativus* at the late boot stage of crop development will probably not affect the number of spikes (heads) per unit area, but increasing the inoculum level at this stage of growth will likely reduce kernel number per spike and kernel weight. Inoculating at a later crop development stage, such as the milk growth stage, will reduce kernel weight, but not kernel number [51]. Mikel et al. [65] and Gregory and Ayers

[66] showed that yield loss due to maize dwarf mosaic virus in sweet corn is related to time of inoculation, with earlier inoculations resulting in greater crop loss. Nutter and coworkers have also shown that the earlier a crop is infected with a plant virus, the higher the yield loss [48]. Reddy et al. [52] inoculated rice with the bacterium *Xanthomonas campestris* at four different growth stages to generate different disease progress curves of bacterial leaf blight in rice. Early inoculations resulted in the highest levels of disease intensity and greatest yield loss.

Timing inoculations to coincide with specific stages of crop development essentially affects the period of time that pathogen and host populations can interact before harvest. Different environmental conditions at the time inoculum is introduced can, however, also dramatically affect the development of the pathogen populations. Romig and Calpouzos [53] created long and short duration epidemics of stem rust (*Puccinia graminis*) of wheat by manipulating the dates of inoculation to coincide with specific crop growth stages. Young and Ross [54] inoculated soybean cultivars with *Septoria glycines* at different growth stages to estimate yield loss. Again in both experiments, the earlier inoculations resulted in greater crop damage. Some researchers have used successive inoculations to simulate disease increase over time [48, 55]. Thus, duration in time (t) prior to harvest that an epidemic is allowed to proceed can be manipulated by bioterrorists to obtain desired levels of disease intensity and greater levels of crop loss.

17.4.4 Choice of Plant Pathogens Based upon Disease Intensity: Yield Relationships

Crop yields often decrease in a linear fashion in response to increasing disease intensity, as in Curve A (Fig. 17.5). Disease intensity:yield response relationships can also have shapes similar to Curve B and Curve C. Obviously, pathosystems with disease intensity:yield response curves similar to B will result in greater yield reductions per unit disease intensity than pathosystems with response curves similar to curve C. Although karnal bunt of wheat has a disease intensity:yield response curve similar to Curve A, it is still a significant economic threat because of phytosanitary trade restrictions that prevent the importation grain from countries where this pathogen has been found.

17.4.5 Use of Geographic Information Systems to Identify Target Areas Favorable for Optimum Pathogen Introduction and Establishment

Weather-based geographic information systems (GIS) data coupled with disease/pest warning models can be used by bioterrorists to geospatially predict (to

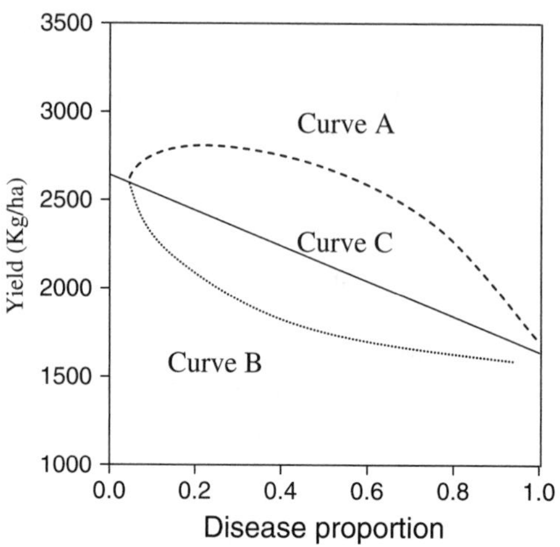

Fig. 17.5 Possible relationships between disease intensity (stimulus) and crop yield (response)

optimize) the probability of successful pathogen infection/establishment [67–69]. Disease-warning systems are management decision aids that are used by farmers because they provide both economic and environmental benefits [38, 68, 69] by increasing the efficiency of pesticide use [68, 70–73]. Leaf wetness duration (LDW) is an important input for many disease-warning systems because the risk of epidemics for many foliar diseases is related to the duration of periods when free water is present on plant surfaces [71, 74]. A reliable forecast of temperature and leaf wetness duration that is provided at least 24 h in advance, could enhance the effectiveness of a bioterrorists attack on crops by enabling perpetrators to take advantage of weather information that would ensure a higher probability of a successful inoculation (infection by the introduced pathogen). Private companies, (e.g., SkyBit, Inc., Bellefonte, PA), provide hourly, site-specific LWD forecasts using models that input forecasted air temperature, relative humidity (RH), and wind speed, for periods up to 72 h into the future. Thus, disease warning (forecasting/advisory) models that are intended for use in disease management can also be used by bioterrorists to determine when environmental conditions will be optimal for a successful inoculation (attack). A good hypothetical example is soybean rust of soybean caused by the fungus *Phakopsora pachyrhizi*. Environmental conditions favorable to optimize infection efficiency of soybean rust to infect soybean requires optimum temperatures between 20 and 23°C and 12 h of continuous leaf wetness (Fig. 17.6). Using weather data from the Midwest Regional Climate Center, the best evening in 2003 to inoculate soybeans with this pathogen (based on these temperature and leaf wetness criteria) occurred on July 4th (Fig. 17.7a). Moreover, conditions were optimal for a small geographic area (See circled areas in Fig. 17.7) that would have wreaked havoc three major soybean-producing states in the U.S.

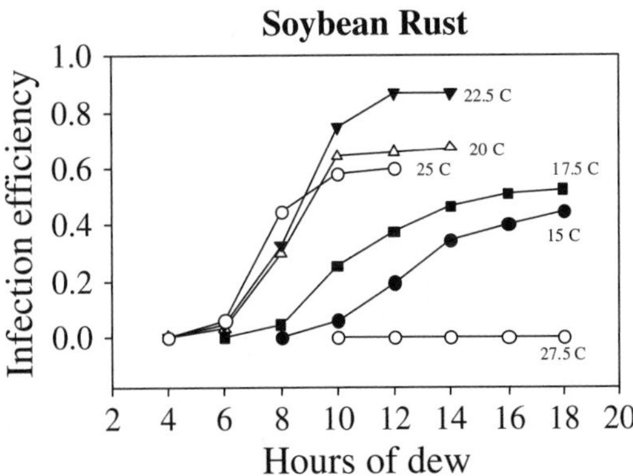

Fig. 17.6 Soybean rust infection index progress curves with relationship between hours of continuous dew (leaf wetness) and infection efficiency at different temperatures

Once a new disease threat is deliberately introduced, it is highly possible for a bioterrorist to predict the local, regional, and long-distance dispersal (transport) of the pathogen/pest. Meteorological conditions influence, and in many cases facilitate the dissemination of plant pathogens and pests. The process of dissemination (release, transport, deposition) is paramount to the development of disease epidemics, for without these processes, there would be no epidemic or outbreak [61, 75]. Atmospheric transport models for plant pathogens provide a link between meteorological conditions and biological and physical properties of the pathogen or pest [76–84]. A number of pathogen, pest, and crop-specific models have been developed to predict the short, meso- and long-distance dispersal of plant pathogens [78–81]. These include the NOAA Air Resources Laboratory Hybrid Single-Particle Lagrangian Integrated Trajectory Model (HYSPLIT) and the MM5 Community Model that was developed at The Pennsylvania State University (http://www.mmm.ucar.edu/mm5/mm5-home.html) and the National Center for Atmospheric Research (http://www.ncar.ucar.edu/ncar/).

17.4.5.1 Post-Introduction Forensics Protocols

Efforts to date to counter agricultural bioterrorism have dealt primarily with preventing the introduction of new and emerging diseases and pests or the development of methods to improve disease/pest detection [13–18]. Until recently, little attention has been given to preparedness after the introduction of a new or emerging plant pathogen or pest has been confirmed [17, 29, 85]. One of the key post-introduction needs will be to determine if a pathogen/pest was introduced (i) accidentally, (ii) by natural means (long distance atmospheric transport, or (iii) by a deliberate act of agricultural bioterrorism. Plant disease epidemiologists will play a major role in post-introduction forensics, just as epidemiologists from the Center for Disease Control and Prevention (in Atlanta) play a major role in post-pathogen introduction forensics and risk assessments for human pathogens. Plant disease epidemiologists trained in

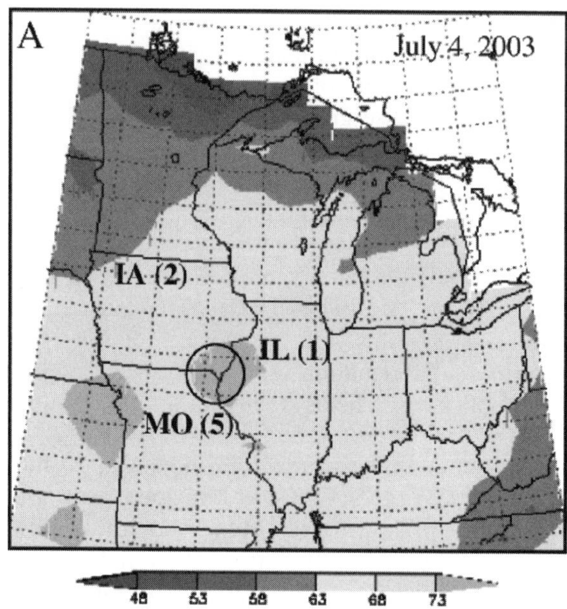

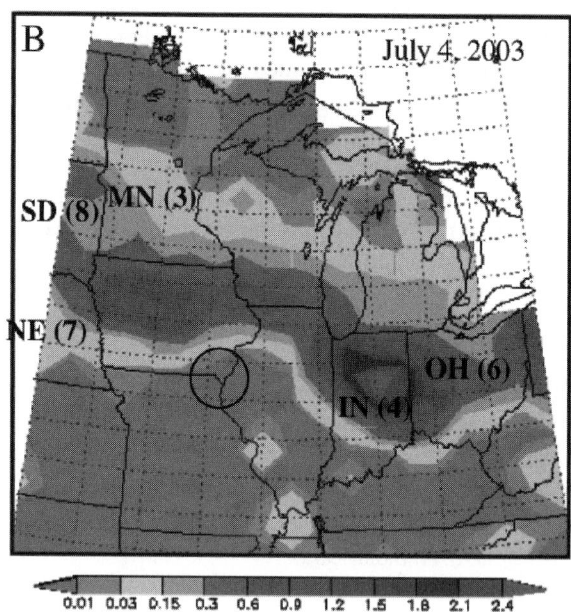

Fig. 17.7 Real-time GIS maps for (**a**) temperature (°F) and (**b**) average precipitation (inches) on July 4, 2003 in the North Central U.S. The area circled for Iowa, Illinois, and Missouri indicates that environmental conditions on this date were highly favorable for infection by the fungus that causes soybean rust. These maps were obtained from the Midwest Regional Climate Center, Illinois State University, Champaign, IL

sampling and disease assessment can provide valuable quantitative and qualitative information concerning: (i) the presence of primary disease foci, (ii) the spatial pattern of primary foci (random, clustered, regular), and (iii) the presence of disease gradients which may indicate the presence of a local or deliberately-introduced source of inoculum [85, 86]. In addition, proper sampling and molecular tools are needed to determine if the introduction consists of a genetically and morphologically homogeneous population or a heterogeneous population of isolates/strains, races, etc. The presence and spatial pattern of the pathogen/pest in neighboring fields (e.g., by mapping the distance of infected/infested fields from major interstate highways using global positioning systems (GPS) and GIS technologies will also important new, quantitative information [86]. Geostatistics can be used to determine if the pattern of diseased fields is random or nonrandom (i.e., deliberate or a natural event).

17.5 Conclusions

U.S. agriculture is vulnerable to attack using plant pathogens as weapons. One of the basic tenets of plant biosecurity is that the presence, actual or predicted distribution, intensity, and economic impact of any yield-reducing factor(s) must be detected early, and accurately identified. As a nation, we must establish coordinated and effective detection, monitoring, and response systems to detect and mitigate terrorists attacks aimed at U.S. agriculture. The development of a real-time, GIS-based (geographic information system) reporting system for new and emerging agricultural pathogens and pests is extremely relevant in the era of agricultural bioterrorism. The goal is to establish a real-time, GIS database network to report, monitor, map (temporally and spatially), the current location(s) and the predicted spread of new and emerging plant diseases and pests. Such networks could also be used to geospatially and temporally monitor endemic pathogens/pests. The integration of remote sensing, GPS, GIS, atmospheric transport models, and weather-based GIS risk prediction models, offers a comprehensive and coordinated system to ensure the production of a safe, affordable, and sustainable U.S. food supply.

References

1. Abelson, P. H. Biological warfare (editorial). Science 286: 1677, 1999.
2. Atlas, R. M. Combating the threat of biowarfare and bioterrorism. BioScience 49: 465–477, 1999.
3. Dudley, J. P., Woodford, M. H. Bioweapons, biodiversity, and ecocide: potential effects of biological weapons on biological diversity. BioScience 52: 583–592, 2002.
4. Harris, S. H. The Japanese biological warfare programmme: an overview. In Biological and Toxin Weapons: Research, Development and Use from the Middle Ages to 1945 (eds. Geissler, E., Moon, J.) Oxford: Oxford University Press, pp. 127–152, 1999.

5. Pearson, G. S. BTWC security implications of human, animal, and plant epidemiology. Rep. NATO adv. Res. Workshop, Cantacuzino Inst. Bucharest 3-5 June. Brief. Pap. No. 23. http://www.brad.ac.uk/acad/sbtwc/briefing/bw-briefing.htm, 1999.
6. Wheelis, M. Agricultural biowarfare and bioterrorism. Edmonds Inst. Occas. Pap. Updated at http://www.fas.org/bwc/agr/main.htm. 2000.
7. Wheelis, M., Casagrande, R., Madden, L. V. Biological attack on agriculture: low-tech, high-impact bioterrorism. BioScience 52, 569–576, 2002.
8. Whitby, S. M. Biological Warfare Against Crops. Hampshire, UK: Palgrave.
9. Condon, M. Implications of plant pathogens to international trading of seeds. In: Plant Pathogens and the Worldwide Movement of Seeds (ed. McGee, D. C.), pp. 17–30. St. Paul, MN: APS Press. 109 pp., 1997.
10. Geissler, E. Biological warfare activities in Germany. In, Biological and Toxin Weapons: Research, Development and Use from the Middle Ages to 1945 (eds. Geissler, E., Moon, J.) Oxford: Oxford University Press, pp. 1923–1945, 1999.
11. Kadlec, R. P. Biological weapons for waging economic warfare. In, Battlefield of the Future: 21st Century Warfare Issues (eds. Schneider, B. R., Grrinter, L. E.) Maxwell Air Force Base, AL: Air University Press, pp. 251–266, 1995.
12. Schaad, N. W., Shaw, J. J., Vidaver, A., Leach, J., Erlick, B. J. Crop biosecurity. http://www.apsnet.org/online/feature/Biosecurity/Top.html, 1999.
13. Meyerson, L. A., Reason, J. K. Biosecurity: moving toward a comprehensive approach. BioScience 52, 593–600, 2002.
14. Moon, J. E. U.S. biological warfare planning and preparedness: the dilemmas of policy. In, Biological and Toxin Weapons: Research, Development and Use from the Middle Ages to 1945 (eds. Geissler, E., Moon, J.) Oxford: Oxford University Press, 215–245 pp., 1999.
15. California Food Emergency Response Team. Investigation of an *Escherichia coli* 0157:H7 outbreak associated with Dole pre-packaged spinach. California Department of Health Services. Sacramento, CA, Final Report 3: 21, 2007.
16. Dingman, D. W. Prevalence of *Escherichia coli* in apple cider manufactured in Connecticut. J. Food Prot. 62, 567–573, 1999.
17. Nutter, F. W., Jr., and Madden, L. V. Plant diseases as a possible consequence of biological attacks. In Biological Terrorism (eds. Greenfield, R. A., Bronze, M. S.) Horizon Scientific Press, Caister Scientific Press, Norfolk, UK, pp. 793–818, 2005.
18. NRC. Countering Agricultural Bioterrorism. Washington, DC: NRC, National Acad. Press, 2002.
19. Geissler, E., Moon, J. Biological and Toxin Weapons: Research, Development and Use from the Middle Ages to 1945. Oxford: Oxford University Press, 1999.
20. Rogers, P., Whitby, S., Dando, M. Biological warfare against crops. Sci. Am. 280, 70–75, 1999.
21. Kadlec, R. P. Twenty-first century germ warfare. In, Battlefield of the Future: 21st Century Warfare Issues (eds. Schneider, B. R., Grrinter, L. E.) Maxwell Air Force Base, AL: Air University Press, pp. 227–250, 1995.
22. Madden, L. V. What are the nonindigenous plant pathogens that threaten U.S. crops and forests. www.apsnet.org/online/feature/exotic, 2001.
23. Monterey Inst. Int. Stud. Chronology of CBW attacks targeting crops & livestock. http://cns.miis.edu/research/cbw/agchron.htm, 2002.
24. Madden, L. V. Plant Pathology fiction: Buzzword. BioScience 52, 619–620, 2002.
25. Madden, L. V., van den Bosch, F. A population-dynamics approach to assess the threat of plant pathogens as biological weapons against annual crops. BioScience 52, 65–74, 2002.
26. Yang, X. B., Dowler, W. M., Royer, M. H. Assessing the risk and potential impact of an exotic plant disease. Plant Dis. 75, 976–982, 1991.

27. Wheelis, M. Outbreaks of Disease: Current Official Reporting. Bradford (UK): University of Bradford, Department of Peace Studies. Briefing Paper No. 21. (20 May 2002; www.brad.ac.uk/acad/sbtwc/briefing/bp21.htm), 1999.
28. Nutter, F. W., Jr. Generating plant disease epidemics in yield loss experiments. Pages 139–160 In, Crop Loss Assessment in Rice. International Rice Research Institute, Los Banos, Philippines. pp. 324, 1990.
29. Fletcher, J., Bender, C., Budowle, B. et al. Plant pathogen forensics: capabilities, needs, and recommendations. Microbiol. Mol. Biol. Rev. 70, 450–471, 2006.
30. Gaussier, H., Yang, Q., Catalano, C. E. Building a virus from scratch: Assembly of an infectious virus using purified components in a rigorously defined biochemical assay system. J. Mol. Biol. 357, 1154–1166, 2006.
31. Cello, J., Paul, A. V., and Wimmer, E. Chemical synthesis of poliovirus cDNA: Generation of infectious virus in the absence of natural template. Science 297, 1016–1018, 2002.
32. Pimentel, D., Lach, L., Zuniga, R., and Morrison, D. Environmental and economic costs associated with non-indigenous species in the United States. BioScience 50, 53–65, 2000.
33. Waibel, H. The economics of integrated pest management in irrigated rice. Springer-Verlag Press, NY. 196 p. Alderman, S. C. and Nutter, F. W., Jr. 1994. Effect of temperature and relative humidity on development of *Cercosporidium personatum* on peanut in Georgia. Plant Dis. 78, 690–694, 1986.
34. Connick, W. J., Jr., Daigle, D. J., Pepperman, A. B., Hebbar, K. P., and Lumsden, R. D. Preparation of stable, granular formulations containing *Fusarium oxysporum* pathogenic to narcotic plants. Biol. Control 13, 79–84, 1998.
35. Bandyopadhyay, R., Frederiksen, R. A. Contemporary global movement of emerging plant diseases. In Food and Agricultural Security: Guarding against Natural Threats and Terrorist Attacks Affecting Health, National Food Supplies, and Agricultural Economics (eds. Frazier, T. W., Richardson, D. C.) New York: New York Academy of Sciences, pp. 28–36, 1999.
36. Streigmaan, A. A Citrus greening continues to spread in citrus growing areas. American Phytopathological Society. Press Release (2007, July 10). http://www.apsnet.org/media/press/07citrusgreening.asp
37. De Graca, J. V. Citrus greening disease. Annu. Rev. Phytopathol. 29, 109–136, 1991.
38. Nutter, F. W., Jr. The role of plant disease epidemiology in developing successful integrated disease management programs In General Concepts in Integrated Pest and Disease Management (eds. Ciancio, A. Mukerji, K. G.) The Netherlands: Springer Publ., pp. 43–77, 2007.
39. Savary, S., Teng, P. S., Willocquet, L., Nutter, F. W., Jr. Quantification and modeling of crops losses: A review of purposes. Annu. Rev. Phytopathology 44, 89–112, 2006.
40. Strange, R. N. Plant Disease Control. London: Chapman and Hall, 1993.
41. Agrios, G. N. Plant Pathology. Academic Press, San Diego, CA., 1997.
42. Fry, W. E. Principles of Plant Disease Management. New York: Academic Press, 1982.
43. Carefoot, G. L., Sprott, E. R. Famine on the wind. New York: Rand McNally. 231 p., 1967.
44. Amsellem, Z., Cohen, B. A., Gressel, J. Engineering hypervirulence in a mycoherbicidal fungus for efficient weed control. Nat. Biotechnol. 20, 1035–1039, 2002.
45. Bailey, B. A., Apel-Birkhold, P. C., Akingbe, O. O., et al. Nep1 Protein from *Fusarium oxysporum* enhances biological control of opium poppy by *Pleospora papaveracea*. Phytopathology 90, 812–818, 2000.
46. Bailey, B. A., Apel-Birkhold, P. C., O'Neill, N. R., et al. Evaluation of infection processes and resulting disease caused by *Dendryphion penicillatum* and *Pleospora papaveracea* on *Papaver somniferum*. Phytopathology 90, 699–709, 2000.
47. Nutter, F. W., Jr. Understanding the interrelationships between botanical, human, and veterinary epidemiology: The Y's and R's of it all. Ecosyst Health 5, 131–140, 1999.

48. Nutter, F. W., Jr., Pederson, V. D., Timian, R. G. Relationship between seed infection by barley stripe mosaic virus and yield loss. Phytopathology 74, 363–366, 1984.
49. Madden, L. V., Nutter, F. W., Jr. Modeling crop losses at the field scale. Can. J. Plant Pathol. 17, 124–137, 1995
50. James, W. C., Jenkins, J. E. E., Jemmett, J. L. The relationship between leaf blotch, caused by *Rhynchosporuum secalis* and losses in grain yield of spring barley. Ann. Appl. Biol. 62, 273–288, 1968.
51. Nutter, F. W., Jr., Pederson, V. C., Foster, A. E. Effect of inoculations with *Cochliobolus sativus* at specific growth stages on grain yield and quality of malting barley. Crop Sci. 25, 933–938, 1985.
52. Reddy, A. P. K., MacKenzie, D. R., Rouse, D. I., Rao, A. V. Relationship of bacterial leaf blight severity to grain yield of rice. Phytopathology 69, 967–969, 1979.
53. Romig, R. W., Calpouzos, L. The relationship between stem rust and loss of spring wheat. Phytopathology 60, 1801–1805, 1970.
54. Young, L. D., Ross, J. P. Brown spot development and yield response of soybean inoculated with Septoria glycines at various growth stages. Phytopathology 88, 8–11, 1978.
55. Gregory, L. V., Ayers, J. E., Nelson, R. R. Predicting yield losses in corn from southern corn leaf blight. Phytopathology 68, 517–521, 1978.
56. Vanderplank, J. E. Plant Diseases: Epidemics and Control. New York: Academic Press, 1963.
57. Campbell, C. L., Madden, L. V. Introduction to Plant Disease Epidemiology. New York, NY: John Wiley & Sons, Inc., 532 p, 1990.
58. Nutter, F. W., Jr., Parker, S. K. Fitting disease progress curves using EPIMODEL. Pages 24–28 In Exercises in Plant Disease Epidemiology, (eds. Francl, L., Neher, D.) St Paul, MN: APS Press, 233 p, 1997.
59. Nutter, F. W., Jr. Quantifying the temporal dynamics of plant viruses: a review. Crop Prot. 16, 603–618, 1997.
60. Patil, V. S., Wuike, R. V., Thakare, C. S., Chirame, B. B. Viability of urediospores of Phakopsora pachyrhizi Syd. at different storage conditions. J. Maharashtra Agric. Univ. 22, 260–261, 1997.
61. Aylor, D. E. The role of intermittent wind in the dispersal of fungal pathogens. Annu. Rev. Phytopathology 28, 73–92, 1990.
62. Allorent, D., Willocquet, L., Sartorato, A., Savary, S. Quantifying and modelling the mobilisation of inoculum from diseased leaves and infected defoliated tissues in epidemics of angular leaf spot of bean. Eur. J. Plant Pathol. 113, 377–394, 2005.
63. Alderman, S. C., Nutter, F. W., Jr., Labrinos, J. L. Spatial and temporal analysis of spread of *Cercosporidium personatum* in peanut. Phytopathology 79, 837–844, 1989.
64. Nutter, F. W., Jr. Detection and measurement of plant disease gradients in peanut using a multispectral radiometer. Phytopathology 79, 958–963, 1989.
65. Mikel, M., A., D'Arcy, C. J., Rhodes, A. H., Ford, R. E. Yield loss in sweet corn correlated with time of inoculation with maize dwarf mosaic virus. Plant Dis. 65, 902–904, 1981.
66. Gregory, L. V., Ayers, J. E. Effect of inoculum with maize dwarf mosaic virus at several growth stages on yield of sweet corn. Plant Dis. 66, 801–804, 1982.
67. Nutter, F. W., Jr., Rubsam, R. R., Taylor, S. E., Harri, J. A., Esker, P. D. Geospatially-referenced disease and weather data to improve site-specific forecasts for Stewart's disease of corn in the U.S. corn belt. Comput Electron Agr 37, 7–14, 2002.
68. Madden, L. V., Ellis, M. A., Lalancette, N., Hughes, G., Wilson, L. L. Evaluation of a disease-warning system for downy mildew of grapes. Plant Dis. 84, 549–554, 2000.
69. Webb, D. H., and Nutter, F. W., Jr. Effect of temperature and duration of leaf wetness on two disease components of alfalfa rust on alfalfa. Phytopathology 81, 946–950, 1997.

70. Wegulo, S. N., Nutter, F. W., Jr., Martinson, C. A. Benefits assessment of fungicide usage on seed corn in Iowa. Plant Dis. 81, 415–422, 1997.
71. Gleason, M. L. Disease-warning systems. In Encyclopedia of Plant Pathology. (eds. Maloy, O. C., Murray, T. D.) Vol I. New York: John Wiley & Sons, pp. 367–370, 2000.
72. Lorente, I., Vilardell, P., Bugiani, R., Gherardi, I., Montesinos, E. Evaluation of BSPcast disease-warning system in reduced fungicide use programs for management of brown spot of pear. Plant Dis. 84, 631–637, 2000.
73. Shtienberg, D., Elad, Y. Incorporation of weather forecasting in integrated, biological-chemical management of *Botrytis cinerea*. Phytopathology 87, 332–340, 1997.
74. Huber, L., Gillespie, T. J. Modeling leaf wetness in relation to plant disease epidemiology. Annu. Rev. Phytopathol. 30, 553–577, 1992.
75. Domino, R. P., Showers, W. B., Taylor, S. E., Shaw, R. H. A spring weather pattern associated with suspected black cutworm moth (Lepidoptera: Noctuidae) introduction to Iowa. Environ. Entomol. 12, 1863–1871, 1983.
76. Fernando, W. G. D., Paulitz, T. C., Seaman, W. L., Dutilleul, P., Miller, J. D. Head blight gradients caused by *Gibberella zeae* from area sources of inoculum in wheat field plots. Phytopathology 87, 414–421, 1997.
77. Leandro, L. F. S., Gleason, M. L., Nutter, F. W., Jr., Wegulo, S. N., Dixon, P. M. Influence of temperature and wetness duration on the ecology of *Colletotrichum acutatum* on symptomless strawberry leaves. Phytopathology 93, 513–520, 2003.
78. Paulitz, T. C., Dutilleul, P., Yamasaki, S. H., Gernando, W. G. D., Seaman, W. L. A generalized two-dimensional Gaussian model of disease foci of head blight of wheat caused by *Gibberella zeae*. Phytopathology 89, 74–83, 1999.
79. Parker, S. K., Nutter, F. W. Jr., Gleason, M. L. Temporal and spatial spread of Septoria leafspot of tomato. Plant Dis. 81, 272–276, 1997.
80. Pedgley, D. E. Long distance transport of spores. In Plant Disease Epidemiology (eds. Leonard, K. J., Fry, W. E.) New York: MacMillan Publishing Company, pp. 346–365, 1986.
81. Smelser, R. B., Showers, W. B., Shaw, R. H., Taylor, S. E. Atmospheric trajectory analysis to project long-range migration of black cutworm (Lepidoptera: Noctuidae) adults. J. Econ. Entomol. 84, 880–885, 1991.
82. Ward, J. M. J., Stromberg, E. L., Nowell, D. C., Nutter, F. W., Jr. Gray leaf spot: A disease of global importance in maize production. Plant Dis. 83, 884–895, 1999.
83. Hadjimitsis, D. G., Clayton, C. R. I., Hope, V. S. Pages 194–201 in The Importance of Accounting Atmospheric Effects in Satellite Remote Sensing: A Case Study from the Lower Thames Valley Area, UK, Reston, VA, Space 2000, American Society of Civil Engineers, 2000.
84. Pendergrass, W. R., Herwehe, J. A. Regional mesoscale meteorological modeling and smoke trajectory/air quality system. http://www.ncrs.fs.fed.us/eamc/project1.htm, 2003.
85. Nutter, F. W., Jr. Developing forensic protocols for the post-introduction attribution of threatening plant pathogens. Phytopathology 94, S77, 2004.
86. Nutter, F. W., Jr., Tylka, G. L., Guan, J., Moreira, A. J. D., Marett, C. C., Rosburg, T. R., Basart, J. P., Chong, C. S. Use of remote sensing to detect plant stress caused by soybean cyst nematode. J. Nematol. 34, 222–231, 2002.

Index

A

Abrin toxin, 183
ACAM 2000 vaccine, 37
Actinobacillus actinomycetemcomitans, 77
Acute fulminant septicemia, 147
Acute stress disorder (ASD), 284–285, 287
Aedes aegypti, 108, 119
Agency for toxic substances and disease registry (ATSDR), 257
Albutilon theophrasti, 347
Aminoglycoside streptomycin
 for *Y. pestis*, 66
Anorexia, 121, 128, 151, 166, 189, 212, 213
Anthrax attacks, 225–226
 crises of, 225, 226, 227
 in United States, 225, 239
Antiqua strains, biovar, 58
Apomorphine and epsilon toxin, 198
Arenaviridae, 108
Arenaviruses, 108, 109, 112, 125, 126, 135
Aspergillis flavus, 345

B

Bacillus anthracis, 6, 209, 211–212, 214–215, 223, 318, 319, 333, 335
 identification of, 318, 319
Bacteremia, 62, 63, 80, 147, 149, 150, 151–152, 177, 333
Ballistic biological weapons, 4
Barley stripe mosaic virus, 348, 362
Bartonella quintana, 162, 177
Bio-agent Detection System (BDS), 330
Biodetection surveillance system, 229
Biological weapons
 biological agents, 239, 254, 279, 280, 283, 285, 286, 291, 292, 331, 336–338, 340–341
 biological and Toxins Weapons Convention (BWC), 10–11
 biosafety level 4 laboratories, 11
 China and U.S usage of, 9
 economic sabotage and, 6
 food supply as target for, 340
 in Iraq, 18
 Japanese experiments on, 13
 living human carriers, 6
 North Korea and U.S usage of, 9, 19, 95
 plant pathogens as, 330
 U.S. agricultural economy as target for, 341
  citrus canker, 342
  citrus greening, 33, 7, 343, 344, 361
  human/animal health, 345
  karnal bunt of wheat, 341, 355
  potato cyst nematode (PCN), 342–343
  safe and affordable food supply, 338, 340, 344
 U.S. program on, 9
 warfare agents, 347
Bioterrorism (BT), 1
 agents, 1, 2, 5–7, 9, 11, 12, 40–41, 57
 agricultural, 335–336, 357, 359
 antigen detection system, 321
 bell-shaped curve for, 298, 310
 biological warfare, 6, 8, 10
 bioterrorism medical action team (B-MATS), 41
 drinking water systems, 207, 209, 211, 217, 221
 environmental issues and, 232
  epidemiologic clues for terrorism related outbreak, 216
 foodborne and waterborne
  biological terrorist agents, 212
  communication among health care providers and public health officials, 219–220

Bioterrorism (*cont.*)
disease recognition as terrorist/ criminal act, 215, 218
and food supply, 205–206
journalism and, 295–296
preparedness, fundings, 226
and public panic, 309
weapon, 18, 20
smallpox virus as, 20, 27–29, 32, 35
Bioterrorism events and psychosocial management
and media role in, 295
mental health response, planning for, 289–290
prevention
planned response, 280, 291
psychosocial consequences, 281
Red Cross disaster assistance, 281
september 11, aftermath of, 262, 267, 280
psychiatric syndromes and behavioral changes
acute and posttraumatic stress disorder, 284–285
maladaptive group panic, 283
neuropsychiatric, 279, 281, 286, 291
peritraumatic dissociation and, 284
public information plan, 287–288
therapeutic interventions
biological agents and responses, 285–286
debriefings, 287
treatment and separate location, 286–287
traumatic stress response
phases, 281–282
somatic symptoms and, 281–282
Borrelia recurrentis, 162
Botulism
adult intestinal toxemia botulism, 94
antitoxin therapy and, 99
as biowarfare event, 95–98
botulinum antitoxins, 85, 106
consultation services, 89
cranial nerve palsies, 89–90, 99
diagnosis and confirmation, 94
clinical samples, 95
mouse bioassay, 94
foodborne, 85, 87–90, 93, 95, 97–98
canning and fermentation, 92–93
infant, 93–94
inhalational, 88
intentional nature, recognization, 97
outbreaks of fish, 88
preparedness and research priorities, 101
preventative measures
immunization, 100–101
isolation and infection control, 100
prophylactic treatment, 100
public health response, components, 97–98
symptoms of, 87, 89, 9–91, 94, 100–101
tensilon test in, 91
therapeutic interventions
supportive intensive care, 98–99
threat, 95–96
toxins
type C and D, 88
types A and E, 87–88, 100
weapon, 87
wound, 93–94
injection drug use, 93
Bronchitis, 145, 266
Bubonic plague, 55, 63–64, 67–68, 70
Bunyaviridae, 108–109, 113, 125–126
Bunyaviruses, 108
Burkholderia pseudomallei, 147

C

Candidatus Liberobacter asiaticus, 337, 344
Candid #1 vaccine, 115, 132
Carbapenems, 152
Center for disease control and prevention (CDC), 17, 18, 19, 23, 24, 35–36, 89, 254, 296, 357
vesicular/pustular rash, smallpox algorithm, 35–36
Cercosporidium personatum, 350
Chickenpox (VZV), 33, 44
Chronic lung disease, 146
Cities Readiness Initiative (CRI), 19
Citrus canker, 342
Citrus greening disease, 337, 343
Claviceps purpurea, 345
Clostridium botulinum
botulinum toxins, 86–88
divisions of, 85–86
retort canning and, 86
spores, 86, 88
toxins
proteolytic and nonproteolytic forms of, 88
types, 87
transmission modes, 88–89
vegetative forms, 85–86
Clostridium Perfringens Epsilon toxin

apomorphine and diazepam, 198
biowarfare disease, 198
category B biowarfare agent, 195
disease diagnosis, 197–198
and gamma-butyrolactone, 198
Human C. Perfringens, 195
natural disease
cerebral edema, 197
fatal necrotic enteritis, 196
intestinal permeability, 197
preventive measures
anti-idiotype vaccine, 199
Freund's adjuvant, 198
N-bromosuccinimide, tryptophan cleaving, 198
type C, 196
Cochliobolus sativus, 353–354
Colletotrichum coccodes, 347
Coma vigil, 167
see also Epidemic typhus fever
Corticotrophin releasing factor (CRF), 283
Council of state and territorial epidemiologists (CSTE), 256–257, 263
Coxiella burnetii, 11, 168
Cranial nerve palsies, 89–90, 99, 130
Crimean-Congo HF (CCHF), bunyavirus, 108, 110, 114, 116–117, 122, 124–126
Ctenocephalides felis, cat fleas, 62
Customs and Border Protection (CBP), 244
Cytomegalovirus (CMV), 39

D
Dengue virus, 119
Department of health and human services of Newark, New Jersey (NDHHS), 259, 260, 262–263, 272
SARS outbreak, 262
Diabetes, 27, 148–149, 154, 226
Diaphorina citri, 344
Diseases, communicable, 244, 251, 255, 258, 259, 263
communicable diseases division (CDD), 259–260, 272
communicable diseases reporting and surveillance system (CDRSS), 258, 263, 264
paper-based reporting and, 264
Disseminated intravascular coagulopathy (DIC), 63, 124, 126, 128
Dryvax vaccines, 28
Dystonia disorder, 96

E
Ebola virus outbreak in community in sub-Saharan Africa, 118
Emergency medical service (EMS), 215, 223, 227, 235, 254, 273
Emergency operations center (EOC), 236
Enteric plague, *See* Pharyngeal plague
Enterobacter agglomerans, 65
Epidemic intelligence service (EIS), 271
Epidemic typhus fever
acute and latent, 159, 166, 167, 168, 170
bioterrorism diseases, 161
Brill–Zinsser disease, 165, 166, 168, 170
diagnosis
clinical syndromes, 166
culture and molecular, 168, 171
laboratory abnormalities, 169–170
serology, 170–171
epidemiology, 164
Pediculus humanus humanus, 162–164
potato famine, 161
preventive measures
and immunization, 174–175
infection control, 173
proteus OX-19 organisms, 161
Rickettsia prowazekii, 161–162
acute *R. prowazekii* infection, 166–167
therapeutic intervention, 171
antimicrobial agents and, 172
transmission modes of, 164–165
typhus vaccines, 174
Erythromycin, 146, 172
Escherichia coli 0157 outbreaks in U.S. spinach and lettuce, 335

F
Filoviridae, 108, 109, 112, 125, 126
Filoviruses, 108, 111, 116, 127, 129, 130, 131
Flaviviridae, 108, 109–126
Flaviviruses, 116, 129
Fomites, 5
Food and Drug Administration (FDA), 34
antiviral drugs, 34
Food and water
attack detection on, 213–215
contamination, 207–211, 213–215, 217–221
terrorism
agent diagnosis, 216–217
response and, 218–219
Francisella tularensis, 211, 213, 215
category A bioterrorism agent, 41, 78
misidentification of, 78

Francisella tularensis (*cont.*)
strain typing of, 79
subspecies of, 78, 326
Fusarium oxysporum, 347

G
Geneva Protocol, 6, 11
Britain and United States, 8
Germany, 7–8
Japan, 7
Global Health Security Initiative (GHSI), 34
Global Outbreak Alert and Response Network (GOARN), 32
Gram-negative bacilli, 56, 59, 65, 145, 152
Gram-negative coccobacillus, 77
Guillain-barre syndrome, 91

H
Haemophilus species, 78
Hantavirus, 116, 124, 130, 205
Hazardous material (Hazmat), 254
Health alert network (HAN), 231, 233, 273
Health and human services administration (HRSA), 226
Health and human services (HHS), 244
Health insurance portability and accountability act (HIPAA), 274
Helicobacter pylori, 321
Hemoptysis, 149
Hemorrhagic fever (HF) virus
bioterrorist attack, 134–135
as bioweapons
animal infection, 118
artificial aerosols/fomites, 120
characteristics of, 112–115
dissemination strategies, 117–120
hospital outbreaks of, 118
infected reservoir/vector, release of, 118–120
person-to-person transmission, 117–118
HEPA filter masks in, 132
infectious dose and route of infection, 117
natural maintenance and transmission, 116–117
temperature, effect of, 133
weaponization of
viruses, 108–116
Hemorrhagic smallpox, 28–32
see also Smallpox
Hepatitis E, 32
Human immunodeficiency virus (HIV), 27–28
Hybrid single-particle lagrangian integrated trajectory model (HYSPLIT), 357
Hypokalemia, 128

I
Immigration and naturalization service (INS), 244
Incident command systems (ICS), 225–226
Indian health service, 146
Infection control practitioners (ICPs), 263, 264, 269, 272
Intimidation, 1, 2, 5
see also Bioterrorism (BT)

J
Junin viruses, 108
Justinian Plague, 57

K
Karnal bunt of wheat, 341–342
Killed whole-cell plague vaccines, 69, 70
Killing Winds, 1
Kyasanur forest disease, 111, 115, 123, 125, 126, 132

L
Laboratory response network (LRN), 32
Lassa fever, 109, 117, 121–122, 125–126, 129, 130
immune plasma and, 128, 129
Lassa fever virus, 32, 109, 117, 121, 122, 125, 126, 129, 130
Legionnaires diseases, 146
Leucopenia, 134
LightCycler system, 325
Lipopolysaccharide (LPS), 82, 147, 158, 170, 190, 201
Liposome/toxoid immunogen, 188
Live vaccine strain (LVS)
Lower respiratory tract infections (LRTIs), 266

M
Macrolides for plague, 66, 172
Marburg virus, 118–120
Medicine and media relationship, 313
Medievalis strains, biovar, 58
Melioidosis
acute fulminant disease, 145
antigen test for, 152
biowarfare melioidosis, 150–151
natural infections
epidemiology, 148

modes of transmission, 148–149
organisms, 147, 148
preventative measures
infection control and immunization, 154–155
pulmonary infiltrates, 145
radiographic diagnosis, 151
biowarfare melioidosis, clinical presentation of, 150–151
hemagglutination test, 152
microbiology and serology in laboratory, 151–152
mortality rate, 153
reactivation fatal disease, 146
therapeutic interventions, 152–154
Meningococcemia, 122, 172
MM5 Community model, 357
Model Acts, 242 248
Model state emergency health powers act (MSEHPA), 241, 244, 245, 248, 249
Modified Vaccinia Ankara (MVA), 20
Monkeypox, 17, 38, 39, 44, 45, 46, 47, 119
in United States and Sudan
cidofovir usage, 46, 47
clinical manifestations of, 44
vaccinations, 41–43
Morbidity and mortality weekly report (MMWR), 252
Morphine addicts, 146
Mousepox, 20–21, 32
Myalgia, 159
Myocarditis, 169
Myopericarditis, 25

N
National electronic disease surveillance system (NEDSS), 258, 264, 268
electronic information systems, 258
National electronic telecommunications system for surveillance (NETSS), 257–258
National notifiable disease surveillance system (NNDSS), 255, 257, 263
National plant diagnostic network (NPDN), 336
Neisseria meningitidis, 7, 78, 194
New York City Department of Health and Mental Hygiene (NYCDOHMH), 262, 267
Nipah virus, 119

O
Occam's Razor, 297
Olympic games biosecurity, 329
OraQuick Rapid HIV-1 antibody test, 28
Orientalis strains, biovar, 58
Orientia tsutsugamushi, 167
Orthopoxviruses, 20–21
treatment or prevention of, 39

P
Papaver somniferum, 347
Parsimony principle, 297
Pediculus humanus humanus, 162–164
Phakopsora pachyrhizi, 337, 348, 356
Pharyngeal plague, 64
Phytophthora infestans, 161
Pichia pastoris, 101
Plague
antimicrobial treatment of, 66–67
biovars strain, 58
biowarfare plague clinical presentation, 64
CDC guidelines, 66, 68
cephalosporins for, 66
diagnosis
clinical presentation, 63–64
giemsa and gram staining for plague bacillus, 65
laboratory, 64–67, 69, 70
radiographic, 64–65
distribution of, 60
flea-vectored transmission, 62
geographical distribution of, 60
hms mutants, 62
immunization
F1 and V antigens, 70, 76
killed whole-cell plague vaccines, 69, 70
monoclonal antibodies, 71, 76
immunofluorescence staining of smears, 66
Indian epidemic of, 55–56
infection control, 67–69
postexposure antimicrobial prophylaxis, 68
life cycle of, 61–62
meningitis, 63–66
pandemic, 57, 58
plasmid-based resistance for, 66
pneumonia, 64, 68
postexposure antimicrobial prophylaxis for prevention of, 68–69

Plague (*cont.*)
- primary plague pneumonia, 64
- rodents and, 71
  - control, 71
- in USA occurrence of, 56
- virulence factors
  - O and pH6 antigen, 59
  - V antigen, 58, 69, 70, 71
- Worldwide incidence of, 61

Plant pathogens
- crop production cycle in, 346, 348
- disease epidemics and, 348–349
  - geographic information systems data, 354–358
  - initial inoculum effectiveness of, 353–354
  - intensity and yield relationships, 355
  - model selection, 349–352
  - monomolecular and logistic growth models, 350
- time of inoculation, 354–355
- usage as biological weapons in war on drugs, 346–348
- weaponization, 338–339

Pleosporum papaveracea, 347
Pneumonia, 148, 149–150
Posttraumatic stress disorder (PTSD), 2, 84
Potato cyst nematode (PCN), 342
Proteus vulgaris, 170
Pseudomonas mallei, 6
Pseudomonas pseudomallei, 147
Pseudo-parkinsonism/akethisia, 286

Public health
- BT preparedness, funding, 226
- centers for public health preparedness, 231
- challenges, 236
- communication, 230–231
- crisis management, 235–236
- department of preventive medicine and community health (DPMCH), 260
- departments of health (DOHs), 225
- disaster medical assistance teams (DMAT), 227
- disaster mortuary assistance teams (DMORT), 227
- environmental issues and bioterrorism, 232
- laboratory services, 232
- law and biological terrorism, 239–249
- medical and hospital preparedness, 233–234
- organizational issues, 226–227
- prophylaxis, delivery, 234–235
- protected health information (PHI), 274
- public health information network (PHIN), 258
- public health laboratory information system (PHLIS) data, 214
- public health security and bioterrorism preparedness and response act of 2002, 337
- restrictions
  - personal liberty, 242
  - privacy, 242, 246, 247–248, 249
  - property, 248–249
  - quarantine and isolation, 242–243
- school of public health (SPH), 260
- syndromic surveillance methodology and, 266
  - classification of, 266
  - electronically-based, 267–268
  - evaluation of, 267
  - ICD-9 codes and, 267
  - role of, 268
- turning point model state public health act (Turning Point Act), 241
- workforce development and needs, 231–232

Public health surveillance for bioterrorism
- active and passive reporting systems, 262–263
- automated electronic data collection, 264, 267
- biosensor technology, 260
- bioterrorism, consequences of, 253–254
- confidentiality
  - personal informations and, 274
- CSTE and included diseases, 257
- data analysis and interpretation
  - aberration detections in, 269–271
  - epidemicity, 269–270
  - sentinel health events, 269
- data reporting and collection, 274
- drop-in surveillance, 262
- feedback and participants, 272
- fundamental surveillance, 255
  - generic surveillance system flow chart, 256
  - infectious diseases and, 255
- health indicator, sources of, 265
- indirect benefits, 260
- infection, laboratory confirmation, 261
- information technology impact, 257
  - computer-based reporting, 257

information dissemination and communication, 271–273
infrastructure, 258
security and, 259, 274
interorganizational communications, 272–273
local emergency departments, 263
outbreak, recognition of, 269
personnel and electronics in, 263–265
real-time outbreak and disease surveillance (RODS), 264
systems of, 255
Puccinia graminis, 355
Puccinia recondita f. sp. *tritici*, 351, 352
Pulex irritans, human fleas, 62

Q

Quarantine and isolation restriction, 242–243
considerations of, 245–246
federal quarantine and isolation law, 244–245
state and local quarantine laws, 243–244

R

Rapid identification assays
antigen–antibody interactions
CANARY system, 321
ELISA test, 320
antigen–non-antibody target interactions, 321–322
diagnostic assays, 328–329
genomic differences and
comprehensive diagnostic test, 322–323
DNA microarrays, 323–324
multiplex assays, 326
real-time probes, 324–325
sample processing development, 327–328
Rhabdomyolysis, 80
see also Tularemia
Ribavirin, antiviral drug
lassa fever and, 127
RVF virus infection and, 129
Ricin, 181
agglutinin properties, 184
biowarfare, 185, 186, 188
liposomally encapsulated toxoid, 188
in castor beans, 182–184
disease
gastrointestinal symptoms and hypersensitivity-like illness, 185
latex allergies, 186
occupational allergies, 185
pulmonary edema and fibrosis, 186
therapeutic measures, 187
ELISA test for, 320
exposure, diagnosis of, 185
formalin-inactivated toxoid, 188
in malignancy treatment, 184
natural, 185–186
preventive measures
microsphere vaccine, 188
monoclonal antibody, 189
polyclonal goat anti-ricin IgG, 188
sodium hypochlorite exposure, 188
as therapeutic agent, 184
toxin, 182–184
Ricinus communis, in oil application, 182–183
Rickettsiae disease, 161–164, 68–69, 71–72, 75
Rickettsia prowazekii infections
bioterrorism-associated, 168–169
Brill–Zinsser disease, 168
category B bioterrorism agent, 161
clinical symptoms of, 166
latency in, 165, 168
mortality rate, 167, 169
Rift valley fever (RVF), 108, 110, 111, 113, 115, 119, 124–126, 129–132
virus, 108, 129, 131
RMSF/Dermacentor tick model, 174
see also Epidemic typhus fever
R. tsutsugamushi disease, 172

S

Salmonella enterica, 59, 101
Salmonella outbreak detection algorithm (SODA) analysis, 214–215
Salmonella typhimurium, 269
Science applications international corporation and biosensor development, 330
Septicemic plague, 56, 63, 64
diffuse alveolar pulmonary infiltrates for, 64–65
Septoria glycines, 355
Serodiagnosis, 320
see also Rapid identification assays
Serratia marcescens drops over San Francisco and urinary tract infections outbreak, 10
Severe acute respiratory syndrome (SARS), 17, 18, 34, 43, 44, 226, 239, 245, 257, 259, 262, 263, 273, 290, 313

Severe acute respiratory (*cont.*)
coronavirus infection, 18
epidemic of, 322
Shigella spp., 212
Simian immunodeficiency virus (SIV), 28
Smallpox
bioterrorist threat, 18
centers for disease control (CDC)
educational training for, 17
guidelines for, 25
and prevention, 35–36
website on, 36
chickenpox comparison with, 33
diagnosis of, 24
hemorrhagic smallpox, 28–29
in hospitals and public health, preparedness, 40–44
international preparedness for, 32–35
patients evaluation, 228, 229
Soviet smallpox weapons program, 18
vaccines
ACAM 2000 vaccine, 37
Atlantic Storm, 35
compensation coverage for vaccine injuries, 42–43
first, second, and third generations, 37–38
Global Mercury, 34
HIV/AIDS and, 27–28
in Hong Kong, 34
myocarditis and/or pericarditis, 25–26
time course of typical skin reactions, 24
and vaccination program, 24
vaccinia and variola virus
comparison between, 21
genetically modified, 20
respiratory droplets and, 21
type 1/type 2 cytokine model, 21
vaccinia immune globulin and antiviral drug development, 38–39
Soviet biowarfare, 8
Staphylococcal enterotoxin B (SEB)
aerosolization and, 191, 192, 194, 198
anti-SEB antibody, 194
catechin and, 193
and corticosteroids, 193
cysteinyl leukotriene antagonists, 193
dexamethasone for, 193
disease
diarrhea, 191
foodborne illness, 191, 196
gastrointestinal symptoms, 192
induced cytokine disease, 193
lethargy and dyspnea, 192
ELISA for, 193, 197
formalin-treated SEB toxoid for, 194
IgY antibody, 194
recombinant mutant toxoid, 194
toxin
aerosolized nonlethal dose of, 190
intoxication, 189, 192
LPS-induced toxicity, 190
as superantigen, 189, 190, 193
vaccine candidate, 190
Staphylococcus aureus, 189
State Research Center of Virology and Biotechnology (VECTOR), 18
Sterile pyuria, 80
Strabismus, 96
Strategic National Stockpile (SNS), 234
Sylvatic plague, 60

T

T-cells, 20, 32, 38
cellular immune response, 20, 21
Terrorist, 2
Thrombocytopenia, 107, 133, 159, 169, 170, 197
TIGER biosensor, 330
Tilletia indica, 341
Toxins and secretion system
targets for real-time detection of, 327
Tuberculosis, 149, 151, 242, 255, 257, 259, 271, 321
Tularemia
agents in, 77
bacteremia, presence of, 81
bioterrorism
outbreak, 77
presentations, 81
ciprofloxacin and doxycycline, treatment for, 81
epidemiology and modes of transmission, 79–80
infection sources, 80
live vaccine strain (LVS), prevention and, 82
oculoglandular, 80–81
outbreak of, 8
preventative measures, 81–82
streptomycin and treatment, 81
symptoms of, 80
therapy, 81–82

tularemic pneumonia, 80
typhoidal, 80 82
ulceroglandular, 79–82
Typhoid, 167, 168, 172, 213

U
Ulceroglandular disease, 80
Uniform Emergency Volunteer Health Practitioners Act (UEVHPA), 241
United States (U.S.)
agriculture, bioterrorist attack on, 341
anthrax attacks
CDC functions and media, 303–305
communication with press during, 305–309
HHS, role in media, 303
lessons from, 313
public health officers and policy-makers, 308
reporters and readers, views, 310
Cuba, infected turkeys with Newcastle disease and U.S., 9
United States National Research Council (NRC), 335–336
Countering Agricultural Bioterrorism, 336
U.S. citizenship and immigration services (USCIS), 244
USDA cooperative agricultural pest survey (CAPS) surveillance program, 342–343
U.S. fish and wildlife service (USFW), 244

V
Vaccinia immune globulin (VIG), 21, 22, 23, 38–40, 46, 47
and antiviral drug development, 38–39
Vaccinia virus, 20, 21–22, 27–28, 37–40, 44, 46
see also Smallpox
Vagabond's disease, 164
V antigen, virulence factors, 58
Varicella-Zoster Virus (VZV), 45–46
Variolation, 5
see also Fomites
Variola virus, 33, 36
in Russia and United States, 32–33
see also Smallpox
Vibrio cholerae, 7
Viral hemorrhagic fever
bioterrorism and, 124–127
clinical aspects of, 125
differential diagnosis of, 127
human infection, 111, 116, 118–120, 129
illness, 120–124
immune plasma and, 128, 129
laboratory findings and diagnosis, 126–127
preventative measures and infection control
contact tracing, 132
environmental clean-up132–133
patient isolation, 131–132
prophylaxis, 131
protein C and, 131
vaccines, 132
surveillance
components of, 133
environmental sampling, 134
human disease, 133–134
therapeutic interventions
antiviral drugs, 128
convalescent immune plasma, 128–129
immunomodulating drugs, 130–131
medications, 128
supportive measures, 128
viruses in, 108–116

W
Water supplies poisoning, 4
Wayson staining for plague bacillus, 65
Weaponization, 338
see also Plant pathogens
Weather-based geographic information systems (GIS) data, 355

X
Xanthomonas axonopodis pv. *citri,* 342
Xenopsylla cheopis, oriental rat flea, 62

Y
Yellow fever, 110, 114, 119, 121, 123–126, 257
Yersinia pestis, 7, 47, 56, 57–58, 68, 213, 215, 225, 321
agglutination testing, 65
automated bacteriological test systems, 65
as biological weapon., 64
clinical forms in humans, 63
ELISAs for early infection, 65

Yersinia pestis (cont.)
F1 antigen
detection of, 65
and encoded by caf operon, 58–59
hemagglutination-inhibition test, 65
genome sequences of, 58
heterologous O antigen in, 59
hms protein, 62
laboratory media for, 65
PhoPQ two-component response regulatory system, 59
plasmids for virulence, 58
second type III secretion system, 58
Yops and F1antigen, transcription and secretion of, 59
Yersinia pseudotuberculosis, 57

Z
Zoonotic virus, 119

Printed in the United States of America